LEAN & STRONG

LEAN & STRONG

EATING SKILLS,

PSYCHOLOGY,

AND WORKOUTS

Josh Hillis

Foreword by Molly Galbraith

ON TARGET PUBLICATIONS
APTOS, CALIFORNIA

LEAN AND STRONG
Eating Skills, Psychology, and Workouts

Josh Hillis

Foreword by Molly Galbraith

Book cover and graphics by Karen Chin

ISBN-13: 978-1-931046-40-4, paperback
ISBN-13: 978-1-931046-39-8, epub
First printing March 2020

On Target Publications
P O Box 1335
Aptos, California 95001 USA
otpbooks.com

Library of Congress Cataloging-in-Publication Data

Names: Hillis, Josh, 1977- author.
Title: Lean and strong : the skills, stages, and psychology of lasting
 fitness / Josh Hillis.
Description: Aptos, CA : On Target Publications, [2019] | Includes index.
Identifiers: LCCN 2019007716 | ISBN 9781931046404 (pbk.)
Subjects: LCSH: Weight loss--Psychological aspects. | Physical fitness. |
 Reducing exercises.
Classification: LCC RM222.2 .H486 2019 | DDC 613.7--dc23
LC record available at https://lccn.loc.gov/2019007716

ALSO BY
JOSH HILLIS

FAT LOSS HAPPENS ON MONDAY

FORTHCOMING

BEATING EMOTIONAL EATING
SPRING 2023

DEDICATION

This book is dedicated to Dan John, who played such an instrumental role in getting my first book deal. First, he helped me sort out my coaching strategy and pushed me to write it up in an ebook. Then, years later, he set up a meeting with our wonderful publisher, Laree Draper, about turning that into a print book. He also guided me in what, from the original, to cut or expand. Finally, he even co-wrote that book.

Getting to write *Fat Loss Happens on Monday* with Dan opened up so many doors. All of the speaking and writing and people I've gotten to work with came out of that. I would never have gotten to make the difference I get to make and help as many people as I get to help if not for his involvement. I'll be forever grateful.

On top of what he has done for me, Dan has continually elevated the effectiveness, professionalism, and wisdom in the fitness field. It's not just that he has so much great information to teach, it's the person he is in teaching it. He shows up for people and shows up for communities. Everyone who knows him is better for it.

For years he has asked me for my "pirate map" for weight loss. It finally exists and is on page 59.

Dan, thanks for everything!

CONTENTS

FOREWORD

Change can be hard.

If you've ever tried to lose weight, get more sleep, pay down debt, or quit smoking, you know firsthand what I mean.

How many times have you gotten really serious about making a major life change?

You think to yourself, *"This is it! I've had enough. I'm going to finally [___insert change you want to make___] once and for all."*

And in the beginning, you believe in yourself because you *feel* how badly you want it to happen.

So you resolve to make sweeping changes and overhaul your life, and you often do. For a while.

Maybe it's for three or four days. Maybe a week. Or maybe it's even a full month.

But eventually life gets in the way.

You might experience extra stress or hardship or a monumental life event like death or divorce or illness, and you slip back into your old ways, exactly as you were before, except this time, you feel worse because you tried and failed…again.

If you're like most folks, this cycle continues for months, years, sometimes even decades. The pattern looks something like this:

Resolve to change → try to overhaul your life → follow a program or change your behavior for a short time → slip back into your old habits and behaviors → feel like a failure → give yourself further "proof" you can't do it → rinse and repeat.

When this happens, we often get down on ourselves for being "weak," not having enough "willpower," or not "wanting it badly enough."

As the co-founder and woman-in-charge of Girls Gone Strong, a health and fitness movement of over 800,000 women from more than 80 countries around the world, I've seen this time and time again (and I even did it myself for years). I know how discouraging it can feel.

But the truth is, change is hard for all of us. It's just that some of us are better at certain things than others. For example, that super fit woman you see at the gym and envy her lean body and muscles? She might struggle with her finances.

Your college roommate who paid down his student loans in under two years and is now debt-free? He might not have a strong relationship with his partner.

Your colleague who seems to have the perfect marriage and kids? That person might be struggling with a tobacco addiction.

Yes, some of us have a knack or predisposition to excel in some areas of our lives. But that doesn't mean we can't achieve our goals in areas where we currently struggle.

It simply means we need the right guide, someone who understands how change happens (and how it doesn't), and what it really takes to make change stick for a lifetime.

This is someone who will take you by the hand and walk you through the process of change, step-by-step, helping you build the skills you need.

That guide is Josh Hillis.

I first met Josh at the Elite Fitness and Performance Summit in Louisville, Kentucky, in 2015. I'd been a fan of his via the internet for years, and was excited to see him present.

Have you ever met someone you've followed online who ended up disappointing you? That is NOT Josh Hillis. He is everything I expected him to be…and more. As I sat in the audience watching him present, he had the room on the edge of our seats, totally engaged by his passion and enthusiasm.

Many presenters stand on stage and talk *at* their audiences. Not Josh. He's interested in talking *with* his audience. He has information to share, yes. But he wants input, suggestions, and ideas. That's who Josh is, someone who values other people, who seeks different perspectives, and who's always looking to learn, grow, and refine his knowledge.

That's how you end up with a book like *Lean and Strong*.

Josh is everything that's good about the fitness field. He's passionate; he's compassionate; he cares about making a difference, and he knows what he's talking about. All of that rings loud and clear in this book. To say Josh is obsessed with learning and honing his craft so he can better serve his clients and readers is an understatement. He's not interested in how change might happen in an "ideal" world—he cares how things work in *real life*.

That's why, in this book, you'll find actionable, practical solutions to losing bodyfat, gaining strength, improving your health and longevity, and reaching your goals. In this book, he gives us what *works*. And he delivers it with a rare blend of frankness, honesty, and compassion.

I'm so happy you picked up a copy of *Lean and Strong*. As you're about to learn, this book delivers exactly what it promises: It will help you get lean and strong. But it does much more than that. It will help you overcome the on-again off-again roller coaster of change so you can finally become the person you want to be.

With Josh in your corner, you'll not only create change, you'll have the skills to sustain it.

For life.

Molly Galbraith
Co-founder and Woman-in-charge
Girls Gone Strong

HOW TO GET LEAN
HOW TO GET STRONG

LEAN

When hungry, eat a balanced meal. Eat slowly enough to notice and stop when full.
Treat eating well like skill practice. Eat three meals per day. Don't snack between meals
because of boredom, stress, or emotions.

STRONG

Do periodized workouts with progressive overload over time.
Practice and develop skill in basic movement patterns.

LEAN AND STRONG

In the long term, increase workout volume. In the short term, adjust workout volume
based on current stress and schedule demands.
Always make eating skills the number one priority.

These are very tight, very complete explanations of how to get lean and strong.

They may be different from what you have seen before. There's no mention of diets or magical foods. There's nothing about burning thousands of calories with punishing workouts. It's just simple work done over time.

This book includes all the eating skills required to do "lean" and is based on skills practice. You'll spend a lot of time practicing. You'll get results while you're practicing, long before anything feels "perfect." Practice is enough.

Your eating skills will increase with practice and as your eating skills increase, everything will change about food and leanness.

This book includes multiple versions of workouts. You can simply do the workouts, in order, and get stronger. You'll get stronger because the workouts are intelligently periodized, and you'll get stronger because you'll develop a new level of skills in each of the movement patterns.

BEHAVIOR CHANGE

Know which skills you're practicing each week, plan for obstacles, and track frequency.
The context for your practice is this: excellence, self-compassion, goldilocksing, and flexibility.

RESULTS FOR LIFE

Results are the natural expression of taking actions in line with your personal values.
The paradox is that you'll get the best results when, instead of focusing on the results, you work on being the kind of person you want to be.

You're going to get the tools to change your behaviors and do the things you need to do to get lean and strong in real life. You're likely going to go deeper into what motivates you than you ever have before.

You'll sort out where fitness fits inside of all of the commitments in your life. When practicing the skills and doing the workouts are an expression of your values, you won't have to worry about "feeling motivated" anymore. Being lean and strong will be part of who you are.

CHAPTER ONE
YOUR FIRST MONTH

This book does something unusual—in the first 20 pages, it will give you everything you need to start. I know that's not how books are supposed to be written. We're supposed to write a book so people have to keep reading until the end to figure it all out.

But here's the thing: I'm a personal trainer. I'm a coach. I just want to improve your performance. I know nothing will make a bigger difference than if you start practicing *this week*.

What's in these first 20 pages is barely enough to get started. It isn't complete, but it's enough. The rest of the book gives the complete picture. For now, just get started.

The most cutting-edge research on learning shows that people learn more if they take a test *before studying*. Of course, they fail the test the first time. And failing the test completely changes the quality of their reading. They study much more intently, with their brains primed to look for the answers to the questions they got wrong.

Then, they take the test again. Maybe the second time they get a "D" or a "C." They study again; this time they know exactly what they know and don't know, and go straight to working on what they got wrong.

These cycles of taking tests and reading—five, six, seven, or even an unlimited number of times—results in everyone learning more. Almost everyone gets an "A" if they just keep studying and test-taking. The process of getting better through repeated, low-stakes testing is well documented, and is called "the testing effect" or "the practice effect." [1,2,3,4,5,6,7]

On top of that, everyone remembers the material and gets higher grades on the final. The students who did repeated testing and studying were also better at applying the material, and adapting it to different situations. It turns out it works in all kinds of scenarios, from teaching people to jump out of planes, to surgeons performing complex surgical tasks, to high jumping in track, to throwing balls with accuracy. [8]

That's how this book is structured. You're going to start practicing the skills this week. The mistakes you make and the failures you have your first week will direct your learning throughout the book. You'll get ten times more out of the book if you're *practicing while you're reading it* than if you wait until the end to start practicing.

The secret sauce is that my clients get the best results in leanness and strength simply because they practice more than everyone else. So let's start practicing.

WHAT TO EAT

The first question people always have is "what do I eat?" This book is going to answer that in the simplest way possible—by looking at a balanced plate. This is the simplest way to guestimate plating healthy and balanced portions:

- 50% of the plate vegetables (and fruit!);

- 25% of the plate protein;

- 25% of the plate carbohydrates;

- About a tablespoon of fat (as a starting guideline).

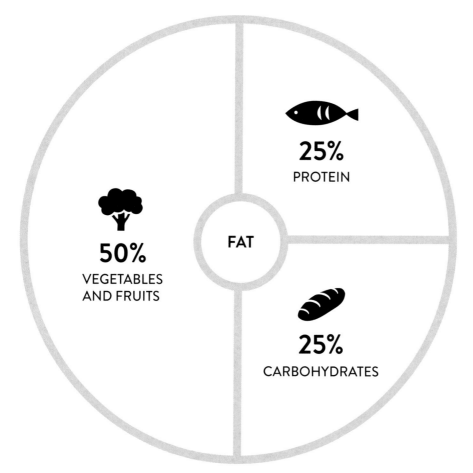

PROTEIN
Chicken, turkey, salmon, mackerel, tofu, tempeh, egg whites, bison, beef, cottage cheese, Greek yogurt

CARBOHYDRATES
Whole grains, brown rice, oats, quinoa, pasta, tortillas, starchy vegetables like potatoes, sweet potatoes, beans

FATS
Extra Virgin olive oil, fish oil, flax oil, avocados, almonds, cashews, walnuts, pure olive oil, canola oil, egg yolks

VEGETABLES
Non-starchy vegetables like onions, bell peppers, tomatoes, romaine, lettuce, arugula, broccoli, carrots, spinach, brussels sprouts

FRUITS
Apples, oranges, bananas, strawberries, blueberries, blackberries, lemons, peaches, pineapple, and mango

*These are examples of what you could include — you are not limited to these.

You've probably seen something like this before. Harvard School of Public Health has a "Healthy Eating Plate" that looks almost exactly like this. You may also notice that these match the plate used for Canada's food guide and are pretty close to the United States' "MyPlate" guidelines from 2019. Dozens of fitness groups have recommended some version of this for decades. Lastly, eating balanced meals is just common sense.

Don't get too hung up on the percentages; it's just a guideline. It's a place to start when thinking about how to put your plate together. Usually people feel the most full for the least calories with a portion of protein, a portion of carbohydrates, two portions of fruit or vegetables, and a portion of fat.

We'll dig into the research on why those particular portions were chosen in the chapter on eating guidelines and in the section "Plating Balanced Portions."

Please don't get too stuck on the idea of a "plate." You can also look for near those ratios stirred into a stew, in a casserole, or on a sandwich. Just use this as a guideline for how to think about putting together a meal.

It isn't a rule; it's a guideline. It's a simple tool to answer the question of "what do I eat?" without having to count anything or eliminate any food groups. When you use a guideline like this to plan your meals, eating for leanness and strength becomes simple.

FOUR KINDS OF EATING SKILLS

LEAN AND STRONG EATING SKILLS MATRIX: BASIC

	DURING MEALS	BETWEEN MEALS
LISTEN TO YOUR BODY	Notice when getting full, and stop	Distinguish true hunger versus cravings, boredom, tiredness, emotions, or thoughts
USE A GUIDELINE	Plate healthy and balanced portions	Eat a meal every four to six hours, without snacking in between

Weight loss is simply:

1. **Having the guides and skills to eat the right amount of food at meals**

2. **Having the guides and skills to not snack when stressed, bored, tired, emotional, and so on.**

We're going to work on eating *guidelines*, which are awesome for creating weight loss and are really useful for when you're tired or stressed.

We're also going to work on eating *skills*, which will transform your relationship to your body, to food, and to fitness.

These are the four areas—during meals listening to your body, during meals guidelines, between meals listening to your body, and between meals guidelines—that we need to work on with your eating skills to hit all of your goals. Each person will have different components of those skills they need.

The lists of component skills follow on the next page.

LEAN AND STRONG EATING SKILLS MATRIX: IN DEPTH

	DURING MEALS	BETWEEN MEALS
LISTEN TO YOUR BODY	Notice when full, and stop • Check in with your stomach mid-meal, notice and speculate about future fullness • Notice that flavor enjoyment is different from fullness • Use five senses mindfulness • Make sure to eat enough • Stop before eating too much • Check in with your stomach one hour after eating	Distinguish hunger from cravings, boredom, tiredness, emotions, or thoughts • Defusion from unwanted thoughts, feelings, and cravings • Flexibility: Saying "yes" to things sometimes, and "no" other times • Notice and wait through normal hunger 30 minutes before eating • Notice when tired and go to sleep
USE A GUIDELINE	Plate balanced portions Plate healthy portion sizes • Put the fork down between bites • Eat without screens • Do something engaging after eating • Wait ten minutes before having seconds or treats	Eat a meal every four to six hours, without snacking in between • Ten-minute wait before snacks or treats • Get engaged with what is going on in the moment • Self-care: coping, self-soothing, fun activities, and hobbies • Turn off screens and lights and go to bed at a certain time

These are all of the skills we could potentially work on. Most people are only *ever* going to use three to seven of these skills (NOT all of them!). As you read through the book, you'll get a sense of which skills you need, and will be able to customize your own program.

First, if you can't make sense of these skills yet, THAT'S NORMAL. I don't expect you to be able to do anything with the information until you've read more.

I just want to make sure you have an overview of the first level of the system we're using. It will make more and more sense each week while you alternate between practicing and reading more from the book.

You'll use the eating skills tracker at the end of this section. I'm going to make it easy by picking the first four skills you're going to practice:

- Plate balanced portions.

- Put the fork down between bites.

- Eat a meal every four to six hours (without snacking in between).

- Distinguish true hunger from cravings, boredom, tiredness, emotions, or thoughts.

You'll fill in your skills tracker by entering the number of times you practice each skill or use each guide. Here's an example of what your tracker might look like halfway through a week.

In the tracker on the following page, you'd enter a '1' if you had one balanced meal that day, a '2' for two balanced meals, or '3' for three balanced meals.

In eating a meal every four to six hours, you'd mark down each *between-meal period* you didn't have a snack. For example, if you had no snacks between breakfast and lunch, between lunch and dinner, or between dinner and going to sleep, enter a '3.' If you snacked after dinner, but not between breakfast and lunch, or lunch and dinner, put a '2.'

For distinguishing true hunger, if you had a craving one time that day and practiced that skill, enter a '1.' But if you had cravings five times that day and practiced that skill every time, use a '5.' If you didn't have any cravings that day, you could put 'n/a' for not applicable.

	DAY:	M	T	W	TH	F	SA	SU
	DATE:							
DURING MEALS	Plate balanced portions	3	0	2	3			
	Put the fork down between meals	1	2	1	3			
BETWEEN MEALS	Eat a meal every four to six hours (without snacking in between)	3	3	3	3			
	Distinguish true hunger from cravings, boredom, tiredness, emotions, or thoughts	1	4	N/A	3			

Remember, the goal is to get practice (reps), not to have "perfect days." It's totally okay to practice each skill one or two times each day—it doesn't have to be every meal. You just need to get practice with some of the skills each day; it stacks up over time. With practice, you'll be able to combine skills and get more frequency. At this point, as long as you practice one of the skills a couple times each day, that practice is significant.

IF/THEN PLANNING

Of the three Meta-skills, we're going to start with If/Then planning. If/Then planning is the most important Meta-skill for behavior change. If/Then planning is simply a matter of planning for:

1. **IF** obstacle _____ shows up,

2. **THEN** I'm going to do _____ to overcome that obstacle.

It's been shown goal setting is much less effective than *obstacle planning*.

In research, this is called an *implementation intention*. Where goal setting has a small-to-medium effect on goal achievement, obstacle planning has a medium-to-large effect on achievement. [9]

People take more consistent action and have more consistent practice if they expect and plan to overcome obstacles, particularly with health behavior.[10] Despite good intentions, goal setting, and feeling motivated about a new plan, most people get crushed by the first or second obstacle in their way. Your plans to overcome the obstacles that always come up are what make the difference in actually achieving your goals.[11,12,13]

Most people fail in behavior change because they repeatedly assume that no obstacles will come up. They don't think things through, so they end up with a really horrible If/Then plan: "IF everything goes perfectly in my life today, THEN I'll practice my skills." Unless you have a charmed life, that's a recipe for failure.

Thinking through obstacles is the most important element of behavior change.

There are two things people typically don't consider:

1. Obstacles are a part of life; we need to accept they're a part of life and expect them.

2. Successful food skill practice isn't a matter of not having obstacles; it's a matter of expecting obstacles and planning for them.

There are two kinds of obstacles we face:

1. **External obstacles:** People bringing pizza to the office, or having a really stressful and draining workday.

2. **Internal obstacles:** Examples might be feeling sad, being tired, having cravings, being angry, or having unwanted thoughts.

Most clients find one of the two obstacles is tougher for them. For some people, their If/Then planning may all revolve around external obstacles:

IF I have a 12-hour workday every Wednesday,
THEN I need to cook Wednesday's dinner
on Tuesday.

IF I get served too much food at the restaurant,
THEN I need to box some up and take it home.

IF I have eight hours of work on my schedule
between lunch and dinner,
THEN I'm going to need a snack halfway
in between.

IF I crave a snack at 10:00 a.m.,
THEN I'm going to check to see if it's been four to
six hours since breakfast.

For other people, they're all internal obstacles:

IF I have a craving for candy in the middle of
the afternoon,
THEN I'm going to check to see if I'm hungry for a
balanced meal.

IF I have a stressful day at work,
THEN I'm going to veg out on TV after I put the
kids to bed.

IF I feel sad,
THEN I'm going to go for a walk.

IF I feel bored,
THEN I'm going to work on a craft.

Or we can look at internal obstacles from acceptance:

IF I have a craving for candy in the middle of the afternoon,
THEN I'm going to remember it's normal to crave candy.

IF I have a stressful day at work,
THEN I'm going to remember it's okay that work is stressful sometimes.

IF I feel sad,
THEN I'm going to remember it's normal and human to feel sad sometimes.

IF I feel bored,
THEN I'm going to remember it's normal and human to feel bored sometimes.

Most people find if they do just a little reflection on the previous week, they can anticipate what obstacles they might find in the upcoming week.

Reflection is a useful tool, and it's totally necessary in your If/Then planning. Consider all of the skills and Meta-skills and take some time each week and reflect on how things are going.

IF/THEN PLANNING ON YOUR SKILLS TRACKER

The second week, we're going to add an If/Then plan to your tracker and plan to overcome an obstacle each week.

		DAY: M	T	W	TH	F	SA	SU
		DATE:						
DURING MEALS	Plate balanced portions	3	0	2	3			
	Put the fork down between bites	1	2	1	1			
BETWEEN MEALS	Eat a meal every four to six hours (without snacking in between)	3	3	3	3			
	Distinguish true hunger from cravings, boredom, tiredness, emotions, or thoughts	2	4	3	3			
VALUES (LIST THREE)	Persistence, compassion, connectedness		X		X			
IF/THEN PLANNING	If: I get stressed at work Then: I'm going to walk a lap around the building		X		X			

If/Then planning is personal—it works better if you come up with your own plan.

THE TEN TURNING POINTS

The Ten Turning Points are ten things my most successful clients always figure out after about a year of practicing the eating skills.

I went through my client notes, mapped them, and now I give them to clients ahead of time. It can still take time to fully internalize, but people now often have massive turning points in their practice in weeks or months that used to take a year.

To start, I'm just going to give you a preview of three:

| THREE OF THE TEN TURNING POINTS ||
WHAT WORKS	WHAT CAUSES FAILURE
Practicing excellence and self-compassion	Practicing perfectionism
Engagement/flow/goldilocksing	Too much or too little all the time
Weight loss comes from self-care	Weight loss comes from punishment

PERFECTIONISM VERSUS EXCELLENCE

There was really interesting research done on "positive perfectionism" versus "negative perfectionism." They found there's no such thing as positive perfectionism; perfectionism *always* has a negative outcome.[281] Perfectionism is about shame, negative self-evaluations, and concern for mistakes.[282,283] Perfectionism is distinguished by quitting, and accompanied by lower wellbeing.[284,285,286]

You know people are perfectionist about their nutrition when any time they "blow their diet," they quit for the rest of the week…or the rest of the month.[287] Sometimes, they quit for the rest of the year. Their perfectionism results in practicing a lot of quitting.

On the other hand, let's look at the pursuit of excellence. Pursuit of excellence is defined by practicing, making mistakes, and practicing more. This represents understanding that excellence requires making mistakes and learning from them. Pursuit of excellence means you keep practicing even after you make multiple mistakes, and continue to make mistakes.

With workouts, pursuit of excellence means doing what you can, whenever you can. Sometimes, that will be full workouts; other times, it's half workouts. Sometimes it's three workouts per week, and other times, it's one or two. It's continuing to get your workouts, even when those workouts aren't as often or as long as you'd like.

The turning point is to notice when you're having perfectionist thoughts. It's okay to *have* perfectionist thoughts; *you just don't act on them by quitting*. Notice those perfectionist thoughts, but continue to practice your eating skills and workout program anyway.

PERFECTIONISM VERSUS SELF-COMPASSION

It turns out, the primary difference between perfectionism and the pursuit of excellence is self-compassion.[14] Self-compassion is what determines whether our pursuits will build us up or destroy us.

Perfectionism has everything to do with living in a fantasyland where we can do everything perfectly. It would be cool if that was possible, but we aren't robots. We're humans. Humans make mistakes. Humans feel bad. Humans are, by nature, imperfect.

Perfectionism is an unwillingness to do work when confronted with our own humanity. It's abdicating responsibility every time we see evidence of being human.

Self-compassion is acknowledging it's normal to make mistakes. It's normal to have all kinds of emotions. It's normal to have cravings. It's normal to make mistakes. It's normal to feel guilty about making mistakes.

Self-compassion is noticing that all of our judgments about ourselves are just thoughts; it's noticing we've had judgmental thoughts, maybe for decades, and that it's a habit. We know we don't need to debate them; we don't need to figure out if they're true or false; we don't need to fight or change them; and we don't need repeat them and beat ourselves up. Self-compassion is noticing these are just thoughts and forgiving ourselves when they show up.

Self-compassion is continuing to practice our eating skills and workouts simply because they're self-care.

Self-compassion is reminding ourselves that no matter how together everyone else looks on the outside, everyone has human issues. People have different easy and difficult things in their lives, but everyone has hard things. Everyone makes mistakes. We're human.

SELF-KINDNESS VERSUS SELF-COMPASSION

A common misconception about self-compassion is that it's "letting yourself off of the hook." Nothing could be further from the truth. Sometimes, but not always, self-kindness is letting yourself off the hook. Sometimes, self-kindness is a glass of wine after a long day at work—and sometimes, that's totally appropriate.

Self-compassion is something else.

Where self-kindness can just be "treat yourself," self-compassion is values-led behavior.

Self-compassion often includes the very hard work of coming to terms with our imperfections, experiencing normal human pain, knowing what really matters to us, and taking actions that take care of our well-being in the long term.

ENGAGEMENT/FLOW/GOLDILOCKSING VERSUS TOO MUCH OR TOO LITTLE

Humans love doing things that are engaging. A meta-analysis of 28 research studies found that the right balance of skill and challenge is a robust predictor of engagement and flow.[15]

- If something is too challenging, we get crushed.

- If something is too easy, we get bored.

- When something is right at the edge of our abilities or just beyond our comfort zone, it's engaging. That's where we find flow.

Most people in the diet world do too much…all the time. They sprint out of the gate, trying something way too hard and unsustainable, then they crash and burn.

Most people in the habit world do too little…all the time. They build such small habits and progress so slowly, and they get bored.

In *Lean and Strong*, we're going to do an approach where we customize your practice to be engaging and challenging. We want to be just at the edge of your abilities.

People have different tolerances for making mistakes. This has a lot to do with our history of success or failure in a certain thing. In general, when we have a history of success with something, we tend to look at mistakes as learning experiences.

On the other hand, when we have a history of failure, we often imagine mistakes as a personal failing. It's normal to have different tolerances for mistakes in different areas of your life. You should expect that the longer you practice skills, the more comfortable you'll get with mistakes as an important part of learning.

Rules of thumb:

- If you don't make mistakes, the endeavor is probably too easy.

- If you make mistakes 10–15% of the time, it's probably right at the level of challenge where it's engaging.

- If you make mistakes more than 15% of the time, you've probably set your practice up to be too hard.

For your food skill practice, it's fine to plan to work on a skill or guideline at just one meal per day if that's how much you can expect to be successful 85% of the time. Some skills are harder than others. Sometimes for an easier skill, we can start shooting for practicing at every meal. Other times, for a harder skill we might practice only three or four times per week. All practice is good practice; just set it up so you're successful 85% of the time.

For workouts, your form should be really tight 85% of the time. Most lifts should look perfect. Once in a while, you're going to push the weight up and things might be a little sloppier that first workout. That's fine as long as you're within a safe range—just stay there until your form is awesome again.

LEAN AND STRONG AS SELF-CARE VERSUS LEAN AND STRONG AS PUNISHMENT

Self-care is a big topic and nearly completely misunderstood in the world of fitness. We're going to cover it in depth in The Ten Turning Points section and go even deeper in The Wise Five section, outlining the three different kinds of self-care.

What you need to know this first month is that the people who are the most successful treat their food skill practice and their workouts as a self-care.

You know people are destined for failure if they treat their diets like punishment for feeling fat. If they think suffering is the key to weight loss, they're never going to last more than a couple months. Weight loss as suffering and punishment is the context for repeated weight loss failure…for the rest of your life.

Similarly, when people use workouts as punishment for something they ate, these are people who are never going to be lean or strong. They're teaching themselves to hate their workouts. I mean, who likes being punished? What's more, it's not an even slightly effective strategy for weight loss (that's what eating skills are for).

I don't know who first said, "Workouts aren't punishment for what you ate; they're a celebration of what your body can do," but no truer words were ever spoken. The people who are the strongest are those who use working out as a way to feel better in their bodies. The people who are the leanest are those who treat their workouts as their time to take care of themselves and to reduce stress.

The people who use workouts as "me time," as something wonderful they can do for their bodies, work out *forever*. People who practice the eating skills because they like the way they feel do their eating skills *forever*.

Our current diet and fitness world is built around the idea of working out and dieting as punishment. The punishment messages are everywhere. You might hear them from friends or read them online, or even hear them from trainers. I don't expect you to stop having those thoughts. It's now a matter of no longer feeding or acting on those thoughts. Instead, focus on your values and take actions in line with them.

Some of the best self-care a person can do is to practice eating skills and to work out. But the context with which you do those things matters. If you do them coming from a place of punishment, you'll fail and quit…over and over again.

If you do it coming from a place of your personal values, you'll find your workouts and skill practice to be the foundation of your personal self-care routine.

	DAY:	M	T	W	TH	F	SA	SU
	DATE:							
DURING MEALS	Plate balanced portions	3	0	2	3			
	Put the fork down between bites	1	2	1	1			
BETWEEN MEALS	Eat a meal every four to six hours (without snacking in between)	3	3	3	3			
	Distinguish true hunger from cravings, boredom, tiredness, emotions, or thoughts	2	4	3	3			
IF/THEN PLANNING	If: I get stressed at work Then: I'm going to walk a lap around the building		X		X			
TURNING POINT	Practicing excellence and self-compassion	X	X	X				

TURNING POINTS
ON YOUR SKILL TRACKER

You're going to start by putting the one Turning Point you're focusing on into your tracker. You can note any time you reflect on that turning point or use it to make a decision about your skill practice in a given week.

VALUES REFLECTION

Of the five elements in The Wise Five, we're going to start with (arguably) the most important: personal values—values are what drive your intrinsic motivation. Intrinsic motivation is one of the most important factors in long-term success with fitness behavior.[16,17]

Values show up in The Meta-skills, The Ten Turning Points, and in The Wise Five. Given how often they show up, here is a short introduction.

Goals: A goal is a destination point. It's something you can measure. It has a clear ending. It's like hitting a certain number of pullups, or hitting a certain scale weight.

Values: A value is a direction. The direction never ends. It's like being a good parent or being a good friend—there's no end; it's an expression of who you want to be. You could also call it character strength.

Values are often made to seem lofty or grand, but in *Lean and Strong*, they're much simpler than that. Your values are just what matters to you, the kind of person you want to be, and what you stand for.

The irony of values and goals is that people who take a values perspective to their food skill and workout practice tend to hit their goals. On the flip side, people who put their body image goals first often struggle to hit those goals or to maintain them for any length of time. Again, there are multiple in-depth explanations of how and why that works later in the book.

For now, just know that being the kind of person you want to be is the most effective way to become lean and strong.

The values exercise on the next page shows up three times in this book. It's the simplest and most accessible of all the values reflections, and it's worth doing *at least* three times. Each time you do it, you'll have a better idea of how it fits into your practice and into your life. The cool thing is, research shows that all we have to do to increase our intrinsic motivation is to reflect on our values weekly.[18]

The Wise Five section of the book will have 12 weeks of values reflections to do in your journal. For now, it's enough to circle a few values and begin thinking how your food skill practice and workouts line up with your values. If they don't, begin to adjust your skill practice so your values are better expressed.

It's funny, but being the kind of person we want to be in the world really is just as simple as clarifying our values and adjusting our actions to match. It's knowing the character strengths we'd like to express in the world, and practicing them. When being lean and strong is simply an expression of your values, you'll be lean and strong for life.

Make sure to write your top three values at the bottom of your eating skills tracker.

28

YOU CAN CIRCLE YOUR TOP ONE TO THREE VALUES FROM THIS CHART OR COME UP WITH YOUR OWN.

Acceptance	Flexibility	Play
Adventure	Freedom	Reciprocity
Assertiveness	Friendship	Respect
Authenticity	Forgiveness	Resourcefulness
Balance	Fun	Responsibility
Beauty	Generosity	Romance
Caring	Gratitude	Safety
Challenge	Home	Self-awareness
Collaboration	Honesty	Self-care
Community	Humor	Self-discipline
Compassion	Humility	Self-expression
Connection	Industriousness	Self-respect
Contribution	Independence	Service
Cooperation	Intimacy	Skillfulness
Courage	Joy	Spirituality
Creativity	Justice	Stewardship
Curiosity	Kindness	Strength
Design	Knowledge	Supportiveness
Dignity	Leadership	Teamwork
Diversity	Learning	Tradition
Encouragement	Love	Trustworthiness
Ethics	Loyalty	Understanding
Equality	Mindfulness	Uniqueness
Excitement	Order	Usefulness
Exploration	Open-mindedness	Vision
Fairness	Optimism	Vulnerability
Faith	Patience	Wellbeing
Family	Persistence	Wholeheartedness
Fitness	Personal Development	Wisdom

SAMPLE SKILLS TRACKER

		DAY:	M	T	W	TH	F	SA	SU
		DATE:							
DURING MEALS	Plate balanced portions		3	0	2	3			
	Put the fork down between bites		1	2	1	1			
BETWEEN MEALS	Eat a meal every four to six hours (without snacking in between)		3	3	3	3			
	Distinguish true hunger from cravings, boredom, tiredness, emotions, or thoughts		2	4	3	3			
IF/THEN PLANNING	If: I get stressed at work Then: I'm going to walk a lap around the building			X		X			
TURNING POINT	Practicing excellence and self-compassion vs. perfectionism		X	X	X				
VALUES (LIST THREE)	Persistence, compassion, connectedness								

SKILLS TRACKER FOR YOUR FIRST FOUR WEEKS

WEEK ONE	DAY:	M	T	W	TH	F	SA	SU
	DATE:							
DURING MEALS	Plate balanced portions							
	Put the fork down between bites							
BETWEEN MEALS	Eat a meal every four to six hours							
	Wait ten minutes before having a snack							

WEEK TWO	DAY:	M	T	W	TH	F	SA	SU
	DATE:							
DURING MEALS	Plate balanced portions							
	Put the fork down between bites							
BETWEEN MEALS	Eat a meal every four to six hours (without snacking in between)							
	Distinguish true hunger from cravings, boredom, tiredness, emotions, or thoughts							
IF/THEN PLANNING	If: Then:							

WEEK THREE		DAY:	M	T	W	TH	F	SA	SU
		DATE:							
DURING MEALS	Plate balanced portions								
	Put the fork down between bites								
BETWEEN MEALS	Eat a meal every four to six hours								
	Wait ten minutes before having a snack								
IF/THEN PLANNING	If: Then:								
TURNING POINT	Practicing excellence and self-compassion								

WEEK FOUR	DAY:	M	T	W	TH	F	SA	SU
	DATE:							
DURING MEALS	Plate balanced portions							
	Put the fork down between bites							
BETWEEN MEALS	Eat a meal every four to six hours (without snacking in between)							
	Distinguish true hunger from cravings, boredom, tiredness, emotions, or thoughts							
IF/THEN PLANNING	If: Then:							
TURNING POINT	Engagement/flow/goldilocksing							
VALUES (LIST THREE)								

YOUR FIRST MONTH OF WORKOUTS

The next pages will show your first month of workouts. There are 12 workouts to do over the course of the month, so you'll do about three workouts per week.

The workouts in this section are at an intermediate level, with medium volume. The intermediate, medium-volume workouts will be the best place to start for the majority of readers.

This book will have workouts in three levels of complexity: beginning, intermediate, and advanced. Those three workouts will have three different levels of volume: low, medium, and high. The "volume" of a workout program is the amount of work you're doing.

We're going to measure the amount of work you are doing by the number of sets. The intermediate workouts are medium complexity, and the volume is the medium total amount of work. It's the best place to start for most people, but the workout section will show you how to customize the skill level and volume for your individual situation.

The workout section starts on page 119. You'll find the workout program options in the appendices, with beginner workouts starting on page 281, intermediate workouts on page 289, and advanced workouts on page 309.

The first page includes all of the odd workouts—1, 3, 5, 7, 9, 11—and the second page has all of the even workouts—2, 4, 6, 8, 10, 12. You'll flip the page every other workout to do the workouts in numerical order.

To be clear:

Do three workouts per week.

Do the workouts in numerical order: 1, 2, 3, 4, 5… just like counting.

It could look like:

— Workout one on Monday

— Workout two on Wednesday

— Workout three on Friday

And so on.

The actual days you do the workouts don't matter, but try to avoid doing two back to back if you can. Sometimes that's unavoidable, and doing two workouts back to back is still better than skipping one.

Adjust the weight on each exercise so the workouts are appropriately challenging. If the workouts seem way too easy, increase the weight. If the workouts seem too hard, decrease the weight. If you blow through the workout in 15 minutes, the weights are too light. If the workout takes you two hours, the weights are too heavy. Adjust the weights of each exercise so all of the exercises are similar in difficulty to the other exercises in the workout.

Notice that the volume of work (the number of sets of each exercise) increases over the course of the month. You'll start off with two sets of everything, and by the end of the month you'll be doing three or four sets of everything.

All of the exercises are grouped either in supersets (two exercises back to back) or tri-sets (three exercises back to back). Either way, do all of the exercises in that group, then rest. In the tri-sets, the first two are strength exercises; the third, in italics, is a mobility exercise.

Do three workouts per week, in numerical order. Week one, do workouts 1, 2, and 3. Week two, do workouts 4, 5, and 6. Use this sheet as a tracker to write down the weight used for each exercise in the box for that workout, underneath the sets and reps.

INTERMEDIATE MEDIUM VOLUME—MONTH ONE, ODD WORKOUTS

	WORKOUT 1	WORKOUT 3	WORKOUT 5	WORKOUT 7	WORKOUT 9	WORKOUT 11
BAND DEAD BUGS	2x10	3x10	3x10	3x10	3x10	3x10
TRAP BAR DEADLIFTS	2x10	3x10	3x10	3x10	3x10	4x10
PUSHUPS	2x max	3x max	3x max	3x max	3x max	4x max
HIP FLEXOR STRETCHES	2x8	3x8	3x8	3x8	3x8	4x8
SINGLE-CABLE ROWS	2x10	3x10	3x10	3x10	3x10	4x10
SPLIT SQUATS	2x10	3x10	3x10	3x10	3x10	4x10
T-SPINE ROTATIONS	2x8	3x8	3x8	3x8	3x8	4x8
ONE-ARM KETTLEBELL SWINGS	1x10	2x10	3x10	4x10	5x10	5x10

When three exercises are grouped together, do those back-to-back as a tri-set. For exercises on one leg or one arm, sets listed are for each side.

INTERMEDIATE MEDIUM VOLUME—MONTH ONE, EVEN WORKOUTS

	WORKOUT 2	WORKOUT 4	WORKOUT 6	WORKOUT 8	WORKOUT 10	WORKOUT 12
PALLOF PRESSES	2x10	3x10	3x10	3x10	3x10	3x10
ASSISTED CHIN-UPS	2x10	3x10	3x10	3x10	3x10	4x10
DOUBLE-KETTLEBELL FRONT SQUATS	2x10	3x10	3x10	3x10	3x10	4x10
T-SPINE ROTATIONS	2x8	3x8	3x8	3x8	3x8	4x8
75° INCLINE DOUBLE-DUMBBELL BENCH PRESSES	2x10	3x10	3x10	3x10	3x10	4x10
ONE-KETTLEBELL COSSACK DEADLIFTS	2x10	3x10	3x10	3x10	3x10	4x10
HIP FLEXOR STRETCHES	2x8	3x8	3x8	3x8	3x8	4x8
ONE-ARM KETTLEBELL SWINGS	1x10	2x10	3x10	4x10	5x10	5x10

OPTIONAL BONUS CONDITIONING: DAN JOHN'S HUMANE BURPEE

WORKOUTS ONE AND TWO	WORKOUTS THREE AND FOUR	WORKOUTS FIVE AND SIX	WORKOUTS SEVEN AND EIGHT	WORKOUTS NINE AND TEN	WORKOUTS ELEVEN AND TWELVE
15 swings 5 squats 5 pushups	15 swings 5 squats 5 pushups	15 swings 5 squats 5 pushups	15 swings 5 squats 5 pushups	15 swings 5 squats 5 pushups	15 swings 5 squats 5 pushups
	15 swings 4 squats 4 pushups	15 swings 4 squats 4 pushups	15 swings 4 squats 4 pushups	15 swings 4 squats 4 pushups	15 swings 4 squats 4 pushups
		15 swings 3 squat 3 pushup	15 swings 3 squats 3 pushups	15 swings 3 squats 3 pushups	15 swings 3 squats 3 pushups
			15 swings 2 squat 2 pushup	15 swings 2 squats 2 pushups	15 swings 2 squats 2 pushups
				15 swings 1 squat 1 pushup	15 swings 1 squat 1 pushup

Let's discuss Dan John's famous "humane" burpee. Believe it or not, lots of people think it's "fun" to do humane burpees at the end of the workout instead of five sets of one-arm kettlebell swings. That's totally an option.

I'm not a fan of normal burpees—they get so ugly, so fast. Most people doing burpees mess them up six different ways:

The squat down is an ugly squat;

The jump back lands really hard;

The low back sags on the pushups;

They're too tight to jump their feet back under them;

They jump with little explosiveness;

And then they land hard and inefficiently.

Pretty much every part of the burpee is terrible.

The humane burpee gets all of the conditioning work of a regular burpee, and yet people are able to do it well. If you can swing, do goblet squats, and pushups, combine those. If you can't yet do full pushups, knee pushups are cool to start. If form starts to come apart, stop and catch your breath.

If that's hard to read, just do it in this order:

Swings x 15, Goblet Squats x 5, Pushups x 5

Swings x 15, Goblet Squats x 4, Pushups x 4

Swings x 15, Goblet Squats x 3, Pushups x 3

Swings x 15, Goblet Squats x 2, Pushups x 2

Swings x 15, Goblet Squats x 1, Pushups x 1

You could also use humane burpees as an optional conditioning day or you could use them on a day when you don't have time to get a full workout. Feel free to substitute humane burpees for any of the conditioning work during any month you like.

HOW TO USE THIS BOOK

Don't Diet

> The first step is to stop doing things that don't work

Eating Skills and Workout Skills

> What skills to practice to get lean and strong

Meta-skills

> How to practice the skills so your practice is successful each week

The Ten Turning Points

> How to think about your skills practice so you don't sabotage your results every eight weeks

The Wise Five

> Understanding intrinsic motivation and how it works

You may or may not need to read this entire book. It's designed to have the most immediately useful material up front and the important long-term concepts in the back. You can start practicing as soon as you start reading, and simply work your way back as much as needed.

PART ONE: DON'T DIET AND DON'T DO ONE-OFF WORKOUTS

This is what 90% of the fitness and diet fields are trying to sell you. You need to know what this means so you can *avoid it*. Most of what you see and hear about diet and fitness on a day-to-day basis is a trap that keeps people in a cycle of failure. Step one is getting out of the failure cycle.

This part is what *not to do*.

Ironically, we're so mired in diet culture, you may have to come back to this step multiple times.

PART TWO: SKILLS AND PROGRAMS

This is where we're going to get into the most effective eating skills and guides. I'm also going to give you the most effective workout skills. If you're someone who's already good at changing habits and behaviors and just needs to know what to do, you might only need to read through this section.

This part is *what to do.*

PART THREE: META-SKILLS

Most people need tools for behavior and habit change. Knowing what to do—even if it's the best techniques—isn't enough. The Meta-skills are your step-by-step roadmap of how to make big changes to eating skills and workouts, even if you've never been successful before.

This part is *how to do it.*

PART FOUR: TURNING POINTS

Honestly, if you practice your skills and Meta-skills for a few years, you will naturally make these important mindset shifts. And when you have these shifts—these turning points—that both catapults you to a new level of results and allows you to keep your results for the rest of your life. Instead of making you practice for a few years to figure them out, I'm just going to tell you.

This part is *what to think* about what you're doing.

PART FIVE: PSYCHOLOGY

Here we are going to look at the psychology of weight loss, motivation, and wellbeing. We're going to build tools for a better body image. This is the section about how to not only hit your goals, but also to create a healthy relationship to your body, to food, and to your workouts. This is where people create a kind of peace around fitness, food, and a body they never could have imagined. We already have a few decades of research on how to do this. It works really well both in research and with clients, but no one else in the fitness field is giving you this information. Here's where you get that information.

This section is where you *transform your relationship* to what you're doing.

READ WHAT YOU NEED

You might not need to read all of this. And you definitely shouldn't wait to start practicing until after you've finished reading.

A person who's great at habit change and food behavior and workouts might only need to read sections one and two. Either way, after reading those sections, everyone should start practicing. In fact, start practicing even before you're done with them.

A person who needs a really powerful strategy to make changes in life related to food or workouts could read sections one, two, and three.

Someone who is doing well with one, two, and three, but still hits roadblocks should read section four.

And people who want to finally be at peace with their bodies can read section five.

Feel free to pick and choose. Skip around. Read what you need. Start practicing immediately.

THE TWO PYRAMIDS OF LEANNESS AND STRENGTH

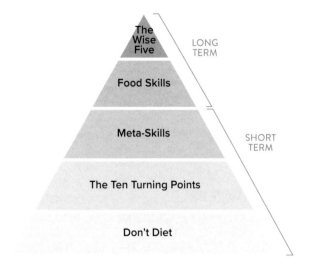

To get lean and strong, your work will mostly be about *not dieting*, practicing *eating skills*, and utilizing the *Meta-skills*. These three should be your biggest focus for your first year of practice.

After one to three years, the pyramid flips:

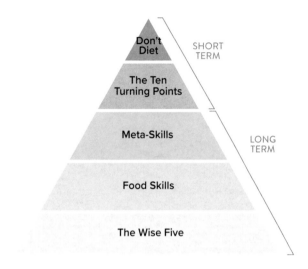

The Wise Five and The Ten Turning Points will be what you use to maintain your leanness and strength for the future. You'll also continue to utilize The Meta-skills. This flip of the pyramid is an important progression to work toward—this is how your practice should grow over the rest of your life.

By the time you get there "lean" and "strong" might take on new definitions for you. You'll see "lean" as being efficient, economical, and agile in pursuit of your goals, and "strong" will show up as doing what matters to you, even when it's hard. We'll dig in on more about that at the very end of the book, on page 244.

MOTIVATION DROPS IN WEEKS THREE AND SIX

After years of working with clients, I know I can predict a motivation drop at either week three or week six. This is where the novelty of a program starts to wear off and the fact it's going to be work sets in. Something comes up at work or with your kids, you just feel tired one day, or you miss doing the food preparation you were doing every week when you were excited about the process. You get the idea: Things come up and you stop "feeling it."

At the same time, it's too early to have seen amazing results. Whatever your goal, you haven't hit it yet. The burst of excitement that comes from seeing big changes hasn't kicked in. Even if you can tell the results are coming, or you've seen small successes, the big goals start to feel really far away…so, so far away. So, you miss a workout, or forget to track your skills for a week. Things just start to slide off.

This is where most coaches give you a silly pep talk. I'm not going to do that. I'm going to let you know everything you're feeling is totally normal. Almost everyone has a dip in motivation at week three or week six—almost everyone.

When most people miss something that week (like a workout or skill practice), they feel like a failure and quit. Other people think if they don't feel motivated, it must be the wrong program…and quit—and then go find another program they will quit at week three.

People quit at predictable times.

I just want you to know and expect this. People do really well if they just keep practicing. They practice even if they don't feel it. They keep practicing even if they sort of wake up and realize they didn't do anything for a week. They just get back to practicing.

If your week three or week six sucks, no prob—you're a normal human being. The people who hit their goals are the people who keep practicing their workouts and eating skills even after these predictable drops in motivation. If you want to hit your goals, keep practicing.

CHAPTER TWO
DON'T DIET

DIETING PREDICTS WEIGHT GAIN

Statistically, dieting is a strong predictor of weight gain.

A meta-analysis of 40 studies on long-term weight loss involving a total of 54,127 normal-weight participants found that dieting *was not predictive of* weight loss. Let me repeat:—Statistically, dieting isn't associated with weight loss in the long term. People lose weight, then gain it all back, or gain it all back…plus more.

In 75% of those studies, dieting strongly predicted weight *gain*.[19] That means if we were betting on whether or not a person would lose or gain weight in the long term, we'd be safe betting that someone who repeatedly diets will gain weight.

The findings of a five-year longitudinal study, "Project EAT-II" published in the *Journal of the American Dietetic Association* in 2007, showed that dieting predicted binge eating in adolescents.

A review in *American Psychologist*, "Medicare's search for effective obesity treatments: Diets are not the answer," showed that two-thirds of all people who diet will gain the weight back in one year. Nearly all of them will gain it back within five years. One-third of all dieters will gain back more than they lost…*each time they diet.*

Dieting seems to predispose people to emotional eating, cravings, and binge eating. Dieting starts a cycle of restricting and overeating.[20]

Many of us have had the same experience, or know someone who's had that experience—they lose 15 pounds, then gain back 17. While it looks like the diet works in the short term, the long-term trend is weight gain.

We're going to call this "The Diet Cycle of Failure."

THE PROS AND CONS OF DIFFERENT DIETS

DIET	PROS	CONS
INTERMITTENT FASTING	Learn that hunger isn't an emergency Simple One less meal to think about and prepare Reduces calories Allows for flexibility in food choices	Makes no difference in weight loss You can just as easily learn that hunger isn't an emergency by fasting four to six hours between meals, even having breakfast Teaches you to ignore true hunger in the morning

DIET	PROS	CONS
PALEO	Protein is good Fruit is good Vegetables are good Fat is good	Makes no difference in weight loss You can have protein, fruit, vegetables, and fat in a less-needlessly restrictive diet Makes people afraid of certain foods, without cause People doing the high volume Lean and Strong programs will do better with starchy carbs that paleo doesn't allow Black-and-white food rules are the top psychological predictor of weight-loss failure
KETOGENIC DIET	Protein is good Vegetables are good Fat is good	Makes no difference in weight loss Any diet that doesn't include fruit is completely ridiculous You can have protein, vegetables, and fat in a less-needlessly restrictive diet Making people afraid of an entire macronutrient should be criminal People doing the high volume Lean and Strong programs will be more effective with the starchy carbs that keto doesn't allow Black-and-white food rules are the top psychological predictor of weight-loss failure

DIET	PROS	CONS
EATING CLEAN	Protein is good Fruit is good Vegetables are good Fat is good	Makes no difference in weight loss The difference between "clean" and "dirty" foods is entirely made up, and the ideas are different depending on whom you ask "Clean" and "dirty" moralizes food in a way that increases emotional eating, increases food reactivity, and it increases binge eating for many people Making people afraid of certain foods should be criminal Black-and-white food rules are the top psychological predictor of weight-loss failure
MEDITERRANEAN DIET	Fish, chicken, and eggs are good Fruit is good Legumes are good Vegetables are good Olive oil and avocados are good Whole grains are good People enjoy it	Makes no difference in weight loss Cuts out more foods than necessary
VEGAN	Fruit is good Vegetables are good Plant-based fat is good May fit ethical or religious beliefs	Makes no difference in weight loss Requires intentionality to get enough protein from plant sources Requires intentionality to compensate for missing nutrients

TRACKING SYSTEMS

DIET	PROS	CONS
CALORIE COUNTING	Reducing calories always causes weight loss	High failure rate Tedious Counting calories is an "after the fact" measure, not an "on the court" measure like skill practice Can cause and/or exacerbate emotional eating, stress eating, and cravings for some people
MEAL PLAN	Reducing calories always causes weight loss It's simple	High failure rate Tedious People don't know what to eat when meal plan meals are not available
POINT SYSTEM	Reducing calories always causes weight loss	High failure rate Tedious Counting points is an "after the fact" measure, not an "on the court" measure like skill practice Can cause or exacerbate emotional eating, stress eating, and cravings for some people
MACRO TRACKING	Reducing calories always causes weight loss Helps people learn to eat balanced meals More flexible than dieting	High failure rate Tedious Counting macros is an "after the fact" measure, not an "on the court" measure such as skill practice

POLITICS, RELIGION, AND CARBOHYDRATES

Talking about carbohydrates these days has become as heated as arguing about politics and religion.

If you're old enough to remember "low fat," you know how sad it is to see people caught up in a new "magic macronutrient" fad. In the 1980s, everyone was sure fat was the evil macro. It's hilarious to see the same fad happen again…with carbs.

Neither one is wrong in the strictest sense:

1. If you eat too much fat, you'll get too many calories, and you'll gain weight.

2. If you eat too many carbohydrates, you'll get too many calories, and you'll gain weight.

A metabolic ward study is the ultimate in nutrition research. In a metabolic ward, study participants are literally locked in and everything they eat is served to them with the highest accuracy. They're monitored to make sure they eat exactly as the study is designed. On top of that, doubly labeled water (water containing two heavy isotopes) is used to measure people's metabolic rate. They measure and compare the elimination of the two isotopes and get a near-perfect measurement of metabolic rate.

A metabolic ward study in the *American Journal of Clinical Nutrition* compared a ketogenic diet (exactly 30 grams of carbohydrates) with a high carbohydrate diet (300 grams of carbohydrates) over four weeks. What was super cool about this study was that they kept the protein and calories the same in both groups. Weight loss was the same between groups.[21]

This is consistent with other longer-term studies. One randomized controlled trial followed 609 participants for a year. They compared a "healthy low carbohydrate" diet with a "healthy low fat" diet, and found no significant difference in weight loss between the two groups.[22]

One randomized controlled trial compared four diets: Atkins (low carbohydrates), Zone (balanced), Ornish (low fat), and Weight Watchers. They found that which diet a person did was insignificant. The only thing that predicted weight loss across groups was adherence.[23]

Another randomized study comparing four different groups with different ratios of protein, carbohydrates, and fat found the same thing: At one year, macronutrient ratios people used made no difference; it all came down to calories.[24]

Finally, a meta-analysis looking at 48 different randomized controlled trials, found this to be consistent across all of them. Over the combined 7,286 participants in all of those studies, people using low fat and low carbohydrate diets both lost the same amount of weight.[25] No matter what marketing you've heard, the only thing that matters is calories.

CARBOHYDRATES, STRENGTH, AND HIGH INTENSITY TRAINING

Generally, low carbohydrates aren't ideal for high intensity training. One study put athletes in groups with matched calories, but different carbohydrate percentages, and had them do high intensity training. The athletes in the ketogenic diet (low carbohydrate) group had 7% less power and covered 15% less distance.[26]

With strength, results are more mixed. It seems that with strength training, whichever group has the highest protein intake gains the most strength, regardless of carbohydrate or fat percentages.

A randomized controlled trial of low carbohydrate versus low fat diets with matched protein showed similar increases in strength.[27] A study of CrossFit™ athletes found no difference in performance between "moderately low" and high carbohydrate athletes, but it should be noted that their "moderately low" carbohydrates were about 12 times more carbohydrates than recommended by the ketogenic diet.[28] In fact, their idea of "moderately low" is pretty close to the one portion of carbohydrates per meal recommended in this book.

The big issue with most studies is that they often compare a ketogenic diet with anywhere between 130–180 grams of protein per day against a high carbohydrate diet with around 80 grams of protein per day.

Of course, 70–80 grams of protein per day is below the protein recommendations for strength training athletes by the International Olympic Committee, American Dietetic Association, Dieticians of Canada, and the American College of Sports Medicine.[29,30] It's likely that for strength, protein is the most important consideration.

STEPPING OVER DOLLARS

The saying "stepping over dollars to pick up pennies" is my favorite explanation of diet rules. And that applies to the minutia of every named diet on the market, even things like "eating clean."

A randomized controlled trial of processed food versus unprocessed food helps us understand this. They were given processed food or whole food in a locked ward where everything they ate, as well as their scale weight, was closely monitored.

The people in the processed food group ate an extra 508 calories per day, and gained weight. Basically, people felt less satisfied and ate more. There was no magic to the processed food; it just wasn't as filling. There was no magic to the whole food; it just helped people feel more full. All of the weight gain or loss in either group was attributable to eating more or fewer calories.[31]

There's no magic. Success is just about eating in ways that make you feel more full and satisfied. Literally every diet you've ever heard of is a waste of time: It's stepping over dollars (behavioral skills and psychology) to pick up pennies (magical foods). You have to give up magical thinking if you want to move forward.

BUT WAIT, MY FRIEND SAID!

Gather 'round children, it's story time. You see, in the 1980s, we were told fat was the evil macronutrient and that avoiding fat would be the magic secret to losing all the weight we wanted to lose. All of a sudden, the words "low fat" popped up everywhere on snack foods. People talked about how "low fat" they were eating, gleeful about how it was the key to everything. If you were born in, say, 1985 or later, I can't fault you for not remembering.

Some people lost weight. It was because fat has calories and reducing fat reduced the calories. When "low fat" snack foods appeared, those same people started snacking between meals again…because fat was the magic ingredient, and calories didn't matter. They all gained the weight back.

So, in the 1980s, we were told fat is evil. In the 2010s, we're told carbohydrates are evil. The low carb craze of the 2010s looks remarkably like the low fat craze of the 1980s. Some people lost weight eating low carb because it lowered their calories. Other people, thinking fat was a magical food with no calories, started adding extra fat to everything (including putting butter in their coffee!) and didn't lose weight. It turns out there aren't any magical foods.

Look—people love magical thinking.

It's way nicer to think there's a magic food that's the key to everything. But that's not real life. If you know someone who lost weight on a low fat diet, it was because it lowered the calories. If you know someone who lost weight on low carb, it was because it lowered the calories.

You have to get past thinking any food or food group has magical properties. This is part of growing up.

WHY DO DIETS WORK FOR SOME PEOPLE?

Diets do work for a minority of people.

If you were one of the people diets worked for, you'd likely not be reading this book. Instead, you've probably tried five or ten or more diets. Some of my clients have dieted more times than they can count. Many tell me they started dieting as young as 12 and have continued to diet all of their adult lives.

If you were in the minority of people whom diets worked for, you'd have already hit all of your goals, *and maintained those results for life.*

It's important, though, to note diets really do work for some people. There's a subset of the population—especially people who've never had any issues with emotional eating or food cravings—for whom dieting works really well.

Dieting works better if:

- You want to lose weight in the short term;

- You have no issues with cravings;

- You don't eat because you're tired;

- You don't eat because you're stressed;

- You don't eat because you have unwanted emotions.

A skills-based approach works better if:

- You want to lose weight and maintain the weight loss over the long term;

- In the past, you've had trouble with cravings;

- In the past, you've eaten when you were tired;

- In the past, you've eaten when you were stressed;

- In the past, you've eaten when you had unwanted emotions.

People who have issues with cravings or eating are less successful with rigid diet rules than are people who don't have issues with cravings.[32]

Rigid diet rules and dichotomous thinking about food—black or white, good or bad, clean or unclean—is related to weight loss failure. One study with 241 people found that thinking some foods were good and some were bad was linked to *weight regain.*[33] A study on eating behavior in 2014 found that rigid dieting predicted weight regain and lower wellbeing.[34]

One study found that calorie counting predicted weight gain, and rigid dieting predicted binge eating.[35]

A one-year weight loss program involving 7,407 people reported in *The International Journal of Eating Behaviors* found that rigid dieting was associated with higher scale weight and increased binge eating.[36] That's a huge sample size, and the results were remarkably consistent.

In a college population, it was found that rigid dieting predicted increased eating, increased weight, and increased loss of control around food in both women and men.[37]

Interestingly, dieting is just as bad for you if you're at a healthy weight. A study looking primarily at normal-weight women found that the women who used rigid dieting showed symptoms of eating disorders, poor body image, and mood disturbances. On the flip side, the normal-weight women who *didn't* use rigid dieting strategies had healthy eating habits, better mood, and better body image.[38]

Three studies looked at how calorie counting apps trigger, maintain, or exacerbate eating disorder symptoms. One study of 493 college students, found that using a calorie tracking app was uniquely associated with eating disorder symptoms.[39] A new study looked at calorie tracking app use by men and found that the app users had higher disordered eating symptomalogy.[40] It's cool they studied dudes, as they often get left out of studies like that, but it sucks that guys are also vulnerable to the negative effects of calorie counting apps.

This isn't to say calorie counting causes disordered eating or is bad for everyone, but in that second study, 40% of calorie counting app users felt it contributed to their disordered eating patterns.

The most damning, a 2004 study in *Behavioral Research and Therapy* found that black-and-white thinking about food, such as rigid diet rules, was "the number one psychological predictor of weight loss failure."[41]

In contrast, all of these studies found that a more flexible approach to managing food intake was more effective for weight loss, weight maintenance, and wellbeing. That's why we'll take a skills-based approach.

One of the most fascinating things found in the research is that people who have issues with cravings and stress eating need more advanced tools than people who don't.[42,43,44,45,46]

Dieting is basically the simplest and dumbest way to lose weight. It works really well when losing weight, and is relatively easy. I'm not saying people for whom dieting works don't work at it. I'm saying they don't have to work as hard as you do.

If losing weight is hard, you need better tools than dieting. Diets may work for your friend, your personal trainer, or your mom. But, if losing weight is hard for you, you need better tools. That's what this book is about—better tools (skills) that make a difference for a much broader group of people.

The diet profession doesn't understand you, and it has underserved you. It's time to get the tools you deserve, tools that will work for you.

GET BETTER: DIETS TO HABITS, SKILLS, AND META-SKILLS

Let's work our way from the least effective to most effective:

	CONCEPT	PROS	CONS
DIETS	Follow these food rules and lose weight	Requires very little thinking	High failure rate
HABITS	You have habits that either propel your behaviors toward your goals or away from your goals. Change bad habits to good habits.	Much higher success rate than diets More accurate look at how behavior is learned	Still sets people up for the feeling of being on or off, which isn't accurate Can be boring and slow
SKILLS	Everything you've ever learned follows a similar pattern of practice. You start out sucking, and you get better with more practice. With enough practice, you master the skills.	More effective than diets or habits Most accurate look at how behavior is learned Lessons learned in the gym can be applied to food, and vice versa	It takes practice to learn skills, and that's hard in the beginning It's outside of your comfort zone

Skills are the most effective. Meta-skills are how you learn the skills. These are the foundation of this book.

I used to use the word "habits," but that isn't as good a metaphor as skills. Habits feel like you're always building or removing something. When things don't feel effortless, people assume they don't "have the habit yet" or they "lost the habit," neither of which is true.

Eating skills, ironically, work similar to workout skills. You can do pushups three times per week and get better at pushups. As long as you're practicing, you get better.

With diets or habits, people assume they have to nail them every meal or they're "off their diet" or "losing their habit." With skills, on the other hand—as long as we practice them regularly—we get better. A person doesn't need to do kettlebell swings every day to get better. Doing kettlebell swings a few times per week will increase the skill of kettlebell swings.

Learning to eat slowly is like learning to do kettlebell swings. You could practice it three times per week and develop the skill. Granted, over time it makes sense to increase the frequency to more meals, but every week you practice, you get better.

If you stop playing your guitar for a week, you don't forget how to play a guitar. Similarly, if you go to Rome on vacation for a week and don't think about your eating skills, you don't forget them. You might even do some of them anyway, just because it feels better to eat using your skills. But even if you ignored the skills completely for a week, you'd still be just as good at them when you got back—you'd just start practicing again.

DON'T DO ONE-OFF WORKOUTS

The workout version of "don't diet" is "don't do one-off workouts." We have a society obsessed with random "workout entertainment." And, that's okay. If your workout goal is *entertainment*, randomness works. It's even fine for conditioning. I'm totally cool with workout entertainment; it just doesn't make you *strong*.

Progress is another kind of fun. Since "strong" is in the title of the book and you bought it, I assume getting stronger is something you want. Many of my clients think the *most fun* part is seeing their strength increase. If strength progress is something you're up for, random workouts aren't a good way to get there.

If someone who has a strength goal tells me, "I love my trainer; we do totally different workouts all of the time!" I know one of two things: Your trainer is either an idiot or is actually giving you intelligently planned workouts and *tricking* you into thinking they're different.

Look, most trainers don't really know how to get results so they basically hammer you with hard workouts, or entertain you with random workouts.

On the flip side, I totally respect trainers who give people smart workouts and trick them into thinking they're random. It's a pretty great way to meet people where they are, and also give them something that works. Maybe the sets and reps stay the same, but they rotate kettlebells one week, dumbbells the next, and barbells the week after that. Or, they change the rep range in a three-day rotating cycle, and it feels random to the client. Lastly, I've seen trainers just change the order of the exercises. All of these can be the same smart program, and just *look* different.

In this program, I'm not going to trick you. I'm just going to give you a really intelligent workout program.

Long-term workout programming is called "periodization," and we know periodized workouts are more effective than non-periodized workouts.[47,48] Also, the advantage periodized workout programs have over non-periodized programs increases over time; each month the performance gap widens.[49] There are several kinds of periodization that work. We're going to use two: block periodization and undulating periodization.

Research mostly points to undulating periodization being more effective for people who have been working out more than a year.[50] It's also a little more complicated, so we're going to save it for the advanced programs. Block periodization is simple, it works, and people love it. In the short term, it's just as effective as undulating periodization,[51] and it's where I like to start clients for their first year.

Again, it's okay to do totally random workouts if you're just doing it for fun and entertainment. It will absolutely bring your general fitness up to being better than if you did nothing at all. Fun and entertainment is cool. But workout entertainment is another book; the workouts in *Lean and Strong* are about getting strong.

If you're interested in getting strong, you'll want to do a periodized workout program.

THIS IS THE FIRST LESSON, AND YOU WILL REPEAT IT

Most people are constantly bombarded with diet and one-off workout messages. Pretty much everything you hear from your friends or read online will be the *opposite* of what you read in this book.

You'll be tempted by many diets. You might even slip and start dieting again. It's okay; just come back to skills.

You'll be tempted to turn the skills and guidelines in this book into diet rules. This is a quick route to a diet cycle of failure. It's okay; just come back to skills.

You might hear the siren's song of magical cleanses or ridiculous elimination programs. It's okay to want things to be that easy and magical and simple, but you know they aren't. Just come back to skills.

You'll see infographics for one-off workouts; you'll hear of friends doing stupid challenges. You may have a coworker who wants you to do some fitness challenge, even though it doesn't fit your goals. You may see a great-looking workout video that promises to destroy you, even though it doesn't fit your goals. It's okay; just come back to your periodized program.

DON'T DO WHAT DOESN'T WORK

Ironically, the most important thing isn't to do things that work (eating skills and periodized workout programs). The most important lesson is avoid things that don't work (diets and random workouts).

Your first mission, should you choose to accept it, is to avoid the diet cycle of failure.

Your second mission, should you choose to accept it, is to avoid silly workout randomness.

CHAPTER THREE
EATING SKILLS

Don't Diet	The first step is to stop doing things that don't work
Eating Skills and Workout Skills	What skills to practice to get lean and strong
Meta-skills	How to practice the skills so your practice is successful each week
The Ten Turning Points	How to think about your skills practice so you don't sabotage your results every eight weeks
The Wise Five	Understanding intrinsic motivation and how it works

THE DIET CYCLE OF FAILURE

A quick recap of the last chapter: The diet perspective is the path to failure. The skill perspective makes the most sense in contrast to what doesn't work.

Most of my clients have failed at five, ten, or more diets. Some of them have failed at so many diets, they've lost count.

The diet cycle of failure looks like this:

1. Rigid diet rules

2. Weight loss

3. Something happens

4. Fall off of rigid diet rules

5. Quit

People will repeat the cycle for years. The worst possible outcome is that people repeat the cycle with even more rigid diet rules. The thinking is, "If the last diet wasn't strict enough, this one will be even stricter!"

The consequence is, they either move faster through the diet cycle of failure, or they hold on longer and fail more spectacularly. They essentially white knuckle the rigid dietary rules until they snap, which is followed by a free-for-all resembling binge eating.

There are some things we talked about in the last chapter about rigid diet rules:

1. They are the number one psychological predictor of weight loss failure.

2. They reduce people's subjective wellbeing (life satisfaction).

3. They are related to a much worse body image.

4. They increase binge eating episodes.

So, rigid diet rules are the path to failure, hating your body, and binge eating. Are you ready to get off the diet cycle of failure?

One study, "Why Diets Fail," found three reasons people fail in the diet phase: dichotomous thinking, thought suppression, and cravings. [52] They defined the "diet phase" as an imposition of rigid rules about food and drastic changes to food intake.

All three of these led to some version of a "binge." I put binge in quotes because they weren't talking about binge eating disorder; they were talking about binge eating behavior purely brought on as a reaction to dieting.

1. *Dichotomous thinking*: This food is "good" and that one is "bad;" this food is "clean" and this one is "dirty."

2. *Thought suppression:* Don't think about wanting that; trying to suppress cravings, feelings, or thoughts.

3. *Cravings:* I see that food I can't have and I want it more.

We can flip the reasons for diet failure and create a skill plan for success:

1. *Continuum thinking:* Food is on a continuum with many shades of gray. Some foods and some balances of foods will keep you full for longer than others. There's no magic.

2. *Thought acceptance:* It's normal to have thoughts. It's normal to have feelings. I can have thoughts and notice them. In noticing my thoughts and accepting them, I'm better able to take care of myself and do things that matter to me.

3. *Flexibility:* Practice saying "yes" to treats sometimes, and practice saying "no" to treats sometimes. Figure out the balance that fits your personal values.

The way most people have been taught to relate to dieting is a perfect plan for failure. The path to success is to notice diet thoughts—in our diet-obsessed culture, you're going to keep having them so you might as well accept them—and then practice the opposite of diet thoughts listed above: *continuum thinking, thought acceptance, and flexibility.*

SKILLS, NOT DIETS

Skills promote better body image, have a higher success rate with weight loss, and increase subjective wellbeing. They're literally the inverse of rigid diet rules.

The benefits of food skill approach:

1. Both short-term and long-term weight loss success;

2. Increased subjective wellbeing (life satisfaction);

3. Better body image;

4. Eliminate the cycle of restricting and overeating;

5. Challenge and mastery experiences related to greater self-efficacy;

6. Challenge is related to engagement and fun;

7. Everyone gets better at skills with practice.

If I have a mission in life, it's to educate people on the pitfalls of rigid diet rules. I want to help people understand the research *all points to rigid diet rules being a recipe for failure and making your life worse.*

And then to flip it—I want to educate people about how a skill-based approach is the most effective way to lose weight and produces the longest lasting results. If you're interested in losing weight once and then being done with it, skills are the only option.

On top of that, the skill-based approach is challenging, fun, and builds self-efficacy. There's something inherently awesome about seeing yourself progress in skill practice. As humans, we're wired to enjoy playing games right at the edge of our skill levels. And we love to see our skill practice improve.

WHAT I LEARNED WITH ONE BY ONE NUTRITION

The coolest part about writing *Fat Loss Happens on Monday* was how many people I got exposed to. In the year immediately following the release of the book, I was interviewed by podcasters and invited to speak all over the country and got to hang out with some of the smartest people in the fitness and nutrition fields.

Steven "Coach Stevo" Ledbetter invited me to speak at the Oakland Motivate Summit about coaching food habits. Georgie Fear, author of *Lean Habits*, was also speaking about coaching food habits. Our talks fit together so seamlessly that afterward, a dozen personal trainers in attendance came up to Georgie and me and asked us if we had a mentorship for trainers.

I'd just met Georgie and her husband, Roland Fisher, the day before, but we were already three peas in a pod. While it seemed a little silly to start a project together the day after meeting, it also totally made sense. We figured if it sucked, we could just walk away. We told the trainers we'd start a mentorship for coaching food habits in a couple months, after we had some time to put it together.

Getting to work with Georgie and Roland on the trainer mentorship over the next year was amazing, and completely transformed how I coach food. The addictive part of being a teacher is that the teacher always learns the most. First, getting to understand something well enough that you can explain it clearly really nails things down. Second, having 30 other coaches using those techniques with their clients and then reporting back multiplied the number of clients we got to test with our ideas. I learned even more hearing how people used the skills with their clients, and what worked and didn't.

I tried the food habits from Georgie's book, *Lean Habits*, and I was sure they wouldn't work. The whole "intuitive eating" vibe of the book seemed a little too good to be true. I really respect Georgie (she's a genius), but I still didn't think people could be taught to regulate the quantity of food they ate (and thus their bodyweight) entirely off of their own hunger and fullness cues.

I started with one of her habits, "Eat three or four meals per day." This made sense on paper—people eat a ton of extra calories snacking between meals and those calories don't provide anywhere near the fullness per calorie that meals do. In her book, Georgie broke down the science and physiology on why—she's a Registered Dietician and has a research interest in the physiology of satiety so she was pretty convincing. Meanwhile, I looked up the psychology of snacking and found that—psychologically—we don't relate to snacks the same way we relate to meals. Aside from the fact that some of the reasons people snack aren't hunger related (boredom, stress, sadness), we assume snacks won't be as filling. We later want food sooner than if we'd eaten the same calories and content in a meal.

Trying "Eat three or four meals per day" with clients was mind-blowing. First, people lost weight with little or no difference in actual hunger. Second, people learned to distinguish between true hunger (in their stomach) and everything else (cravings, habit, boredom, stress, emotions, and so on).

The part about distinguishing true hunger from cravings was so totally game-changing, I was in for trying the rest of the habits.

Georgie, Roland, and I spent that first year together working with some wonderful trainers in the mentorship and continually swapping ideas and strategies about food habits.

While discussing more autonomy and less rigid ways to coach habits, we started bouncing around the idea of working together. We reincorporated One by One Nutrition as partners, and worked together for two years.

It was one of the most amazing learning experiences of my life. I transitioned partially out of the gym, and started doing significantly more nutrition habits phone coaching. We put together groups and taught them hunger and fullness skills. I'm forever grateful for how much I learned working not just with Georgie, but also coaches Sarah Campbell, Maryclaire Brescia, and Kara Buetel.

That year working together in the mentorship plus two more years with One by One Nutrition had a huge impact on me, and directly informed some of the listen-to-your-body skills in this book, like eating a meal every four to six hours and waiting until hungry before eating. Ultimately, that project ended and we went our separate ways, but it had a major impact on my effectiveness as a coach.

SKILLS, NOT HABITS

I had been giving workshops in gyms, relating the things we were working on back to gym movements. Sometimes, I'd started to say "skills" instead of "habits." It was a better metaphor—eating skills are like workout skills. A skill like "eating slowly" is similar to a skill like a kettlebell swing.

In the habit perspective, you're working on actions for weight loss, but there's always a concern whether your habit is getting stronger or weaker, or if old habits are still too strong, and so on. You worry about how many days per week your current habit is as a percentage of your habit success. The idea was close, because it was working on the *actions* of weight loss, but it wasn't entirely correct.

"Skills" are more accurate. Think about a kettlebell swing again—if people practice the kettlebell swing three days per week, the movement gets better. They don't "lose" the kettlebell swing skill on the days they aren't practicing. They aren't "out of the habit." Those are just days they didn't practice. Eating skills are like that. Eating skills are like every other skill you've ever learned—the more repetitions you get of a skill, the better you are at that skill.

LIKE PLAYING A CLARINET

If you ever learned to play a musical instrument, or if your kids learned to play a musical instrument in school, it was similar. The more repetition of practice, the better you got. If you took a day off, you didn't get reps in, but you didn't lose the skill. You can practice any skill; you get faster or better the more reps you get in. But there isn't a penalty for not getting a rep. The habit metaphor for food action made it feel like any meal you didn't practice, you'd get penalized, but it doesn't work like that in real life.

It works like a skill.

Going back to the clarinet—think about the evolution of playing:

- Playing the recorder in elementary school: lots of mistakes, lots of practice—often more missed notes than right notes

- Playing the clarinet in junior high: lots of missed notes—often missing just as many notes as in elementary school, but on more complex songs or with better timing

- Playing the clarinet in high school: significantly fewer missed notes on the kinds of songs played in elementary school or junior high; the notes are played with better timing and more expression—still misses notes when practicing new and significantly more complex songs

One thing you'll notice:

At every stage there were missed notes.

In the beginning, there were tons of missed notes, even in basic songs. Then, *after years*, those songs are near mastery and have few missed notes, along with better timing and expression. New and more complex songs would still have missed notes. This is what eating skills are like.

THE MISTAKE OF DIET PERFECTION VERSUS CLARINET PRACTICE

People approach food with diet rules that require perfection. It's sort of like being asked to play for the New York Symphony Orchestra on day one. It's amazing that people can white knuckle it for even a couple months.

Then, when they "miss a note" eating wise, they feel like a massive failure. They "blew their diet." And they polish that off by eating a bunch of junk food and way too much…until next week, next month, next year, whenever.

Until we realize there's only one way to learn skills—with practice—we're going to repeat the diet cycle of failure over and over again.

Practice requires three things:

1. Getting it right sometimes;

2. Making mistakes sometimes;

3. Learning from both getting it right and making mistakes.

If you try to practice without making mistakes, you'll never be successful with either eating or strength training skills.

GYM SKILLS AND EATING SKILLS

The trainers I've mentored really like the skill perspective. The clients I work with really like the way workouts and food work the same way—it's just skill practice.

A lot of my clients have had a background in kettlebell training or yoga, and were familiar with a "skill practice" approach to fitness as opposed to a "suffering and fatigue" approach. They had already seen how working from a skill-based approach made dramatic differences in their fitness practice, and were hyped to take that same approach to their food skill practice.

And that's why I call them skills now, instead of habits. Habits were a major evolution from diets and calorie counting, but the concept was only halfway there. Food skill practice is the next level.

THROWING IT ALL OUT
AND STARTING OVER

After writing *Fat Loss Happens on Monday*, I mostly coached from those habits—habits revolving around helping people get better at tracking, planning, shopping, and cooking.

Working with One by One Nutrition, I coached from those habits (later, skills), mostly around teaching internal hunger and fullness cue-based eating.

After leaving One by One Nutrition, I realized I wasn't bound by anything I'd done before. I could throw it all out, and start with a blank slate. I got the crazy idea that maybe the paradigms I had for coaching might be holding back what was possible.

I started by literally throwing away everything I'd used before, and went back to the research. I read research on intuitive eating, and found out how amazing it is for changing people's relationship to their bodies, their relationships with food, and how it reduces emotional eating.[53,54,55,56,57] Given how powerful and consistent an effect it has on people's wellbeing, intuitive eating skills have to be included. These became the *listen-to-your-body skills* in this section. To be clear, these aren't *exactly* intuitive eating skills. We're borrowing what's effective from intuitive eating to hone your natural hunger and fullness cues.

As far as intuitive eating skills and weight loss, the research is a mixed bag. Some studies show it works well for weight loss.[58,59] Others found that intuitive eating isn't as effective for weight loss as are guidelines and mindful decision making.[60,61]

I went back to the research on mindfulness and eating, and found there's a distinction between mindful eating and mindful decision making, and that mindful decision making is more effective for weight loss.[62,63] Mindful eating is more or less intuitive eating. Mindful decision making means mindfully making choices ahead of time, based on your values, and it looks a lot like the guidelines in this book. Mindful decision making is really effective for weight loss, and should absolutely be a part of your program if weight loss is your goal.[64,65,66,67,68,69] These became the guidelines in this section.

I did a research review on emotional eating and found people who have emotional eating issues need different skills and guidelines than people who don't (as reviewed in the "Don't Diet" section on page 41). I looked at the research on perfectionism, and found that perfectionism is the opposite of the pursuit of excellence (as covered in the section on "perfectionism versus excellence" on page 23). I went back to my client notes over the previous year, and discovered there are ten things all of my most successful clients figure out. These became The Ten Turning Points.

Lastly, reading research about Self Determination Theory (SDT) and contextual behavioral science (CBS) with health behavior, I found that any book on behavior change that doesn't include the basic tenets of SDT and CBS is wicked incomplete. In the long run, those elements are what make people successful, and are what changes their lives. That became the Wise Five in the last section of this book.

Speaking of psychology, going back to school for psychology has had a profound impact on this book. I'm really lucky to have amazing professors like Dr. Cynthia Erickson, who taught me not just about statistics and research methods, but also about the most cutting-edge, evidence-based teaching methods, like the testing effect. Consider Dr. Maureen Flynn's Second Wave Positive Psychology class, where I got an in-depth look at Acceptance and Commitment Therapy, and the evidence on how important it is to feel all human feelings, positive and negative.

Dr. Richard Kessel taught me about creating frameworks to hang ideas on so people can learn them more effectively. Dr. Harvey Milkman's class teaching addictions and cravings was where I learned how to use self-care, mindfulness, meaningful engagement of talents and effortful activities to increase self-efficacy and beat cravings. Dr. Courtney Rocheleau taught me how to read and evaluate research and in whose class I got to write a literature review on behavioral weight loss for people with emotional eating. All of these professors, in different ways, contributed either to the content of this book, the way I was able to research it, or how the book was structured so you can get the most out of it.

One of the biggest things I found, which you'll see in this section, is that intuitive eating skills and eating guidelines aren't mutually exclusive. I've never seen a book or research paper that used both at the same time—they almost always contrast them. This is totally anecdotal and just comes from my experience working with clients, but here it is: The clients who do the best use *both*. They sometimes more trust their body skills, and sometimes they use more eating guidelines, but they almost always use a combination of both. I think it's kind of ironic, but people learn the body skills faster and are more successful with them when they can use some guidelines as a framework for their practice.

That's the evolution of the eating skills and guidelines in this section.

HOW DOES INTUITIVE EATING WORK?

This is where this program really pulls ahead of everything else in the field. We're going to look at the research on intuitive eating and then use the *Lean and Strong* method to systematically teach you how to do it.

First, let's look at what intuitive eating is.

Intuitive eating is:

- **Unconditional permission to eat when hungry** and whatever food is desired at the moment—by not ignoring hunger signals or classifying food into acceptable and non-acceptable categories;

- **Eating to satisfy physical hunger** rather than to cope with emotional fluctuations or distress;

- Reliance on (reflecting an awareness and trust of) **internal hunger and satiety cues** to determine when and how much to eat.[70,71,72,73,74]

If that sounds crazy to you, let's take a look at what weight gain and weight loss look like in terms of actual behaviors:

Weight gain—in actions:

1. Eating when not hungry;

2. Eating unbalanced meals;

3. Eating past being full;

4. Snacking when bored or to procrastinate;

5. Snacking or eating treats or drinking alcohol when stressed or emotional;

6. Cycles of resistance of certain foods and treats, then exploding and overeating them.

Weight loss—in actions:

1. Eating a meal when hungry;

2. Eating balanced meals;

3. Stopping when full;

4. *Not* snacking between meals due to boredom or procrastination;

5. *Not* having treats because of emotions or stress;

6. Using healthy, non-food ways to cope with emotions and stress;

7. Having a serving of treats once in a while.

You can look at those lists and see that all of the things related to weight gain are *actions*. It doesn't matter what magical diet you're on if you're snacking between meals due to boredom or emotions.

On the flip side, it's easy to see that any person taking the actions in the weight loss list would have a healthy weight forever. Again, there are no evil foods to avoid… mostly, just "eating like an adult," as strength coach Dan John would say.

To be clear, the *listen-to-your-body skills* in this book aren't exactly intuitive eating. Many intuitive eating programs are completely against the idea of weight loss as a goal. That's a bummer, because those skills work really well. We're borrowing skills from intuitive eating to tap into our hunger and fullness cues, and using them in a way that's super effective for weight loss.

EATING SKILLS

The biggest mistake most people make with intuitive eating is that after a lifetime of ignoring hunger and fullness cues, they attempt to just "hope it all works out."

Most people spend their lives:

- Eating when they are bored or stressed, even though they aren't hungry;

- Dieting and ignoring hunger;

- Calorie counting and ignoring hunger;

- Working too much and ignoring hunger;

- Eating while distracted and missing their fullness signals;

- Eating too fast and missing their fullness signals;

- Giving up on diets and ignoring fullness;

- Having free days and ignoring fullness.

If you've spent *decades* ignoring hunger and fullness, you can't expect to be an expert at it the first day you decide to try.

You need to work on the component skills that make up listening to hunger and listening to fullness, and noticing the difference between emotions and hunger. Fortunately, that's what this section is about.

EATING GUIDELINES

The eating guidelines are at the opposite end of the spectrum. Sometimes this is distinguished between mindful eating (aka intuitive eating) and mindful decision making. In these cases, mindful decision making leads to faster weight loss.[75]

One study rated people on intuitive eating using a pasta taste test. They were allowed to eat as much pasta as they wanted, but were randomly divided into two groups: One group got a 12-inch plate, and the other group got an eight-inch plate. The people with the smaller plates ate less. Interestingly, and contrary to what the researchers had predicted, the difference was the biggest with people who scored highest on intuitive eating. The guideline of plate size made a huge difference in their intuitive skill use.[76]

Other times, it's been compared as intuitive eating versus flexible restraint, in which case flexible restraint also leads to faster weight loss. There's an interesting look at the difference between three things: intuitive eating (similar to the "trust your body" skills), flexible dietary control (like guidelines), and rigid dietary control (dieting):

- Intuitive eating: Best for body image

- Flexible control: Best for weight loss

- Rigid control (dieting): Worst for body image; good for short-term weight loss[77,78]

The potential pitfall is turning the guidelines into diet rules: If you turn them into hard rules, you're screwed. If you have black-and-white thinking about foods, that some foods are "good" and others are "bad," you're similarly screwed.

We're going to work on four kinds of skills:

	DURING MEALS	BETWEEN MEALS
LISTEN TO YOUR BODY SKILLS	Notice when getting full, and stop when full	Distinguish true hunger versus cravings, boredom, tiredness, emotions, or thoughts
USE A GUIDELINE	Plate healthy and balanced portions	Eat a balanced meal every four to six hours, without snacking in between

You'll use a mix of both guidelines and skills. Guidelines will help, especially when you're just learning the skills, or when you're in times of intense stress.

In the end, you probably want the one skill from each box that makes the biggest difference for you. That'll leave you with two *listen-to-your-body skills* and two *guidelines*. You'll use the "trust yourself" skills most of the time; the guides you'll use in times of stress. Simple.

Dan John talks about having a "pirate map" to a goal. Essentially, it's the clearest and simplest steps to follow. For weight loss, the pirate map looks like this:

1. Eat a balanced meal every four to six hours.

2. Distinguish true hunger from cravings, boredom, tiredness, emotions, or thoughts.

3. Plate healthy and balanced portions.

4. Eat slowly. Notice when getting full and stop.

As long as you can keep them flexible—as guidelines—you're cool. They're super effective; just hold them lightly. It comes down to using them as a target...but not freaking out when things aren't exactly perfect. These are guidelines, not rules.

This is Dan's idea of "eating like an adult." These four things are how I'd nail down what eating like an adult looks like in steps.

We'll break those down into sub-skills, but that's the whole game. It's those four things, and nothing but those four things. Whenever you feel lost or stuck, all you need to do is come back to these four things, and see which you're missing.

SKILLS ARE FASTER

The biggest misconception about habit-based or skills-based weight loss is thinking it's slower.

It's not.

Skills always win. It's the tortoise and the hare.

Sure, it sounds cool when your friend loses ten pounds in a week...but your friend has probably been losing and regaining that same ten pounds for a decade or two.

On the flip side, losing a half-pound to a pound per week and having that handled forever is much, much faster. Do it right, once, and be done with it. Sure, your friend may lose and re-gain ten pounds twice in the time it takes you to lose ten. But then, while you're losing another ten pounds, your friend will have lost and regained that same ten pounds another time or two. Fast results create an illusion of progress…but if you're losing and regaining the same weight every other month, there's no progress at all—it's just a cycle of failure.

The hare always loses because the hare starts and quits over and over again. Doesn't that sound like the diet cycle of failure? Start really fast, then quit?

The tortoise always wins, always goes faster because of continual steps in the direction of what matters.

PROBLEM SOLVING:
THE FOUR SKILLS MATRIX

The big evolution for this system was realizing that skills fit into a matrix to solve problems we have with eating too much.

If you eat too much between meals—
work on *between-meal skills.*

If you eat too much during meals—
work on *during-meal skills.*

If you want to transform your relationship to your body and to food—
work on *listen-to-your-body skills.*

If you're new to *listen-to-your-body skills,*
you're tired, or you're stressed out—
work on *eating guidelines.*

First, we want to distinguish whether your issues are mostly between meals or during meals. Often, I find clients have been working diligently on their meals, but they never addressed boredom or stress snacking between meals. Working on "between meals" makes all of the difference for them.

People always have the most food enjoyment, best body image, highest wellbeing, and most sustainable weight loss results when they use *listen-to-your-body eating skills.*

Listen-to-your-body eating skills can take a year or two to master. In the meantime, people get better results by practicing a combination of *listen-to-your-body skills* and *eating guidelines.*

Lastly, when people are tired or stressed out, it's always harder to use *listen-to-your-body skills.* In these cases, people can just rely on *eating guidelines.*

THERE ARE ONLY FOUR THINGS YOU NEED TO DO TO LOSE WEIGHT.

We have a four-way matrix of *Lean and Strong Eating Skills* and *Guidelines:*

	DURING MEALS	BETWEEN MEALS
LISTEN TO YOUR BODY SKILLS	Notice when getting full, and stop	Distinguish hunger from cravings, boredom, tiredness, emotions, or thoughts
USE A GUIDELINE	Plate healthy and balanced portions	Eat a balanced meal every four to six hours, without snacking in between

Next, we'll break these down into component skills.

	DURING MEALS	BETWEEN MEALS
LISTEN TO YOUR BODY SKILLS	Notice when full, and stop Check in with stomach mid-meal, notice/speculate about future fullness Notice that flavor enjoyment is different than fullness Five senses mindfulness Make sure to eat enough Stop before eating too much Check in with stomach one hour after eating	Distinguish hunger from cravings, boredom, tiredness, emotions, or thoughts De-fusion from unwanted thoughts, feelings, and cravings Flexibility: Saying "yes" to things sometimes, and "no" to things other times Notice and wait through normal hunger: 30 minutes before eating Notice when tired and go to sleep
USE A GUIDELINE	Plate balanced portions Plate healthy portion sizes Put the fork down between bites Eat without screens Do something engaging after eating Wait ten minutes before having seconds or treats	Eat a meal every four to six hours, without snacking in between Ten-minute wait before snacks or treats Get engaged with what is going on right now Self-care: coping, self-soothing, fun activities, and hobbies Turn off screens and lights and go to bed at a certain time

Most people after years of dieting are completely disconnected from their hunger and fullness cues. They've taught themselves to ignore true hunger, basically trying to starve themselves through diets. During all the years of dieting, they've practiced not eating when hungry, and are out of practice distinguishing true hunger.

Simultaneously, they've eaten when they aren't hungry due to boredom or emotions. Or, they've had "free days" and eaten way past fullness. To make matters worse, every time they've gone through the diet cycle of failure, they've filled their feelings of failure with a totally off-the-rails free-for-all (because, screw it), again eating way past fullness.

They've essentially been practicing not eating when they have true hunger and eating when they don't have hunger. Their signals are all messed up. They're out of practice.

Fortunately, skills are about practice. It's time to start practicing noticing what's really going on when you have the thought, "I should eat something." Let's find out if it's about hunger…or not.

SKILL DETAILS: USING A GUIDELINE BETWEEN MEALS

The National Food Consumption Surveys in 1977 and 2007, surveying 15,000 households—a large-scale study looking at eating habits over 30 years—concluded that increased snacking has contributed more to the obesity epidemic than increased portion sizes. They attributed less than one-third of the cause of weight gain due to eating too much at meals, and more than two-thirds to increased snacking.[79]

Studies comparing identical twins are always intriguing given that we can compare people with the same genetics. A study in *The European Journal of Nutrition* evaluated the eating habits of twins. They found, if the twins had differing weights, the twin who weighed more had a higher frequency of snacking.[80]

Calories from snacks are often mindless and totally unrelated to true hunger.

USE A GUIDELINE BETWEEN MEALS	Eat a meal every four to six hours, without snacking in between
	Ten-minute wait before snacks or treats
	Get engaged with what is going on right now
	Self-care: coping, self-soothing, fun activities, and hobbies
	Turn off screens and lights, and go to bed at a certain time

EAT A MEAL EVERY FOUR TO SIX HOURS

Most people's issue with getting lean or losing weight isn't what they eat *at* meals; it's what they eat *between* meals. Basically, they snack or graze all the time…for reasons that have nothing to do with actual hunger. Eating every four to six hours gives us a guideline we can follow to see if we're eating from true hunger, or because we're bored or craving treats.

Snacks don't provide much in the way of fullness; they're usually lower quality food choices, and they're often eaten in the absence of hunger.[81] People tend to eat a higher quality of food at meals than they do at snacks.[82]

A group of researchers looked at the CDC's National Health and Nutrition Examination Survey, reviewing the eating frequency of 18,965 people. They found that eating three meals per day was related to the lowest weight, and that eating snacks beyond the three meals was related to increased weight.[83]

A literature review in *Physiology and Behavior*, "Energy intake and obesity: Ingestive frequency outweighs portion size," looked at dozens of studies on portion size and number of meals per day. The findings consistently showed that snacks don't have much effect on fullness.

Multiple studies show a link between snacking between meals and bodyweight. As our bodyweights went up in the United States, timing between feedings has decreased to only three hours between feedings. They note that while portion sizes have increased by 12%, snack frequency has increased by 29%. The authors concluded that while portion sizes have also increased, it's actually frequency of snacking that's a bigger problem with weight gain.[84]

A review in *The Journal of Nutrition* looked at eating frequency and fullness throughout the day. They found that eating five or six times per day didn't increase fullness any more than eating three times per day. They did find that people eating one or two times per day were hungrier than people eating three times per day. Their conclusion was that there's no benefit related to increased eating frequency for feeling more full.[85]

Interestingly, studies have shown that simply labeling something as a "snack" makes it less filling than a "meal," even when the calories are matched. Participants were divided into four groups and all given the same 516 calories of pasta. Two of the groups were told their pasta was a meal, and two groups were told it was a snack. They then divided those two groups into sitting at a table with silverware versus eating standing up with a plastic container.

After eating, the participants were given a fake taste test with M&M's candies. Against the researchers predictions, eating standing or sitting made no difference. On the other hand, simply being told "please eat the *meal*" or "please eat the *snack*" made a huge difference. People who had been told they ate a snack ate significantly more M&M's in the taste test.[86] This means psychologically we'll eat more later if we believe we've had a snack.

Other studies have similar findings: Snacks have a low effect on fullness. People will eat the same amount at the next meal, whether they had a snack earlier or not. If you end up eating the same amount at your meals, the snacks are just extra calories.[87]

THE MAIN GUIDELINE FOR BETWEEN MEALS

If you're eating balanced meals with a sufficient amount of food, you shouldn't need to snack. Eating breakfast, lunch, and dinner is a totally reasonable proposition for leaning up, and puts your meals about four to six hours apart.

If you aren't snacking, you eat balanced meals, and you get your portion sizes right, you'll find you get truly hungry about 30 minutes before the next meal, which is right when you should get hungry.

If you find you're getting hungry two hours after a meal, you know something is off. It's possible your previous meal was too small or unbalanced, and you actually *are* hungry. Or, it's possible you aren't actually hungry—you're bored, tired, stressed out, or "eating your feelings."

In the *listen-to-your-body between-meals skills* discussion, we'll get into skills for differentiating between hunger, cravings, or stress eating based on trusting your body. For now, the guideline is simply to consider that if you want food sooner than four to six hours, it might not be actual hunger.

Eating every four to six hours will usually put you at three meals per day. Sometimes it will put you at three meals and one snack.

HOW TO START

If you're a person who's used to having multiple daily snacks, putting everything on a plate is a good way to start the "meals, not snacks" skill. If you normally have three snacks and three meals, put the snacks on a plate with your meal.

For example, if you normally have eggs and toast for breakfast, chips mid-morning, then a sandwich for lunch, put the mid-morning snack of chips on your plate with your sandwich at lunch. It really works to start the practice with the same amount of food, but combine it into three mealtimes. This will allow you to distinguish non-hunger snack cravings between meals, and to notice when getting full if everything is on one plate.

THE DELIBERATE ONE SNACK PER DAY

Eating every four to six hours will usually put you at three meals per day. Sometimes it will put you at three meals and one deliberate snack. That deliberate snack may come up as needed. For example:

If lunch has to be at 11:30 a.m. and dinner has to be at 7:00 p.m., that's seven-and-a-half hours between meals, which is too long, so putting a snack in between makes sense. Or, sometimes you have to add a snack to make a workout work. There's a massive difference between adding a snack so you don't go longer than six hours between meals, and having a snack out of habit or boredom.

Everyone has had a time when they had a long gap between meals, then overate at the next meal because they felt starved. Sometimes, our real-life schedules don't allow for a meal every six hours, so we have to add a snack. That's a smart play.

We sometimes need to have a snack to make our workout schedule work. That's okay too. If you do your morning workout before breakfast, you might need a snack beforehand. If you do an evening workout and are hungry after work, you may need a snack before your workout. These are smart reasons to deliberately add a snack to make your workout schedule work.

The biggest thing we're trying to remove with snacks is the mindless and low-quality snacking that adds a ton of extra calories to your day. We want to remove the stress snacking, habit snacking, seeing-food snacking, tired snacking, and procrastination snacking.

The deliberate "I need this to make my workout work" snacking is totally cool. Using a snack to bridge the gap when meals are going to be more than six hours apart is a great plan.

WHAT ARE BETTER OPTIONS FOR ONE DELIBERATE SNACK?

A meal, ideally, has four things: protein, vegetables, carbohydrates, and fat. An ideal snack has any two of the four. Examples might be some almonds and an apple, some deli meat and a banana, or a Greek yogurt.

While we've made a pretty solid case against snacking, if a deliberate snack makes sense, quality matters. You probably won't be shocked that low-nutrient and high-calorie snack foods are related to less fullness and a higher bodyweight.

Also unsurprisingly, high-nutrient and low-calorie snacks are related to more fullness and a lower bodyweight. Examples would be fruit, reasonable portions of nuts, Greek yogurt, or vegetables.[88]

A review of snacking literature, including longitudinal (long-term) and experimental, found that some people snack and remain lean, and other people snack and gain weight. There were three big differences between the two groups.

People who snacked and were lean:

1. Snacked at deliberate times. They never snacked mindlessly or because they saw food that looked good.

2. Snacked on obviously healthy foods.

3. Adjusted their subsequent meals to be smaller because they had snacked.

People who snacked and gained weight did the reverse:

1. They snacked when they had an urge to snack.

2. They snacked on sweet or salty snack foods.

3. They ate normal-sized meals, even after snacking.[89]

If you are going to have a deliberate snack, make sure you do it in a way that doesn't cause weight gain. Snack deliberately; make it something that's obviously healthy, and adjust other meals accordingly.

COUNT THE SNACKS MOST PEOPLE FORGET

Anything you put in your mouth that has calories is a snack. Coffee with cream counts as a snack. Coffee with butter or MCT oil counts as a snack—and sometimes a meal, given how much people are adding these days. Full-sugar soda counts as a snack. Fruit counts as a snack. The five M&Ms you stole from your friend across the cubical counts as a snack. Those two chips you ate count as a snack. All of the little bites and all of the beverages that have calories count as snacks.

COUNTING YOUR SNACKS

Many people will initially notice they're having three to five snacks per day, between their coffee with cream (or butter or oil), their full-sugar soda, their muffin in the break room, and the couple pieces of candy on the conference table. The goal of this guideline is for you to notice all the little snacks popping up in your day.

Ideally, bring the number of snacks down to zero or one. If your meals are adequately filling and spaced evenly apart, it's pretty cool to have three meals and no snacks. Three meals per day is a reasonable expectation for a human. Three meals per day is totally sustainable and intelligent.

On the other hand, if you have gaps longer than six hours between meals or if you need a snack so you aren't starving before or after a workout, then one deliberate snack is smart. Don't stress too much trying to decide if you should have a snack.

If you use four to six hours as a guideline, it's really simple, as you'll see in the chart on the following page.

GUIDELINE	EAT A MEAL EVERY FOUR TO SIX HOURS, WITHOUT SNACKING IN BETWEEN
WHY EAT A MEAL EVERY FOUR TO SIX HOURS, WITHOUT SNACKING IN BETWEEN	Many people find their actual issue isn't that they eat too much at meals; it's that they eat too much between meals because they're bored, tired, stressed out, or "eating their feelings."
WAYS TO GOLDILOCKS EATING EVERY FOUR TO SIX HOURS, WITHOUT SNACKING IN BETWEEN	"I'm going to eat breakfast at 7:00 a.m., and so I'll have lunch between 11:00 a.m.–1:00 p.m., without snacking in between." "I'm going to eat lunch at noon, so I'll have dinner at 6:00 p.m., without snacking in between." "I'll have dinner at 7:00 p.m., and go to sleep between 11:00 p.m.– midnight, without snacking in between." "I'm going to eat breakfast, then I'm not going to eat again until I'm ready to eat lunch. When I feel hungry for lunch, I'll eat lunch." "I know I always crave something sugary in the afternoon. Since I don't feel hungry for a balanced meal, I know it's not actual hunger." "When I'm hungry, I'm going to eat a full, balanced meal."

GET ENGAGED WITH WHAT'S HAPPENING

This one might seem weird as a food skill, but it's actually a useful way to curb snacking. We often crave snacks simply because we're disengaged. We're bored.

We're not *really* doing what we're supposed to be doing, but we aren't taking a break either. People love to mindlessly snack while they're disengaged.

Doing something engaging and fully participating in it is a great way not to give in to cravings. That could be as simple as fully immersing yourself in your work. It could be being fully present in a conversation.

The "five senses experiencing" part is a way to be engaged when there isn't something to actively do. You might notice the trees or the sky out the window. Or, maybe you really *listen* to the music that's playing.

You could pay attention to what someone is saying, without thinking of what you're going to say next. Perhaps you just take a second to really feel the weight of your feet on the ground.

It's normal for our minds to wander at times. Noticing something with one of your five senses—sight, smell, touch, hearing, or taste—is an easy way to re-engage with the present.

The flip side also becomes true: When you notice you can't engage, you can take a break.

Everyone has a limited attention span. We can be engaged at work for an amount of time, then we can either take a break, or we sort of disengage anyway. We can be absorbed in a movie, or we can be half paying attention to a movie that sucks.

We can be fully paying attention to a conversation, or we could be kind of checked out. In many cases, we'd be better off alternating between fully engaged and taking break than half paying attention. It's typically that half paying attention place where we mindlessly eat.

The mistake would be to think mindful engagement is a way to distract yourself, and make the feelings and cravings go away. While it might sometimes work as a distraction, other times you'll find it doesn't work—the cravings still persist. Unfortunately, there's no magic way to make cravings go away.

The alternate and more effective way to look at this is that the mindful engagement is just what you do because it's the kind of person you want to be.

And you can be that person you want to be, whether the cravings fade or whether they stick around for a while. You get engaged and present with your life because it's good to be engaged and present with your life.

Engage with your five senses not to suppress or distract yourself from cravings, but just to be aware of what you're doing. You'll notice you can have a craving for something and not eat it, and that cravings come and go in their own time.

Cravings build, build, build, and then faaaaaaaaade away. That's the natural path of cravings; they do that all on their own. Meanwhile, just engage with what matters to you.

Engagement isn't about a constant, perfect attention. It's simply the process of coming back—noticing a craving, then coming back to what you're doing…noticing a stressful thought, then coming back to what you're doing.

SKILL	BE FULLY ENGAGED OR PRESENT WITH FIVE SENSES
WHY TO BE FULLY ENGAGED OR PRESENT WITH FIVE SENSES	People mindlessly eat when they're half checked out. Being fully engaged in what you're doing is a powerful way to reduce snacking, or fully disengage and take a break.
WAYS TO GOLDILOCKS YOUR WHY TO BE FULLY ENGAGED OR PRESENT WITH FIVE SENSES PRACTICE	"If I get really stressed out, I'm going to stop for a second and look at the trees outside." "If I get overwhelmed by an emotion, I'm going to stop for a second and just feel the pressure of my feet on the ground." "At work, I'm going to be fully engaged for 25-minute chunks, then I'm going to take a five-minute break." "I know when I crave a snack at work, I usually just need a break. I'm going to use snack cravings as a signal that I need to go for a quick walk around the building, then come back and be fully present in my work." "If I'm bored by the TV show I'm watching and start to think about snacking, I'm going to find a really great movie to watch or a good book to read." "At dinner with my friends, instead of being half-checked out and mindlessly snacking on chips, I'm going to really listen to what my friends are saying, and be engaged with them."

GUIDELINE: WAIT TEN MINUTES BEFORE A SNACK OR A TREAT

This is amazingly useful and unbelievably simple.

Most of us get into a habit where we have a craving for a treat, and we eat it almost mindlessly. There's no gap to do any kind of thinking or make a choice because it happens so fast. This guideline slows you down long enough to choose. It's a great way to smash the pattern of mindless snacking.

The wait doesn't even have to be ten minutes. The length of time isn't nearly as important as breaking that pattern of wanting something and immediately having it. Wanting something and then instantly eating it is a habit that keeps us eating almost mechanically, with very little enjoyment and no choice.

When we add a gap between stimulus and response, we have time to think. We have time to choose. If I want to eat a cookie and I wait ten minutes, I have time to notice if I really want it, or if I'm just bored. I can check in with myself, and see if I'm reacting to stress. Or, I can see if I only want it because of a fleeting thought.

The cool thing is, if after ten minutes you decide to have it, you get to have it—but you've taken the time to *choose*. You've had time to *think*. You've had time to *check in with your body*. If after checking in, you really want it, eat it.

Most people find that sometimes they still want the snack, and sometimes they don't. That's amazing! That's so useful! People start to think through whether it's one of their favorite foods, or if it's just "there." People figure out if they're actually hungry for a meal and need to have a meal. People discover all kinds of things when they slow their roll with snacking.

We'll dig into it more as we discuss the Meta-skill of flexibility. For now, just be thinking, if after ten minutes you're always saying "yes" to the snack or treat, something is wrong. On the flip side, if—after ten minutes—you're always saying "no" to a snack or treat, something is also wrong. If you *always have the same answer*, it means you probably aren't really checking in and thinking about it. Go ahead and say "yes" if it's truly going to be amazing. Say "no" if you're just eating out of habit.

Often, clients start off shooting for 50/50. Fifty percent of the time, they'll say "yes" to treats, and 50% of the time, they'll say "no." That's another great way to break out of the pattern of not thinking. Over time, you can adjust that ratio based on your values. Eventually, when you get good at stopping, thinking, and checking in with yourself, you can completely discard all ratios, and just think for yourself. The ten-minute wait and the 50/50 concept are both just training wheels for you to start thinking things through.

If you really struggle with snacking, try to kick it up to a 20-minute wait. As you get better at this skill, you can reduce the waiting time. Many people find, as they get more practice and get better at it, they only need to wait one minute. Super-advanced folks only have to wait ten seconds.

GUIDELINE	WAIT TEN MINUTES BEFORE A SNACK OR A TREAT
WHY PRACTICE THIS GUIDELINE	Most people don't actually know if they want the treats they eat; they eat them out of habit, because of a craving, or because they're bored.
WAYS TO GOLDILOCKS THIS GUIDELINE	"When I want a treat in the afternoon, I'm going to wait (and work) for another ten minutes before I have it." "If I want a treat, I'm going to stop for one minute and check in with myself about whether I want it or whether I'm tired." "If I want a treat at work, I'm going to go for a walk for five minutes to see if I really wanted a treat, or if I just needed a break."

DELIBERATE SELF-CARE

We all need self-care, but we tend to actually give ourselves very little of it.

Essentially, if food is your only coping strategy when you feel sad, frustrated, tired, angry, or lonely, you're going to end up using food a lot. Trying to "fix feelings" with food is a dead end. That's why we all need to have healthy coping strategies. We need to have ways to soothe ourselves other than with food. The issue isn't food itself; the issue is that we need to soothe ourselves somehow.

We also want to feel good and do things that are pleasurable. Again, if food is the only pleasurable thing you have in your toolbox, you're going to use it a lot. We all want a treat sometimes, but food isn't the only kind of treat there is.

If there's a magic bullet for not snacking after dinner, it's having a hobby. I know it's not what most people typically think of when trying to eliminate snacking and treats, but people are often just bored and under-stimulated. You want something nice, so find something nice to do.

Also, it's really effective to do something that's good for you while you're feeling hard emotions. This isn't about pushing emotions away or distracting yourself—it's about doing something that fits your values, is good for you, and takes care of you, *while you're feeling your feelings*. If you feel bad, get a hug. If you don't have a person handy to hug, hug a pet. Work on a craft. Take a warm bath. Do something to soothe yourself, but have a strategy to cope that isn't food.

Mostly, we have an image of self-care as scented candles and relaxing bubble baths. Worse, sometimes we're told self-care is a trip to Bali (because everyone can afford that). Essentially, we're told self-care is about pleasure, and self-care takes lots of money and time.

We've been given only *one* of the three kinds of self-care. That one kind of self-care can be great, but it isn't practical all of the time. It also neglects the truth that what we often need is one of the other two kinds of self-care.

Three kinds of self-care:

- Relaxation is important, but it's often much simpler and cheaper than what the world is trying to sell us. The other two kinds of self-care are often more important.

- Effortful and skill-based self-care might be some of the best things we can do for ourselves. Practicing skills like playing an instrument or knitting are phenomenal for wellbeing. These are things that give us pride as our skills develop over time.

- Taking care of things is really important self-care. Often, we're great about taking care of some things, like our family or career, and terrible about taking care of other things, like setting boundaries or having a tough conversation.

It's good to know all three kinds of self-care, and to pull from the appropriate one you need at a given time.

If you're a nurse who just worked a 12-hour overnight shift, you probably want relaxation self-care. If you're a parent who came home from a tough day at work to handle a challenging situation with one of your children, you might also need relaxation self-care.

If you have a little free time at the end of the night and aren't totally wiped, you might be surprised at how much you get out of some skill-based or effortful self-care. Doing something that builds skills outside of your life responsibilities can be super fun and engaging.

Sometimes, though, the most effective self-care is taking care of something. If you normally struggle with setting boundaries, setting and holding a boundary might be ten times more effective than any amount of relaxation.

Or, if you have a crushing deadline, renegotiating that deadline might be what you need the most. Self-care could be saying "no" to the really great project or volunteer opportunity, or even doing something for a friend when you actually don't have the bandwidth. It could be asking for help when normally you do everything on your own.

People almost never think of the third one—taking care of things—as self-care. First, given how often people eat to procrastinate, this is an important one to consider. Second, we often use relaxation or hobbies as a band-aid for not dealing with an underlying issue. Pull from the right kind of self-care at the right time. Know all of your options.

THE THREE KINDS OF SELF-CARE WITH EXAMPLES

TAKING CARE OF THINGS SELF-CARE	SKILL-BASED AND EFFORTFUL SELF-CARE	RELAXATION SELF-CARE
Setting healthy boundaries	Singing	Taking a walk
Saying "no" to things	Gardening	Watching TV
Having hard, but important, conversations	Woodworking	Playing with a pet
Planning for the future	dancing	Taking a bath
Reflecting on what you've accomplished, learned, or noticed	Hiking	Getting a massage
Going shopping for food for the week	Working on your car	Aromatherapy
Practicing eating skills to take care of yourself	Playing guitar	Hanging out with a friend
Cooking good food to take care of yourself	Rock climbing	Listening to music
Working out to take care of yourself	Taking Brazilian Jiu Jitsu classes	Going to a concert
Paying the bills	Practicing Tai Chi	Going to an amusement park
Going to the doctor, when you need to	Meditation	Going to a movie
Cleaning the house	Taking an alignment-based yoga class	Going out to a nice restaurant
Going to bed on time	Investing	Playing frisbee in the park
Working out	Painting	Going on a picnic
Doing the laundry	Skiing	Going for a hike
Calling a family member you love	Snowboarding	Taking a hatha yoga class
Volunteering for a cause that matters to you	Backpacking	Reading a book
If you're religious, going to religious services	Mountain Biking	Reading comic books
Going to sleep on time	Knitting	Reading magazines
	Making balloon animals	Playing board-games
	Working out	Playing cards
	Cooking	Cuddling, Making out
	Writing fiction	Having sex
	Writing non-fiction	Taking a nap
	Blogging	Looking at the ocean
	Writing poetry	Watching a sunset
	Journaling	Watching a campfire

Especially in the beginning, it may feel like these skills don't "fix" your cravings or your feelings. *They aren't supposed to.* Self-care doesn't numb feelings the way food does. They're just ways for you do something good for yourself.

GUIDELINE	DELIBERATE SELF-CARE
WHY PRACTICE THIS GUIDELINE	Most people don't do very much actual self-care. Instead of taking care of themselves, they substitute snacks.
WAYS TO GOLDILOCKS THIS GUIDELINE	"When I'm stressed out, I'm going to go outside and watch a tree blow in the wind." "If I have a rough week at work, I'm going to go for a hike." "If I'm bored after dinner, I'm going to work on a craft." "As a treat for myself, I'm going to play videogames." "I always feel good after working in the garden."

TURN OFF SCREENS AND LIGHTS AND GO TO BED AT A CERTAIN TIME

If there are two magic bullets for food, they're sleep and exercise. Most people make better food choices when they exercise during the week. Everyone makes better food choices when they get more sleep.

Most of my clients are pretty good about exercise… but they're terrible about sleep.

It often shocks people to discover this, but sleep is a necessity. Our culture often lionizes working too much and not sleeping enough, but there's actually nothing all that great about not sleeping.

When we're sleep deprived, we feel hunger more often and more intensely. Meta-analyses show that if we look at multiple studies on sleep and hunger, the results are consistent: People consume more calories when they've had less sleep.[90,91]

When we're sleep deprived, we're less resilient to stress. When we're sleep deprived, we have a harder time coping with uncomfortable and hard emotions.[92] We're even more likely to misread social situations and get in more arguments.[93]

Let's review—sleep deprivation makes you:

- Feel hungrier;

- Crave high-calorie, low-nutrition foods;

- Crave snacks more frequently;

- Be less strong and resilient in the face of stress;

- Be less strong and resilient in the face of uncomfortable emotions.

It's easy to see that increasing sleep has a massive impact on *every food skill* you could practice. Many clients find that the majority of their issues with snacking between meals or emotional eating were due to sleep deprivation. I've had clients in whom sleeping enough fixed *all* of their food issues.

It's really common for people to discover their issue with late-night snacking doesn't actually have anything to do with snacks; it has to do with being exhausted. You might be tired, at the end of your rope, but semi-hypnotized by the television…and *eating to keep yourself awake.*

Look, the fix for being tired isn't food. It's sleep. Take care of yourself by going to sleep.

The thing is, we can't actually control how much we sleep. Sometimes you go to bed and fall right to sleep; other times you go to bed and lie awake for a while. That's okay. We're going to focus on what we can control: turning off screens, turning off the lights, and going to bed.

It's well known that screens are great for keeping us awake. If you *want to stay awake* far, far past your level of tiredness, just keep looking at a screen.[94] On the flip side, the easiest place to start for getting more sleep is to pick a time to turn off screens.

When you turn off screens, feel free to do something analog: read a book (fiction), play a board game, talk to your partner, read a magazine, do a craft, do a puzzle. Do anything where you aren't looking at a hypnotic blue light.

Often people complain, "I want to watch TV because I'm too tired to read!" If you're too tired to do anything other than stare at a screen…that's a red flag you're exhausted and you really need sleep. Another option is to turn off the lights and go to bed. Turning off the lights and getting into bed really works because that's how people go to sleep.

You can't control when you fall asleep, but you can totally control when you go to bed. And going to bed is enough. Focus on the part you can control.

GUIDELINE	TURN OFF SCREENS AND LIGHTS AND GO TO BED AT A CERTAIN TIME
WHY PRACTICE THIS GUIDELINE	Most late night snacking is really tiredness. Instead of fixing the tiredness problem by going to sleep, people eat. On the flip side, when people go to sleep, they not only miss the treats they'd eat at midnight, but they crave fewer treats the next day.
WAYS TO GOLDILOCKS THIS GUIDELINE	"I'm going to turn off screens and read my favorite book series at 10:00 p.m." "I'm going to turn off screens and knit at 9:00 p.m." "I'm going to turn off screens and read a comic book at 11:00 p.m." "I'm going to turn off the lights and get in bed at 10:30 p.m."

Note: If you're having a lot of trouble getting to sleep, look into a great ACT-based program called *Sleep School*, created by Kat Lederle, Claire Durant, and Guy Meadows. They have an online program at *thesleepschool.org*. Dr. Guy Meadows also has a book, *The Sleep Book*.

SKILL DETAILS: USING A GUIDELINE DURING MEALS

USE A GUIDELINE DURING MEALS	Plate balanced portions
	Plate healthy portion sizes
	Put the fork down between bites
	Eat without screens
	Do something engaging after eating
	Wait ten minutes before having seconds or treats

PLATE BALANCED PORTIONS

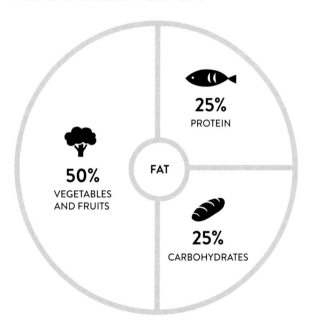

This is the simplest way to guestimate plating healthy and balanced portions:

- 50% of the plate vegetables (and fruit!);

- 25% of the plate protein;

- 25% of the plate carbohydrates;

- About a tablespoon of fat (as a starting guideline).

You've probably seen something like this before. Harvard University's T.H. Chan School of Public Health has a "Healthy Eating Plate" that looks almost exactly like this. You may also notice that these match the plate used for Canada's food guide and are pretty close to the United States' "MyPlate" guidelines from 2019.

The biggest differences in this plate versus the above guidelines relate to fat. Though not on their plate graphic, USDA's "MyPlate" posts allowances for two-and-a-half to three tablespoons per day of unsaturated fat for women, and three to three-and-a-half tablespoons per day for men. MyPlate also recommends eight ounces of seafood per week, to get the Omega-3s in fish oil. Harvard School of Public Health "Health Eating Plate" put healthy plant oils specifically on their plate recommendation to make a point that healthy fats are an important meal component. The big difference is that the "Healthy Eating Plate" puts no precise limit on how much or what percentage of a meal is fat, so long as it's healthy fat and fits within your total calories. They also gave fish oil a double thumbs up. "MyPlate" and "Healthy Eating Plate" both recommend choosing fats that are liquid at room temperature—hurray for olive oil!

So, the *Lean and Strong* plate guideline actually matches both, in various ways, even if the graphics for the other plates look different at first glance.

The thing is, balanced meals make people feel full. Protein and fiber (vegetables and fruit) both play an extra special role in fullness.[95] Vegans and vegetarians can play the protein game also; it doesn't make a difference if your protein comes from animal or plant sources. Protein increases fullness either way.[96]

The percentages are guides, not absolute rules, but this guideline may be helpful for you as a starting place. If you're making a meal like a stew or something stirred together, it's the same—just use those in the same ratio. Here's the deal with plating healthy and balanced portions:

1. Balanced portions make it easier to notice when you're full.

2. Healthy portion sizes make it easier to notice when you're full.
   Balanced meals are more filling. That's the magic.

In practice, plating a balanced portion usually means:

- Increasing vegetable intake;

- Consistently having a portion of protein;

- Reducing the carbohydrate intake to one portion—in the United States, people often have five portions;

- Reducing fat intake to one tablespoon—people often have more servings of fat than they realize because it doesn't look like a lot on the plate.

If you aren't losing weight after plating balanced meals, 95% of the time, it's food you're eating between meals or after dinner that's the issue. The other five percent of the time, it means you should use a smaller plate.

Don't be afraid of carbohydrates! Yes, you can put bread, pasta, rice, potatoes, or whatever you want in that 25% of the plate.

The reason people gain weight isn't because they have *one* portion of carbohydrates; they gain weight because they have *five*.

ARE FRUITS A CARBOHYDRATE OR A VEGETABLE?

This is kind of a funny question I hear a lot. Fruits are carbohydrates. Yes, they're carbohydrates.

That being said, I usually have people put fruit in the "vegetable" portion of the plate. If someone has never eaten vegetables, it can be much easier to start by adding fruit rather than vegetables, and that's a huge positive step. Fruits are super healthy; they have lots of amazing fiber and, let's get real—no one ever gained weight because they had an extra apple.

Depending on the meal, you can use fruit in either the carbohydrate portion of your plate or the vegetable portion. At breakfast, if you aren't doing a scramble, it can often be easier to get fruit than vegetables. And when travelling, often fruit is easier to get than vegetables. It's a totally cool switch sometimes, even though yes, fruits are carbohydrates.

SPECIFIC NUTRIENT RESEARCH FOR LOSING WEIGHT AND GETTING LEAN

It's really easy to overdo fat intake. One study put women into three groups consuming different percentages of their meals from fat. The first group consumed 15–20% fat, the second consumed 20–35% fat, and the third group consumed 35–50% fat. The group that consumed 35–50% fat automatically consumed 15.4% more calories and gained a significant weight.[97]

One study looked at fat consumption during a meal and then subsequent fullness. They found that people given access to extra fat in meals will naturally consume twice as many calories from fat…with no extra increase in fullness.[98] If you can double your fat intake without feeling any more full, it makes it super hard to lose weight.

There's nothing magic about certain percentages of macronutrients. A study in a metabolic ward where people were locked in and fed perfect percentages of food found no difference in weight loss when calories and protein were matched. The fat content varied from low at 15%, to intermediate at 40% or 45%, to high fat at 75%, 80%, or even 85%. No one lost more weight with any different ratios of carbohydrates or fat—and this was in a metabolic ward with absolutely perfectly measured meals fed to them.[99]

Protein is awesome for increasing fullness. A review of macronutrient literature noted that protein has a bigger impact on fullness than either carbohydrates or fat.[100] This finding that protein creates the most fullness has been replicated multiple times.[101,102,103,104,105,106]

One particularly cool study on protein and fullness created a market where 50 participants had to buy all of their food for six months. They were given no information about the quantity of calories they were "buying," and could get as much or as little as they wanted. Participants were randomized to one of two groups, either 12% protein or 25% protein. Whatever meals they got each week, a computer system made sure each group got that specific percentage of protein. To make sure they were actually eating the precise amount of protein, the amount of nitrogen in their urine, which is an accurate way to measure protein intake, was measured every seven days. The 25% protein group naturally consumed fewer calories (they believe due to increased fullness) lost significantly more weight, and had a bigger reduction in waist measurements.[107]

Fruit and vegetable intake is the least controversial. Pretty much everyone knows it's healthy to eat fruits and vegetables and that they help with fullness. In the interest of research, two large scale reviews showed that increasing fruit and vegetable intake can increase fullness and help reduce calories, resulting in weight loss. They

both caution that there's nothing magical about fruit and vegetable intake; it just helps with reducing calories and that reduction causes weight loss. Eating fruits and vegetables relates to lower weight.[108,109]

SPECIFIC NUTRIENT RESEARCH FOR GETTING STRONG

As of this book's writing, people are uncomfortable with carbohydrates. You have to know—if you're reading this book because you want to get stronger—you need to eat carbohydrates, and it really helps if some of them are grains. An article in the NSCA's *Journal of Strength and Conditioning Research* stated that, along with hydration, having carbohydrates for fuel is a primary determinant of muscular fatigue.[110]

A randomized crossover study put athletes into two groups, either a ketogenic diet at less than 50 grams of carbohydrates per day or a high carbohydrate diet of 2.7 to 4.5 grams of carbohydrates per pound of bodyweight. All of the athletes participated in both conditions: half started with keto and moved to high carb; the other half started with high carb and then moved to keto. They had the athletes perform high intensity interval training for four days under both conditions. Regardless of which diet they started or finished with, all of the athletes had a significant drop in power while doing the keto diet. In the ketogenic condition, they had a 7% loss of power in one of the interval tests, and they covered 15% less distance in a bike sprint test.[111]

A literature review, *Diet composition and the performance of high intensity exercise,* found that a drastic reduction in carbohydrate causes a significant drop in high intensity exercise performance. Attempting to remove carbohydrates completely (5% of energy from carbohydrates) caused a whopping 10–30% drop in performance.[112]

Reducing carbohydrates reduces performance in power and speed tests. It's unlikely you'll be able to work out at an optimal level for strength or power without eating bread, rice, pasta, and grains. Regardless of the ridiculous scare tactics many diet companies use in relation to these foods, no one ever had trouble getting lean eating *one portion* of carbohydrates at meals. And that portion is necessary for optimal workouts.

Everyone knows protein is the basic building block of muscle, and it's tough to gain strength or recover from workouts without it. A few large reviews and meta-analyses give us a clear picture of the research: Total protein intake has a significant effect on strength gain.[113,114,115,116]

For people into measuring, .73 grams of protein per pound of bodyweight (1.6 grams per kilogram of bodyweight) per day is recommended for optimal strength gain in those analyses. A palm-sized amount of protein, or about 25% of your plate, could fall anywhere between 25 and 30 grams of protein. Depending on bodyweight, you might need more portions of protein per day for optimal strength gain:

- Six portions of protein are optimal to gain strength for someone who is 234 pounds.

- Five portions of protein are optimal to gain strength for someone who is 195 pounds.

- Four portions of protein are optimal to gain strength for someone who is 156 pounds.

- Three portions of protein will be optimal for strength for someone who is 117 pounds.

If you're thinking of a portion of protein being palm-sized, you might need one portion, 1.3 portions, 1.7 portions, or even two portions of protein at each meal.

If your primary goal is weight loss, three portions of protein per day will probably be sufficient. If your main goal is strength, you're going to want more, based on how much you weigh. For someone who has mixed goals of getting both lean and strong, you may find your protein portions should fall in between.

The other thing to keep in mind is, there's a huge difference between "optimal" and "required." We don't live in a perfect world, and we really don't need to hit optimal most of the time. The majority of my clients are normal folks who want to lose weight. If they can get to three portions of protein per day, they're doing awesome. They lose weight, and they all get stronger. They don't care if getting stronger takes slightly longer because they aren't hitting "optimal" in their protein intake. They're getting enough, and they get stronger over time.

One research review, *A Critical Examination of Dietary Protein Requirements, Benefits, and Excesses in Athletes,* looked at minimal versus optimal amounts of protein. This review also put optimal daily protein intake at .7 grams of protein per pound of bodyweight, and put *minimal* required protein for strength gain at .55 grams of protein per pound of bodyweight. Looking at the minimums for strength gain:[117]

- Four portions of protein meets the requirements for anyone 218 pounds or under.

- Three portions of protein meets the requirements for anyone 163 pounds or under.

The people who hit optimal tend to be my clients who are athletes, personal trainers, and kettlebell instructors. Getting stronger is a high priority for them and it's worth getting to optimal for them. The majority of my clients just hit the minimum, and they also get stronger. You get to choose for yourself.

PLATING SUB-SKILLS

- Increase protein: Protein is magical for increasing fullness. Many people get hungry between meals because they aren't eating enough protein.

- It's also the building block of muscle—if you want to be lean and strong, you need to get enough protein. It can be really helpful just to work on increasing protein for a few weeks.

- Increase vegetables: Vegetables are a magic bullet for fullness. Slowly working your way up to one or two portions of vegetables (half a plate) will be helpful and sometimes even necessary for people to be able to notice they are full between meals.

- Reduce fat intake: The thing about fat is it's really easy to over-do. For starters, it doesn't take much fat to add up to a lot of calories. It's easy to have five servings of fat on a plate (like egg yolks, and olive oil, and avocado, and bacon) and not even notice. Based on quantity, just the guacamole and sour cream at your favorite restaurant might add up to five servings. Also, while fat is amazing for

keeping you full between meals, it doesn't have a big impact on your ability to notice how full you are during a meal. If you've ever felt pretty good during a meal but too full an hour later, that was probably too much fat.

- Reduce carbohydrate intake: Right now, low carbohydrate diets are all the rage (again), and many people have been taught to be scared of carbohydrates. This is stupid. We know that if you're someone who works out, your strength and performance will be significantly greater if you eat adequate carbohydrates. The reason people gain weight is because they have five servings of carbohydrates. No one gains weight eating one serving of carbohydrates. Feel free to eat a portion of bread or a portion of rice. There's a world of difference between one and five portions.

GUIDELINE	PLATE BALANCED PORTIONS
WHY PRACTICE THIS GUIDELINE	Plating healthy portions makes it easier to notice and stop when you're full.
WAYS TO GOLDILOCKS THIS GUIDELINE	"I'm going to plan dinners that are one-quarter protein, one-quarter carbohydrates, one-half vegetables, and a tablespoon of fat." "When I go out to lunch, I'm only going to order one serving of carbohydrates." "I'm going to have protein at every meal this week." "I'm going to eat two servings of vegetables at lunch and dinner this week." "I'm going to have fruit with breakfast this week." "When I make something in the crock pot, I'm going to use one-quarter protein, one-quarter carbohydrates, and one-half vegetables."

PLATE HEALTHY PORTION SIZES

It makes it easier to stop at a healthy place with food when you plate healthy portion sizes.

Unit bias is on your side with plating! Maybe you heard of the studies where they gave people different amounts of snack foods, and people ate whatever unit they were given. One study tested this with soft pretzels, M&M's, and Tootsie Rolls left in the lobby of a large, upscale apartment building. With the Philadelphia-style soft pretzels, they supplied either whole pretzels or half pretzels. When there were whole pretzels, people ate the whole pretzels, and when there were half pretzels, people ate half pretzels. With the M&M's, people ate more when serving themselves with a bigger scoop versus a smaller scoop. With Tootsie Rolls, people ate the same number of Tootsie Rolls whether they were large (twelve grams) or mini (three grams) candies. In all conditions, people ate whatever serving "unit" was presented.[118]

It turns out people are amazingly terrible at estimating how much food is "enough." They've done studies reducing people's breakfast by 40% and reducing lunch by 50%, and people didn't actually notice or eat more later.[119] Other studies have shown that portion sizes we think are "normal" range from 70–190% of a portion. Anything within the perceived-to-be-within-normal portion range would be eaten.[120]

Basically, we have a tendency to think the amount of food put in front of us is the right amount. Most restaurants serve twice as much food as we need and this works against us. If we don't pay attention, we'll eat more than we need because we assume what's in front of us is the right amount—though we'll probably feel too full later.

However, we can use this to our advantage: By plating healthy portion sizes, we're more likely to think the healthy amount we plated ourselves is the "right amount."

Thanksgiving dinner is an example most Americans are familiar with. If all the food is on the table in front of you, you're far more likely to keep serving yourself more, never really knowing how much you've had. If, on the other hand, it's the day after Thanksgiving and you make yourself a turkey sandwich, you're likely to eat that sandwich and feel like it was just right.

Note: Please don't ever try to lose weight on holidays like Thanksgiving. Just be social and be with your family. Part of what's cool about skills is that you don't "lose your skills" if you don't worry about them for a day. Just chill and have fun and enjoy the food and be with people when you have special occasions with people you love. That also doesn't mean you need to force-feed yourself because "it's a free day." Just eat normally. Eat what you want, then stop when full. Enjoy the food. Be with family.

That's it. That's all there is. There's no magic. It's easier to stop when you're full if you plate a portion of chicken and a portion of pasta and two portions of vegetables than it is when you plate twice that much.

PLATING PORTION SIZES GUIDELINES
(THESE ARE NOT RULES)

- Protein: Often a quarter of your plate, or the palm of your hand, or more. Adjust based on your own needs, fullness, and strength goals.

- Vegetables and fruit: Usually about half of your plate, or two fistfuls.

- Fat: One tablespoon is a good starting guideline. This could also be one serving of nuts (often 15–25 nuts, depending on which kind) or one-third to two-thirds of an avocado. If you are using your hand as a guide, you can think about the size of your thumb. Some people might do double that or half that, depending on their individual needs.

- Carbohydrates: One quarter of your plate, or about the size of your fist. Adjust based on leanness goals or activity needs—more active athletes might need more.

The best portion sizes are different for everyone. Feel free to put more or less on your plate, or use bigger or smaller plates. I can't emphasize enough that these are just guidelines, not rules. They're a place to start thinking about this and begin experimenting.

The caveat is this: Most people don't need to adjust their meals nearly as much as they need to not snack between meals. If you're snacking between meals, there's really no way to know if your portion sizes are correct, because the snacking always adds so many useless calories.

In terms of portion sizes, you'll adjust those until you get as lean as you want. What you eat for portion sizes might be different than someone else. For example, if you have a significant other, and one of you is 6′2″ and the other is 5′2″, the person who is shorter will need smaller portion sizes than the taller one. Those are just the facts.

One last note in terms of plating healthy portion sizes: Many people who have a history of dieting always plate *too little* food. They never plate *enough*, and they always go back for seconds or snack between meals. Going back for seconds or snacking between meals always adds up to way more total calories than if they'd just portioned a healthy amount of food in the first place.

These people need to increase their portion sizes at meals until they aren't snacking between meals or going back for seconds.

Note:

This is usually the *last* skill I have people work on.

If people have done many of the other skills like eating balanced meals and noticing when they're hungry or full, portioning often isn't necessary.

It comes down to this—if you're doing most of the other skills and your scale weight hasn't come down, you're eating too much food. There could be a bunch of reasons for this:

1.   You notice you're full, but you keep eating anyway;

2.   You're really stressed out, so you feel hungry for more food than you need;

3.   You aren't getting enough sleep, so you feel hungry for more food than you need;

4.   You've ignored your hunger and fullness cues for decades, and you aren't in touch with how much food your body needs.

In any of those cases, it's totally okay to put less food on the plate, and see what happens.

Almost universally, people report that at 20 minutes to an hour later, they're totally satisfied. And they don't get truly hungry again until 30 minutes before the next meal.

The coolest thing about adjusting portion sizes is that you can always self-check with the *listen-to-your-body skills.*

- You know you're plating the right amount when you get truly hungry about 30 minutes before the next meal.

- If you get truly hungry in an hour or two (not cravings), you know you plated too little.

When adjusting your portion sizes, remember to keep your plate balanced. Make sure you include enough protein and vegetables.

Note: People almost never eat too much protein. Protein is so great for increasing fullness, I usually urge people to increase protein. It's carbohydrates and fat we often have to reduce to one portion per meal.

Go ahead and have as many vegetables as you want. Veggies are great; just watch how many servings of fat you put *on* them.

CUSTOMIZING PORTION SIZES

Not everyone will eat the same amount of food. Not everyone's portion sizes will be the same.

- Someone who is six feet tall will plate more; someone who is five feet tall will plate less.

- Someone who works construction will plate more; someone who works at a desk will plate less.

- Someone who is 250 pounds will plate more; someone who is 150 pounds will plate less.

- Someone who is a lifetime athlete will plate more; someone who is just getting back into working out will plate less.

You'll need to adjust the portion sizes based on your individual situation. Most of us just aren't that active, and we often don't need as much food as most restaurants serve. And, as mentioned earlier, usually the problem is what we eat mindlessly between meals. That being said, if you've got your between-meals snacking handled (you've stopped doing it), you'll want to adjust your portion sizes.

You can keep the same ratios (50% vegetables, 25% protein, 25% carbohydrates, a tablespoon of fat), and scale that up or down, depending on which way the scale is moving. Some people get smaller plates, and you could, but you could also just serve yourself a smidge less.

SKILL	PLATE HEALTHY PORTION SIZES
WHY PRACTICE THIS GUIDELINE	Plating healthy portions makes it easier to notice and stop when you're full.
WAYS TO GOLDILOCKS THIS GUIDELINE	"I'm going to use a smaller plate." "I'm going to plate portions of protein and carbohydrates that are about the size of my fist, two fists of vegetables, and about a tablespoon of fat." "I'm not going to have four servings of fat on my salad—olive oil, avocado, bacon, and eggs. I'm going to pick one serving and have that." "I'm not having three servings of carbohydrates with lunch—rice, beans, and a tortilla. I'm going to pick one and have that." "I'm going to measure my food for a week and recalibrate my idea of portion sizes."

EATING WITHOUT SCREENS

Eating without screens is a simple skill: Eat without watching TV or looking at your phone. Most people already know they eat more while watching TV. It really surprises people to learn that the research we'll talk about next shows that if you eat while watching a screen, you not only eat more at that meal, you also eat more at the *next meal*. Or, if you watch TV while eating dinner, you're more likely to eat a late night snack later.

This guideline is amazing because you can get leaner without making any changes to your food content. All you have to do is *pay attention to your food*. It's a super reasonable guideline. It's also another guideline where people report enjoying their food more. It's silly, but people sometimes lose five or ten pounds just eating without screens and putting the fork down between bites. That's it.

Studies have shown that people eat more if they eat a meal while watching TV.[121] People snack more while watching TV.[122] Television watching increases the amount of food eaten significantly more than other distracted eating conditions like social eating or driving.[123] Television increases consumption of pizza by 36% and macaroni and cheese by 71%, whereas listening to music does not.[124] Television viewing at lunch increases afternoon snacking.[125]

Interestingly, researchers think it may have something to do with memory. Two studies showed that watching TV not only increased the amount of food people ate at their next meal, but it also reduced their memory of eating.[126] Weirdly, they got the same results when they had people eat meals in the dark, unable to see their food.[127] The other aspect of eating while distracted is that it reduces our willpower to eat less.[128]

One study had people with extreme amnesia consume two lunches in a row. The first lunch was 1,000 calories, and they were allowed to eat as much as they wanted. When they were done, they rated how much they liked it and how full they felt. All of the evidence of having eaten was removed, and then 15 minutes later, a second 1,000-calorie identical meal was brought in, and they were again told it was lunch time. They ate the second meal, the same as the first. Some reported feeling uncomfortable and said they liked the second lunch significantly less, but they didn't realize they were full. The researchers concluded that our memory of the meal might be required for us to understand that the fullness signals coming from our bodies are, in fact, that we're full.[129]

What you should take away from this is that eating without screens may be the simplest way to reduce calories. Any time we have a way to feel more full, enjoy our food more, and consume fewer calories, that's awesome. If we can have all of that without changing the content of the food or having to count anything…astronomically cool. This may be one of the most powerful tools we have for eating less and feeling full.

SKILL	EATING WITHOUT SCREENS
WHY PRACTICE THIS GUIDELINE	When you eat without screens, you eat less at that meal; you snack less after the meal, and you eat less at the following meal.
WAYS TO GOLDILOCKS THIS GUIDELINE	"I'm going to talk to my family at dinner." "I'm going to listen to music instead of watching TV at dinner." "I'm going to pay attention to my food instead of looking at my phone at lunch." "I'm going to eat lunch sitting on a park bench by work."

PUT THE FORK DOWN BETWEEN BITES

This is my favorite guideline. It's simple, actionable, and makes a difference for almost every client.

It usually doesn't surprise people that eating slowly reduces total calories consumed, increases fullness, increases enjoyment, and lowers bodyweight. Since most people can relate to this already, we'll just jam through the research:

- A meta-analysis of 22 studies showed that eating slower reduces caloric intake without actually effecting hunger. [130]

- An eight-year longitudinal study showed that people who ate faster gained more weight. This result held constant, even controlling for other variables like age, exercise, and previous body-weight. Eating speed turns out to be a major determinant of weight.[131]

- Healthy women who ate slowly ate fewer calories, but were more full later. Healthy women who ate faster ate more calories, and were hungry later. Eating slowly is a double awesome of both eating less and being more full.[132]

- A nationwide survey of middle-aged women found that the women who self-reported they ate quickly had higher bodyweight than women who reported eating slowly.[133]

Putting the fork down between bites is the *action* of eating slowly. We know eating slowly gives people a chance to notice they're getting full. Many people who are used to eating quickly report that in eating more slowly, they were able to notice they were getting full while eating—for the first time in their lives.

If you eat a meal in five to ten minutes, you have no chance of noticing you're getting full. You also have no real chance of tasting or enjoying your food.

By extending a meal (20 minutes is often a guideline given to work up to), we find we simultaneously eat less total food (which helps for weight loss), notice we're getting full (which helps for satisfaction and sustainability), and we enjoy the food more (which helps sustainability and enjoying our lives).

Unfortunately, just watching the clock and trying to hold on as hard as possible to eat slowly doesn't work. We need actions. One action we can take is to put the fork or sandwich down between bites. Some people have simply *not* put a bite into their mouths while they're still chewing the previous bite of food. Another popular option is to take a sip of water between bites. These are things people who eat slowly do naturally. By practicing these actions, we can reverse-engineer eating in a way that has us self-limit meal quantity to the amount of food our bodies need…and how much we enjoy.

If you're going on vacation, I recommend this as the *only* skill to practice while away. Slowing down meals on vacation always means you enjoy them more. The double-whammy of enjoying your food more and noticing when you're full makes for a really enjoyable vacation. On vacation, you can eat like you're wine tasting, enjoying and savoring every bite.

If you know that you typically eat quickly, this is probably the most important guideline to work on. Start with this one.

IMPORTANT NOTE: WHAT IF I DON'T HAVE TIME TO EAT SLOWLY?

If you're a parent of young children and don't have time to eat slowly because getting your kids fed is a part-time job, that's okay.

If you're a nurse and don't have time to eat slowly because you have rounds to do, that's okay. This skill isn't an issue when you don't have time to eat *because you don't have time to get seconds either.*

This is a really effective skill for reducing the amount of food consumed because you have time to notice. For the people who barely have time to get some food in their mouths, it's unnecessary. If your work or home life preclude you from eating slowly, it's totally okay. Instead, focus on plating a decent meal and eating that meal however you can.

Often, for people with limited time, the issue is never plating a real meal; instead, it's about having snacks…or eating while cooking, or eating the kids' food after serving meals. Just try to plate a legit, balanced meal, and eat it in whatever time frame you can. Then stop.

GUIDELINE	PUT THE FORK DOWN BETWEEN BITES
WHY PRACTICE THIS GUIDELINE	The most powerful skill for noticing when you're full is to eat slower. Putting the fork down between bites is the simplest action you can take to slow down your eating.
WAYS TO GOLDILOCKS THIS GUIDELINE	"I'm going to put my fork down between bites at dinner." "I'm going to put the sandwich down between bites at lunch." "I'm going to put the fork down between bites all the meals I eat while I'm on vacation."

GUIDELINE: WAIT TEN MINUTES BEFORE GETTING SECONDS OR DESSERT

This guide is amazingly useful and unbelievably simple. It perfectly mirrors the between-meals guideline of waiting ten minutes before getting a snack or treat.

Most of us get into a habit where we want seconds, and we eat it mindlessly. There's no gap to do any kind of thinking, or make a choice because it happens so fast. This guideline is about slowing down long enough to choose for yourself.

The biggest reason most people get seconds is they don't plate enough food to begin with; the guideline of *plating enough food* is required to use this guideline. You *have to* plate enough food that you don't need seconds.

Whenever a client is struggling with having seconds, we always increase the amount of food on the first plate. If you are plating a silly little amount of food, of course you're always going to want seconds.

The next reason most people get seconds is they eat too fast to notice when they've had enough. In that case, slowing down will help. The guideline of *putting the fork down between bites* is awesome for that. That being said, if you mess up and eat too fast, you can use *waiting ten minutes before getting seconds* to fix it.

Even if you've eaten too fast, you can still wait until the meal has had some time to settle before having seconds. If you inhaled your food, just wait 20 minutes before having seconds. Most of the time, you'll find you had enough, and just need to wait for your body to catch up.

Beyond that, we need to work on smashing the pattern of immediately getting seconds. When we add a gap between stimulus and response, we have time to think. We have time to choose. If I want to have seconds but wait ten minutes, I have the time to notice if I really am hungry for more food or if I'm just in the habit of getting seconds. I can also check in with myself, and see if I'm just reacting to stress.

The cool thing is, if after ten minutes you choose to have it, you get to have it. But you've had time to *choose*. You've had time to *think*. You've had time to *check in with your body*. If after checking in, you really are still hungry, have more food.

Most people find that sometimes they're still hungry, but most of the time—if they plated enough food to begin with—they're actually fine. Waiting is an awesome way to learn to check in with your body and then trust yourself.

It works best not to just wait ten minutes while staring at an open container of food. If you can, leave the kitchen. Go watch TV or work on a hobby. Read. Do something fun. If we don't immediately do something else, we run the risk of eating out of boredom or just because we're still sitting there staring at the food.

Similar to the *wait 10 minutes before eating a snack* guideline, this can be lengthened or shortened depending on how well it's going. If you're struggling with not getting seconds or having a hard time deciding if you're satisfied, you can extend it longer. You could do 20 minutes or even an hour. As you get good at this skill, you might be able to shorten it to one minute. Super ninja level is ten seconds.

Always remember, after your waiting period, if you're truly hungry, you should eat more. If that's the case, remember that next time and plate more food so you don't get in the habit of getting seconds. For most people, most of the time, it's more that we're enjoying the flavor, and want to eat more rather than still being hungry. Waiting is an opportunity for us to notice the difference.

GUIDELINE	DELIBERATE SELF-CARE: COPING SKILLS, SELF-SOOTHING, AND FUN ACTIVITIES
WHY PRACTICE THIS GUIDELINE	Most people don't actually know if they want seconds; they eat seconds out of habit.
WAYS TO GOLDILOCKS THIS GUIDELINE	"When I want seconds after dinner, I'm going to go watch TV for 10 minutes before I have it." "If I want a seconds, I'm going to stop for 10 minutes and check in with myself to see whether I'm actually hungry. During that 10 minutes, I'll read a good book." "If I accidentally eat too fast, I'm going to wait 10 or 20 minutes before having seconds so I give my body time to catch up and see if I'm full."

SKILL DETAILS: LISTEN TO YOUR BODY BETWEEN MEALS

LISTEN TO YOUR BODY BETWEEN MEALS	Distinguish hunger from cravings, boredom, tiredness, emotions, or thoughts De-fusion from unwanted thoughts, feelings, and cravings Participation in, and five senses experience of, what's going on around you right now Notice and wait through normal hunger: 30 minutes before eating Notice when tired and go to sleep

DISTINGUISH TRUE HUNGER FROM CRAVINGS, BOREDOM, TIREDNESS, EMOTIONS, OR THOUGHTS

True hunger:

1. Is in your stomach;
2. Builds over time;
3. Is for a balanced meal.

Cravings, boredom, stress, tiredness, emotional eating:

1. Is not in your stomach;
2. Builds, then fades;
3. Is for a specific treat.

The coolest thing about distinguishing true hunger is this: When you're hungry, *you should eat.*

My clients are often amazed that I want them to eat when they're hungry. **OF COURSE YOU SHOULD EAT WHEN YOU'RE HUNGRY.**

You just need to know the difference between hunger and all of the other reasons people eat.

It's not eating when you're hungry that causes most weight gain—it's the eating when you're *not* hungry.

I'm re-typing this because we have to repeat it multiple times in food coaching…over months:

- When you're truly hungry, you should eat a meal.

- When you're bored, stressed, tired, or craving something, we should find a way to either accept that those are normal human feelings, or we should add some self-care and healthy coping strategies that address the actual feelings.

TRUE HUNGER	CRAVINGS, BOREDOM, STRESS, TIREDNESS, EMOTIONAL EATING
Is for a balanced meal	Is a craving for a specific snack or treat
Builds, and continues to build over time	Builds, but often begins to fade after 20 minutes
Is a physical sensation you can feel in your stomach	Is related to boredom, stress, tiredness, an emotion, or unwanted thoughts

We need to stop filling non-food needs with food. We need to eat meals when we're hungry for meals.

The guideline of eating a meal every four to six hours is often a helpful starting place for this skill. If you're eating sooner than four hours, it's probably a craving and not true hunger. If you're waiting more than six hours, that's usually too long, and you'll roll into the next meal too hungry.

Most people have spent their lives ignoring their natural hunger and fullness cues. They starved when they were hungry, then they snapped and ate when they had emotions. I get it; you've been practicing ignoring your body for decades. It's time to flip that.

Again, repeat after me:

- Lean and strong people eat a meal when they're hungry.

- Lean and strong people don't eat to fix non-hunger issues.

- Lean and strong people address non-hunger issues with acceptance and self-care.

Ironically, it's a simple skill to practice. If you find yourself wanting food and it's been less than four hours between meals, ask yourself three questions:

1. Is this hunger a physical sensation I can feel in my stomach?

2. Did this hunger build over time?

3. Am I hungry for a balanced meal?

If you notice yourself saying "no" to the questions above, check in with yourself and find out what's going on:

4. Am I bored? Stressed? Tired? Feeling an emotion? Having an unwanted thought?

Often, "Am I hungry for a balanced meal?" is people's favorite question. It's just so simple. If a meal of green-chili chicken with Spanish rice and a salad doesn't sound good but the candy in the candy jar does, that's a pretty good indicator you aren't actually hungry.

For many people, this is the skill that makes the difference in their afternoon or after dinner snacking. When you discover something isn't food related, you can handle the actual issue. For many people, something as simple as going for a short walk fixes most non-food issues.

SKILL	DISTINGUISH BETWEEN TRUE HUNGER AND CRAVINGS, BOREDOM, STRESS, TIREDNESS, AND EMOTIONS
WHY PRACTICE THIS SKILL	Most people who have trouble staying lean, have trouble because they are eating for non-hunger reasons. Being able to distinguish between true hunger and non-hunger cravings often is the most important skill people need to get lean.
WAYS TO GOLDILOCKS THIS SKILL	"Between lunch and dinner, I'm going to notice if I feel hunger in my stomach, or if I just have a headache." "If I need a break mid-morning, I'm going to go for a ten-minute walk around the building instead of snacking." "Between breakfast and lunch, I'm going to notice if I'm truly hungry, or if I'm just bored." "Between lunch and dinner, I'm going to notice if I feel hunger in my stomach, or if I just need to take a five-minute break from work." "After dinner, I'm going to notice if I'm truly hungry, or if I'm just bored. If I'm bored, I'll do a craft." "If I know I'm craving a treat because I'm stressed out after work, I'm going to go for a walk."

NOTICE AND WAIT THROUGH NORMAL HUNGER BEFORE MEALS

Noticing and waiting through normal hunger is one of the most powerful self-checks you can do for plating and stopping when full. The ability to recognize hunger can be practiced and learned.

Research shows that people who eat when hungry have a lower bodyweight than people who don't pay attention to hunger.[134] Eating in response to hunger is associated with lower caloric intake. One hundred and eight-one people who were trained in recognizing hunger for seven weeks and then practiced on their own for another 12 weeks found that simply eating when hungry lead to a *one-third* decrease in calories.[135]

On top of that, paying attention to hunger signals has wide-ranging wellbeing benefits. Learning to eat based on actual hunger is related to better body acceptance, better self-esteem, less depression, lower anxiety, and decreased body dissatisfaction.[136]

People who learn to notice their natural hunger cues are also more effective at noticing what *isn't* true hunger, such as stress, cravings, or emotions. In that way, noticing hunger is a phenomenally effective tool against emotional eating, boredom eating, stress eating, and tired eating.

Let's review how we distinguish between the two:

TRUE HUNGER	CRAVINGS, BOREDOM, STRESS, TIREDNESS, AND EMOTIONS
Is for a balanced meal	Is a craving for a specific snack or treat
Builds, and continues to build over time	Builds, but often begins to fade after 20 minutes
Is a physical sensation you can feel in your stomach	Is related boredom, stress, tiredness, an emotion, or unwanted thoughts

You may notice this is the perfect mirror to the previous skill, distinguishing hunger from cravings, boredom, stress, tiredness, and emotions.

The first step is to notice it is in fact true hunger. Often, this is described as a "hollow" feeling in your stomach. The same three questions apply to this skill:

1. Is this hunger a physical sensation I can feel in my stomach?

2. Did this hunger build over time?

3. Am I hungry for a balanced meal?

The initial reason the waiting part is cool is that it's normal. It's normal to be hungry for about a half-hour before meals. Many clients are scared to death of feeling hungry, and often eat bigger meals or snack preemptively to make sure they never feel hunger.

If you never feel hunger, it will be impossible to lose weight.

But you don't want to be hungry for hours. If you're hungry for an hour, you should definitely eat. This isn't about starving between meals. In fact, when people are hungry for hours, they almost always overeat at the next meal. That's not the goal. The goal is to be hungry for a reasonable amount of time.

The second reason this is cool is as a self-check for your other guidelines and skills. If you aren't hungry 30 minutes before your next meal:

- It could be you plated too much at the previous meal.

- It could be you didn't notice when full, and stop then.

- It could be this meal is too soon, earlier than four hours.

- It could be you snacked between meals.

All of those are great learning experiences. The goal isn't to nail any of this stuff perfectly. The goal is to use a skill, and learn about the skills you used at the previous meal. Unfortunately, there's an enormous amount of trial and error in learning all things.

Going back to the clarinet example—in the beginning of learning to play a clarinet, most people hit more wrong than right notes. Still, a couple years down the road, they can play much more accurately, even while playing more complex songs.

Similar to the clarinet, eating skills and guides are a practice. You practice, and then you self-check with your "noticing hunger" skill.

Working Backward

This is a skill you may often have to work from backward. If you look at your schedule and notice you'll have a longer-than-normal gap between lunch and dinner, you may eat more at lunch to get you through until 30 minutes before dinner. Similarly, if you have a shorter than normal gap between lunch and dinner, you might eat less at lunch so you get hungry before dinner.

Stress and Hunger

Stress can screw with people in different ways. Some people when extremely stressed may have the experience of hunger before they actually need food. On the other hand, some people when extremely stressed may not feel hunger at all. Under extreme stress, it's often better to trust guidelines instead of skills like this one.

Breakfast Does Not Apply

Because of sleep and the long gap between dinner and breakfast, many people don't feel hungry at breakfast time. That's okay. Go ahead and eat breakfast anyway. Breakfast is good for you. Just eat breakfast at whatever time makes sense in your schedule. Then you can practice this skill at lunch and dinner.

SKILL	NOTICE HUNGER 30 MINUTES BEFORE A MEAL
WHY PRACTICE THIS SKILL	It's normal to feel hungry 30 minutes before meals. It's required to be hungry 30 minutes before meals to lose weight.
WAYS TO GOLDILOCKS THIS SKILL	"I'm going to try eating a little less at lunch this week to see if I get hungry 30 minutes before dinner." "I'm normally starving before dinner, so I'm going to try eating a little more at lunch to have hunger land 30 minutes before dinner." "I'm never hungry before lunch, so I'm going to drop my mid-morning snack to see if I'm hungry 30 minutes before lunch. "I'm going to notice when I get hungry, and I'm going to eat dinner 30 minutes after I notice."

DE-FUSION—FEEL YOUR FEELINGS AND THINK ABOUT YOUR THOUGHTS

Defusion means separating your thoughts from your actions—to literally de-fuse the two.

Fusion is when your thoughts and actions are fused: You have a craving for a cookie in the afternoon and you eat the cookie.

Defusion is the opposite: You have a craving and you don't eat the cookie.

I'll alternate between using "de-fusion" and "defusion." In contextual behavioral science, it's always written as "defusion," so I'll use it like that. That being said, when people read "de-fusion," they more quickly get what it means and how to use it.

Most people fight their thoughts and feelings, avoid their thoughts and feelings, or emotionally numb their thoughts and feelings with food. De-fusion means accepting those thoughts in such a way that they don't bully you, and you can take the actions that matter to you.[137]

You've probably heard advice about trying to change or control your thoughts. Studies have shown that when people are presented with the option of trying to change their thoughts to create weight loss, this approach makes the most sense, and is the most appealing strategy.[138]

Unfortunately, some of those same researchers found that those strategies can backfire, especially for people who struggle with emotional eating. They had participants carry a clear bag of chocolates with them 24 hours per day for a week, and used one of two strategies: changing thoughts or defusion. They found that for people with low and medium emotional eating issues, changing thoughts and defusion both produced similar results. For people with *high* emotional eating issues, changing thoughts produced far worse results and caused people to eat *more* chocolate. On the flip side, defusion was a really effective strategy for all groups, especially for the people with high emotional eating issues.[139]

There have been tons of similar experiments; apparently having people carry chocolates is a super popular study design! One used specifically overweight women and found that defusion was more effective than thought control.[140] Another also broke out the results by emotional eating scores and again found that people with higher emotional eating issues did better with defusion.[141]

Rebound is a big thing too. A study that tracked both chocolates consumed during the week and chocolates consumed in a fake taste test "after the study" found that people who used thought suppression techniques ate four times more chocolates than people who used defusion.[142] If you've ever had a huge rebound after trying to control cravings or emotional eating, you know what that rebound is like.

This is an introduction to the enormous skill of defusion—I'm currently writing an entire book about it. What we'll cover here is enough to get you started.

Defusion is about separating or "de-fusing" from thoughts. When we're "fused" with thoughts, we think our unwanted thoughts are true, urgent, shouldn't be there, or are commands. [143]

An example of an unwanted thought: "I feel fat. This isn't working."

THOUGHT	ACTION WHEN FUSED WITH THAT THOUGHT	DE-FUSION AND ACTION
"I feel fat."	Immediately starts a new crash diet	Recognizes and accepts it's normal to have negative body thoughts in our diet-obsessed culture. We all have a diet "inner critic." Goes back to practicing Lean and Strong skills
"This isn't working."	Immediately starts looking for new crash diets to try	Recognizes and accepts it's normal to have impatient thoughts. We all have a diet "inner critic." Goes back to practicing Lean and Strong skills

THOUGHT	ACTION WHEN FUSED WITH THAT THOUGHT	DE-FUSION AND ACTION
"I blew my diet."	Eats all the leftover pizza and doughnuts	Recognizes and accepts it's normal to have perfectionist thoughts. We all have a perfectionist "inner critic." Goes back to practicing Lean and Strong skills
"I'll never get good at any of these skills."	Gives up	Recognizes and accepts it's normal to feel like you aren't making enough progress. We all have inner "doubt monsters." Goes back to practicing Lean and Strong skills
"Most people just follow a diet and get results. I'm broken somehow."	Gives up or finds a new diet to try	Recognizes and accepts it's normal to feel like you aren't good at things you haven't practiced before. We all have inner "thought monsters." Goes back to practicing Lean and Strong skills

Defusion doesn't mean fighting your thoughts. It isn't about fixing your thoughts and it doesn't mean having different thoughts or better thoughts.

It's just about *recognizing them as thoughts.*

Recognize that in our diet-obsessed culture, we're going to have a lot of unhelpful thoughts. It's normal to have those thoughts with all the diet talk and diet media and diet marketing that surrounds us. Some people call these your diet "inner critic" or your diet "thought monster."

People often report that after a year or two of practice noticing those thoughts as just thoughts, it turns down the volume on those thoughts. The thoughts seem far less compelling and less "true."

But that takes a year or two of practicing the skills while you still have those thoughts.

People always read this as, "I must fight the thoughts!" DO NOT FIGHT THE THOUGHTS.

It doesn't work, and you don't have to do it. It's easier to just notice the diet thoughts as being normal in our culture.

You win by practicing *Lean and Strong* skills in spite of the thoughts.

Accept the thoughts.

Recognize the thoughts as thoughts.

Remember these thoughts are normal in our diet culture.

Notice many aren't even from you—they're things people told you or things you read or saw on TV.

Remember having thoughts doesn't mean they're true or false. Instead, thoughts are helpful or unhelpful. Debating the truth of a thought is a huge pitfall.

THOUGHTS AND FEELINGS COME AND GO LIKE THE WEATHER

We don't really have control over our thoughts and feelings any more than we have control over the weather. We have control over our *actions*.

It might be sunny, and we drive to work. Or, it may be rainy, and we drive to work. We can't control whether it's rainy or sunny, but we can still drive to work.

Sometimes you have rainy feelings: "I feel sad." Other times you have sunny feelings: "I feel happy!"

You can't really control which you get, when, or how long they last. But just like rain and sun, they come and go in their own time. Unless you live in Seattle, the rain always eventually goes away. You drive your car in the direction of your goals anyway.

Sometimes you have rainy thoughts: "I'm so tired of having to work this hard on my food," or "I totally deserve a candy bar."

Sometimes you have sunny thoughts: "I feel so strong today!"

It's not about having more sunny thoughts than rainy thoughts. Just like the weather, you don't get to control the sun or the rain. Your job is just to drive in the direction of your goals.

CONTROL WHAT YOU CAN; ACCEPT WHAT YOU CAN'T

I *can't control* the weather,
but I can control driving to work.

I *can't control* my thoughts and feelings,
but I can control practicing my eating skills.

Just notice if the thought is helping you *take actions* in line with your values. If a thought isn't helping you take actions in line with your values—as with most diet thoughts—just notice and accept it. Allow that thought to be there while you take actions in line with your goals.

Defusion is *allowing the thoughts to be there*.

We're going to have two ways you can approach defusion in *Lean and Strong*: thought/emotion labeling and noticing thoughts and emotions come and go.

THOUGHT LABELING OR EMOTION LABELING LOOKS LIKE THIS

— Say to yourself, "I notice I'm having the thought that _____" and actually noticing the difference between being the one who has the thought or observes the thought versus thinking the thought is you or is a command.

— Label the thought as your "inner critic."

— Label the emotion according to the feelings wheel.

— Journal about your thoughts and feelings. See how getting them out on the page gives you a little distance from them. You clearly see them as thoughts and feelings.

NOTICING THAT THOUGHTS AND FEELINGS COME AND GO

- Use the weather metaphor. Notice how the weather always changes. Sun comes and goes in its own time. Rain comes and goes in its own time. Emotions come and go in their own time.

- Think about the movie *Inside Out,* which I'll describe more later for those who haven't seen it, and notice how it's normal to have emotions show up at different times. Sometimes you get joy; sometimes you get sadness. It's healthy to let them come and go in their own time.

All of these tools allow you to be with your thoughts and emotions, to let them be, but give you enough distance you can still practice your eating skills and do your workouts. When you stop trying to control your thoughts and emotions, it's easier to control what actions you take out in the world.

If you can separate from your thoughts—if you can think about your thoughts—they won't control you, and they won't seem as intense. In the research, sometimes this is called defusion, and sometimes it's called metacognition. The ability to think about your thoughts, to step back, gives you power.

There's a world of difference between:

"I feel fat."

versus

"I notice I'm having the thought that I feel fat again. I totally get that social media has taught me to always feel fat. I can recognize I'm having that thought and where it came from. Even though I'm having that thought, I can still practice my eating skills; I can still work out; I can still do the things that matter to me. I know thoughts and feelings come and go like the weather."

In the first example, the thought is unexamined. Just because it popped into your head, you assume it's something you have to engage. Often people assume a thought is something you need to fix immediately…with food.

In the second example, they think about their thoughts. They realize it's okay and normal to have that thought. They realize just because that thought is normal doesn't mean it's helpful and because it isn't helpful, they don't take actions because of it. Instead, they take actions that fit their goals and values, and just let that thought be.

EMOTIONAL LABELING

Two studies published in *Psychological Science* found that when unable to differentiate what emotion they're feeling, people will be less likely to effectively cope. The first study found that if people lack skills at differentiating emotion, they won't be effective with *any* emotional coping mechanism. The second study found that for people who don't differentiate emotions well, coping effectiveness depended on which strategies they used. Coping strategies like rumination on the emotion, suppressing the emotion, and sharing about the emotion made people feel worse. Coping strategies like looking at a different perspective about the emotion and distraction from the emotion were neutral. Only emotional acceptance was effective for people with low emotional differentiation.[144]

Emotional differentiation is like hydration. Hydration doesn't produce magical results for sports performance, but if you're dehydrated, performance tanks. Similarly, emotional differentiation doesn't create effective coping strategies, but without emotional differentiation, you'll be ineffective with all or most coping strategies.

The way to know you suck at emotional differentiation is if you say you feel the same all the time. If you say you feel "bad" about everything, you're probably not differentiating between different feelings, like sadness or anger. If you say you "feel fat" all the time, you're probably substituting "fat" for figuring out if you feel frustrated, tired, lonely, or sad. If you feel "tired" all the time, you might investigate if that's a lazy alternative to doing the work of differentiating.

The easiest way to start differentiating and giving yourself a stronger shot at coping with emotions without food is to use a feelings wheel. In the beginning, it's easier to pick from a menu than to try to come up with the answer from nothing.

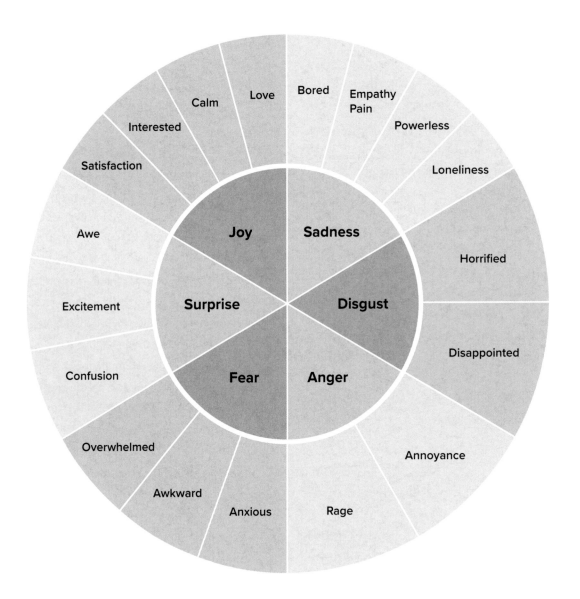

This feelings wheel is inspired by both English teacher Kaitlin Robb's feelings wheel and emotion researcher Robert Plutchik's emotions wheel. I also borrowed many of the emotions from the emotions distinguished in research by Alan Cowen and Dacher Keltner.

Don't get too caught up in the categorizations; just look at the wheel and pick out a word (or two or three) that describe how you feel. If you feel sad, you can just say "sad;" you don't need to pick something on the next ring. Similarly, if "loneliness" is a better fit, use that. And yes, I know "bored" doesn't fit well under "sad." Again, it's not that I was trying to create a perfect organization of emotions; I just wanted to create a menu. If you prefer, you can use Cowen and Keltner's emotions, which I made into a menu on page 230. Most of my clients really like the wheel, so here it is.

Lastly, if you get stuck, notice you might be feeling more than one emotion. Emotions aren't binary; it's normal to feel different things at the same time or in short succession.

This is an introduction to defusion; my book on just this skill is currently in process. In the meantime, if you want to dig into this while waiting for it, I recommend *A Liberated Mind* by Steven Hayes.

DEFUSION EVERY MONDAY MORNING

People often get freaked about this skill, thinking it's impossible. It's actually already common in your life; you probably just aren't applying it to food.

Many people think every Monday morning, "I really don't want to go to work today" or "My bed is so warm; I just want to stay in bed for another hour." And then… they get up and go to work anyway. That's defusion. You're already doing it literally every Monday morning.

That's all it is.

You aren't pretending like you're really stoked to go work at that moment. You aren't suppressing how much you don't want to go to work. You don't have to change your thoughts about wanting to go to work…*you just go.*

You've accepted it's normal and okay not to want to go to work on Monday morning, and go anyway. It's normal to have thoughts about wanting to stay in bed. But you know your values and the kind of person you want to be include going to work even when you have thoughts that you don't feel like it.

GIVE IT AT LEAST A MONTH OF PRACTICE

One thing to note about defusion: It takes practice. It's a high-level skill and you shouldn't expect it to work awesomely the first time you try it. Some people find it actually makes cravings and emotional eating *worse* for the first couple weeks.

Other clients found they thought about practicing it a lot, but weren't actually using it as a strategy in the moment. Of course, like most skills, just thinking about using it isn't as effective as actually using it. Practice is noticing and accepting your thoughts *in the moment.*

If you struggle with doing this in the moment, try journaling your thoughts. In your journal, write it out like, "I'm noticing I'm having the thought that _____." Writing it out as a thought you notice yourself having gives you separation—seeing it on the page gives you a little more distance. The act of journaling about the thought in this way makes it easier to see the thought as being separate from you.

That separation gives you the power to choose your actions. It's a powerful place to stand with your skill practice: Brains have thoughts, your brain is currently having thoughts, and you can take actions in this moment completely contrary to your thoughts.

Give it some time. Put in real practice, in the moment. In months, you might find it to be the most important and effective tool in your toolbox. It's worth the practice and time required.

Multiple studies have shown, at three, six and twelve months, defusion not only worked well for weight loss, but also increased people's quality of life.[145,146,147]

Three things to remember about thoughts, emotions, and cravings:

1. They are things you have—they are not *you.*
2. They are normal.
3. They come and go in their own time.

If defusion starts to feel complicated or super hard, remember it's just separating your thoughts from your actions. Remember it's okay for thoughts to come and go. All you need to do is take actions in line with your values.

You could also look at defusion as "taking action in line with your values, even when it's hard."

SKILL	DEFUSION
WHY PRACTICE THIS SKILL	Most people get bullied by their thoughts. They try to fight their thoughts and feelings, and even if they're successful, the thoughts and feelings rebound, and they emotionally eat later. The only way is through.
WAYS TO GOLDILOCKS THIS SKILL	"When I have unwanted thoughts, I'm going to journal about them." "When I have intense feelings, I'm going to look at a feelings wheel and identify my feelings." "I'm going to use the "Driving in the Weather" metaphor to remember it's okay to have rain. I just need to drive in the direction of my values." "I'm going to notice my diet thoughts and remember where they came from. I'm going to accept them as being normal in our day and age, and practice my skills even when I have those thoughts."

SKILL DETAILS: LISTEN TO YOUR BODY DURING MEALS

LISTEN TO YOUR BODY DURING MEALS	Notice before getting too full, and stop
	Notice if you're still hungry, and eat more if you are
	Check in with your stomach mid-meal, then notice or speculate about future fullness
	Notice flavor enjoyment is different from fullness
	Practice five-senses mindfulness
	Make sure to eat enough
	Stop before eating too much
	Check in with your stomach one hour after eating

NOTICE BEFORE GETTING TOO FULL, AND STOP

Noticing before getting too full and stopping has several sub-skills. Given that each of the skills in this category is a distinct sub-skill, we're going to do a quick overview, discuss stopping, and then go into how each sub-skill works.

- Notice if still hungry, and eat more if you are
- Check in with your stomach mid-meal, notice or speculate about future fullness
- Notice flavor enjoyment is different from fullness
- Practice five-senses mindfulness
- Make sure to eat enough
- Stop before eating too much
- Check in with your stomach one hour after eating

SKILL	NOTICE WHEN FULL, AND STOP BEFORE EATING TOO MUCH
WHY PRACTICE THIS SKILL	Most people eat too much at meals because they never check in with their bodies and their stomachs to see how much they actually need.
WAYS TO GOLDILOCKS THIS SKILL	"When I check in with my stomach mid-meal, if I feel full, I'm going to stop." "When I put my fork down between bites, I'm going to check in with my stomach. If I feel like it's the right amount, I'm going to stop."

NOTICE WHEN STILL HUNGRY, AND EAT MORE IF YOU ARE

Eating less than enough is just as unsuccessful as eating more than enough.

The pitfall of working on noticing when full and stopping is that people start working on eating less and less. Then, if they feel hungry later—a half hour, an hour, or two hours later—they try to suffer through.

The issue with eating too little at meals is that people almost always end up snacking later. Then they get in a cycle of eating too little of their balanced meal and too much of whatever shows up as a snack when they're super hungry. The snacks always end up being more calories and less nutrition than what they would have gotten at the earlier meal. The snacks also don't provide as much fullness as if they'd just eaten a little more at the meal. They think they have an insurmountable problem with snacking, but really the problem was they're eating too little at meals.

A simple fix: If you finish what you've plated, wait another ten or twenty minutes to see if you feel satisfied. If you're still hungry, eat some more.

Checking in with your stomach after eating is the only way to really learn the right amount to eat at a meal. If you've put your fork down between bites, you've enjoyed the meal with five-senses experiencing, and if it was a balanced and whole-food meal, you should be able to learn how to tell when you've had the right amount. If you still feel hungry ten minutes after your meal, eat some more.

Note: Don't just white-knuckle waiting ten or twenty minutes. Talk to your family. Watch TV.

Don't stare at the food and wait, because people who are food reactive—they want food when they see it—will have the experience of wanting it even if they don't feel hungry.

SKILL	NOTICE WHEN STILL HUNGRY AND EAT MORE IF YOU ARE
WHY PRACTICE THIS SKILL	Many people who have trouble with snacking between meals are eating too little during meals.
WAYS TO GOLDILOCKS THIS SKILL	"If I finish eating and want seconds, I'm going to wait ten minutes to see if I'm still truly hungry. If I am, I'm going to have more."

CHECK IN WITH YOUR STOMACH MID-MEAL—NOTICE AND SPECULATE ABOUT FUTURE FULLNESS

This idea is cool because it's a relatively simple way to start practicing noticing when full. All you do is check in with your stomach halfway through the meal. See how your stomach feels. Start to speculate about your future fullness.

Take a look at the food on the plate and try to guess if it's the right amount, or too much or too little. The issue most people have with food volume is a lack of awareness.

They can't tell they're getting full because they've never actually checked in with their stomachs.

Many people never check in with their stomach because they're watching TV and eating really fast, making food a thing that happens in the background. They always end up eating too much because they never check in before the food is gone.

Other people have been heavily dieting for years and don't check in with their stomachs because they base everything they eat on external counts like macros, or calories, or the meal plan. Because everything is always coming from outside, they never check in with their stomachs. Sometimes they under-eat because that was the meal plan. Or sometimes they over-eat because they had calories left over for the day.

Trusting your body to tell you the right amount of food takes a lot of practice. The practice looks like this:

1. Check in with your stomach mid-meal and speculate on how full you're going to be.

2. Check in at the end of the meal to see how your stomach feels.

3. Check in with your stomach sometime before the next meal to see if you got it right.

Steps one and two are basically guesses. Step three is where you self-check.

Over time with more self-checking, you'll see how well you did at your guesses during meals. After a couple months of practice, you'll notice you've gotten really good at guessing most of the time. Your confidence in your mid-meal guess will build with the experience of self-checking.

SKILL	CHECK IN WITH YOUR STOMACH MID-MEAL, NOTICE AND SPECULATE ABOUT FUTURE FULLNESS
WHY PRACTICE THIS SKILL	This is a simple and actionable way to start checking in with your stomach and being mindful about fullness.
WAYS TO GOLDILOCKS THIS SKILL	"I'm going to remember to check in with my stomach about halfway through the meal, and guess about future fullness." "I'm going to draw a line down the center of my plate with my fork, and when I get to the line, I'm going to check in with my stomach, and guess about future fullness." "I'm going to set a timer for ten minutes and when the timer goes off, I'm going to check in with my stomach, and guess about future fullness." "I'm going to check in with my stomach halfway through the meal, three-quarters of the way through the meal, and at the end of the meal." "I'm going to check in with my stomach an hour after the lunch, and see if I guessed right." "I'm going to check in with my stomach an hour before dinner, and see if I guessed right at lunch."

NOTICE FLAVOR ENJOYMENT IS DIFFERENT FROM FULLNESS

Noticing diminishing returns is about noticing when flavor enjoyment begins to diminish.

There are basically two ways to use diminishing returns:

1.   Similar to noticing when full, notice when you're no longer enjoying your food…and stop eating.

2.   Noticing flavor enjoyment is totally different from fullness, where flavor enjoyment might continue long after you're full. In this case, you'll be noticing when you can't rely on flavor enjoyment diminishing as a time to stop.

We've all had times when something we were eating started to lose the enjoyment it gave us, but we kept eating. Maybe we keep eating because there's more on the plate. Or maybe we keep eating because the box is still open. Regardless of the circumstances, we've found ourselves eating something long after we stopped enjoying it.

Noticing diminishing returns is pretty simple—just check in with yourself and see if you're still enjoying what you're eating. If you're no longer enjoying it, stop.

Other times, we might find certain foods that feel like the flavor enjoyment could go on forever. That might be chocolate, or it might be pizza. Whatever it is for you, you have some foods where if you relied on flavor enjoyment, you'd eat way, way, way past full.

In those cases, we use the skill in the opposite way—we recognize fullness and flavor enjoyment are independent. This way, we aren't surprised that after three slices of pizza, a fourth sounds good. We can know (often ahead of time) that "just one more" will always sound good, even if that's going to leave us feeling gross and overfull later.

This can be a powerful distinction. For example, I know I'm always going to want "just one more chocolate chip cookie" because they're awesome. It's better to decide ahead of time that three cookies will be enough, and then stop after that. Even though the flavor enjoyment is still high, I know more will leave me feeling stuffed. More doesn't fit my values.

Sometimes even delicious balanced meals fall into this category. Many of my clients make really amazing food. These balanced meals with delicious vegetables, protein, carbohydrates, and fat can be similar; after one plate, it's still delicious and you want more. Of course you want more; you made it delicious!

You can work with this flavor and fullness discrepancy either by paying attention to fullness or by plating appropriate portions. Either way works. The trick is not to be surprised if you still want more of something that's super delicious.

Usually the "waiting before having seconds" and "doing something engaging after eating" guidelines work well for this. Whichever way the skill shows up, check in and notice how the flavor enjoyment is proceeding.

SKILL	NOTICE FLAVOR ENJOYMENT IS DIFFERENT FROM FULLNESS
WHY PRACTICE THIS SKILL	This is a simple and actionable way to start checking in with yourself to see if you're enjoying your food.

SKILL	NOTICE FLAVOR ENJOYMENT IS DIFFERENT FROM FULLNESS
WAYS TO GOLDILOCKS THIS SKILL	"I'm going to remember to check in with myself at about three-quarters of the way through the meal to see if I'm still enjoying it." "If I'm eating my favorite food, I'm going to keep in mind enjoyment and fullness are different things." "If I notice I'm not really enjoying what I'm eating, I'm going to stop eating and go do something else." "If it's super delicious but I've already had one plate, I'm going to wait 20 minutes and check in with fullness, before getting seconds."

FIVE-SENSES MINDFULNESS

One of the clearest accesses to mindfulness is "five senses" experiencing. With food, that's as simple as taking a second to:

1. Look at your food;

2. Taste your food;

3. Smell your food;

4. Listen to your food (think crunchy food);

5. Touch your food.

We have a ton of evidence that five-senses experiencing of your food makes you enjoy your food more, be more satisfied with your food, and be full longer. Recent research has shown that much of fullness is psychological. We know that if people pay attention to the sound crunchy food makes, they eat less and feel more full and satisfied.[148]

Similarly, a meta-analysis of 24 studies showed that if you can see your meal, you feel full and more satisfied during the meal. Even weirder, if you don't look at your food, you're also likely to eat more at *the next meal*.

When you think about it, it's actually pretty odd to be glued to the TV and not see your meal, but that's fairly normal, at least in American culture. Again, that leads not only to more food consumed at that meal, but also more late night snacking later.[149]

Consistent with that meta-analysis, another randomized controlled trial found that paying more attention to lunch increases your memory of eating it and decreases snacking in the afternoon.[150]

Research on mindful eating and serving size has found that attentional awareness reduced portion sizes of energy-dense food.[151]

You would think tasting the food would be a thing people do, but they really don't. Most people guzzle their food pretty quickly, often while watching a screen; they barely notice their food. For contrast, watch a cooking show on TV. Notice how the judges taste the food—they look at it; they smell it; they notice the texture (feel) of the food in the mouth, and they try to pick out all the flavors.

Picking out flavors is an actionable way to start noticing taste. See if you can pick out the seasonings.

Notice the difference between the taste of the sauce versus the taste of what the sauce covers. Taste the difference between the protein and the vegetables.

Five-senses mindfulness can have a huge impact on your feelings of fullness between meals. On top of that, everyone reports *enjoying their food more.*

SKILL	FIVE-SENSES EXPERIENCING
WHY PRACTICE THIS SKILL	Paying attention to some or all of your five senses while eating increases both food enjoyment and fullness.
WAYS TO GOLDILOCKS THIS SKILL	"During lunch, I'm going to stop every time I put my fork down and pay attention to how my food tastes." "During dinner, I'm going to stop twice and pay attention to how my food looks." "During dinner, I'm going to stop three times and notice how my dinner smells."

CHECK IN WITH YOUR STOMACH ONE HOUR AFTER EATING

This is the self-check for the *listen-to-your-body skills.*

Simply checking in with your stomach one hour after a meal lets you know how well you did with the other *listen-to-your-body skills.* If you nailed *noticing when full and stopping,* you should feel pretty good one hour after eating. If you undershot, you might be a little hungry. If you overshot, you might feel too full.

On the flip side, this skill can be a super helpful first skill if you're struggling with any of these *listen-to-your-body skills:*

- Checking in with your stomach mid-meal;
- Noticing flavor enjoyment is different from fullness;
- Noticing when full, and stopping if you are.

Many people have trouble at first with the skills "noticing flavor enjoyment is different from fullness," "checking in with your stomach mid-meal," or "noticing when full, and stopping if you are." They often say they always feel hungry during meals and when they stop eating. If that's the case, you can set those skills aside for now and just use this self-check one hour after eating to see if you ate too much or too little.

Simply use this skill—check in with your stomach one hour after eating—to adjust your plate guidelines.

I've had clients who reduced the total amount of food on their plates by a third and realized they were full and satisfied an hour later. They found they had gotten in the habit of eating more food than they needed.

It's actually a pretty weird experience to realize you've been eating more food than you need just because you got used to serving yourself or ordering a certain amount. It's extraordinarily cool to discover you can eat fewer calories without counting them, and without actually feeling starved between meals.

Note: The goal is to check in *with your stomach*. This isn't checking in to see if you'd like to eat something else, if you're bored, if you're stressed, or if you want a treat. You're checking in with your stomach to *see if you're hungry in your stomach*.

If you're having trouble distinguishing this, pair it with the "distinguish true hunger versus stress, boredom, tiredness, or emotions" skill. Here's a quick recap of the three questions in that skill:

1. *Do I feel a "hollow" feeling in my stomach or do I feel something else (tired, headache, bored, stressed)?*

2. *Am I hungry for a complete meal or a specific treat?*

3. *Does the hunger build over time, or build and then fade?*

If you feel legitimately hungry, eat a snack that's clearly healthy, like a banana and a dozen almonds to get you through to the next meal. If you aren't hungry, that's awesome! That means you did well plating your last meal, both in terms of quantity and balance.

SKILL	CHECK IN WITH YOUR STOMACH AFTER EATING
WHY PRACTICE THIS SKILL	This is the self-check for the other during-meal listen-to-your-body skills.
WAYS TO GOLDILOCKS THIS SKILL	"I'm going to check in with my stomach an hour after lunch to see if I guessed right." "I'm going to check in with my stomach an hour after lunch to see if I guessed right about fullness at breakfast." "I'm going to check in with my stomach an hour before dinner to see if I guessed right at lunch."

QUICK REVIEW: ALL THE SKILLS FIT INTO THESE FOUR BOXES

	DURING MEALS	BETWEEN MEALS
LISTEN TO YOUR BODY	Notice when getting full, and stop when you are	Distinguish true hunger versus cravings, boredom, tiredness, emotions, or thoughts
USE A GUIDELINE	Plate healthy and balanced portions	Eat a balanced meal every four to six hours, without snacking

GUIDELINES ARE NOT RULES

A guideline is a tool to streamline decision making. Guidelines are *not mandatory* and they are *not rules*.

People typically want to turn food skill guidelines into rules. Don't do that.

A guideline is there as a tool to make eating easier for you and to help make decisions easier. In general, if you're feeling like you have to choose between listening to your body and using a guideline, listen to your body.

The caveat is if you're stressed out, emotional, bored, or tired, it might be harder to listen to your body. It may be tough to distinguish what's going on in your head versus what's going on in your stomach. In those cases, using a guideline can be helpful. Those tend to also be the situations in which you have the least energy to make decisions or to distinguish between true hunger versus cravings, boredom, stress, and emotions.

MINDFUL DECISION-MAKING, MINDFUL EATING

If it helps in not turning guidelines into rules, you can just think of them as mindful decision-making. They can simply be a filter to help think your food decisions through, really fast.

The more mindfulness you put into making a food decision, the less you need a guideline. If you're willing to think things through, you can make all your food decisions simply by thinking through your values. I've had clients rock the mindful decision-making that way; it just takes more "thinking" work.

Guidelines are simply a way to streamline mindful decision-making.

On the flip side, skills aren't rules either. They're skills. They could be looked at as mindful eating or intuitive eating.

The research into mindful eating and mindful decision-making shows that these have an impact on both scale weight and wellbeing. Mindful eating may have a slight edge on wellbeing, while mindful decision-making may have a clear edge on weight loss.[152] It's believed the mindful decision-making edge on weight loss is because mindful eating can take up to a year of practice to really get good at, and most studies are shorter than that.

Intuitive eating (IE):

- The purpose of IE is to create a better relationship to food and to body image.

- IE is likely the opposite of disordered eating.[153]

- Half of the studies show IE creates weight loss, and half show it creates a stable weight maintenance, especially for people who are already at a healthy weight.[154]

- Research consistently shows IE increases psychological well-being, creates a better relationship to food, and better body image (see citations above).

Mindful decision making (MDM):

- The purpose of MDM is to create weight loss.

- Some studies use MDM to increase self-compassion.[155]

- Research consistently shows that MDM creates effective weight loss (see citations above).

- In the only two studies I could find that directly compared IE and MDM, MDM was more effective for weight loss.[156,157]

My experience with clients is that combining both—intuitive eating *and* mindful decision making—is more effective for weight loss than either one in isolation.

HOW TO USE COMBINATIONS OF SKILLS FOR MORE EFFECTIVE SKILL PRACTICE

We have 16 skills in four categories. You'll probably find it helps—at least in the beginning—to use a combination of internal and external focus skills for whatever you're working on.

You might work on snacking between meals:

Guideline
Eat three or four meals per day

Listen to your body
Distinguish hunger versus cravings, boredom, tiredness, emotions, or thoughts

Here you could use the external structure of eating three or four meals to notice when you had a craving for a specific food—not for a full meal—or if you were eating because of thoughts between meals even while knowing you ate enough at the last meal.

You might work on meal size:

Guideline
Eat every four to six hours

Listen to your body:
Notice and speculate about fullness
at halfway through the meal

In this case, you could use the external structure of four to six hours between meals to help you work on noticing and speculating about fullness halfway through the meal. In the middle of the meal, you'd guess if the amount of food you're eating is sufficient to get you to the next meal four to six hours away.

You could do double internal:

Guideline
Notice hunger for 30–60 minutes

Listen to your body
Stop before eating too much

Similar to the last idea, you can work on stopping before eating too much. As you're getting to the end of the meal, begin to speculate if you're in the range of being satisfied with the meal or if it will be too much and it's time to stop. Then, you can self-check with hunger. If you don't get hungry 30 minutes before the next meal, you know the previous meal was too much. If you get hungry hours before the next meal, you know the previous meal was too little.

You might work on meal size again:

Guideline
Eat a meal every four to six hours

Listen to your body
Make sure to eat enough

Eating a meal every four to six hours is a skill of not snacking between meals. Eat satisfying meals when you eat. When you aren't ready to eat a meal, don't eat anything. This cuts down boredom snacking, food cravings, emotional eating, and so on. Many people initially fail with that gap between meals simply because they're eating too little at meals. Usually, they've eaten bird-sized diet-rules meals, but the meals are not enough to get them to the next meal, so they invariably snack on candy or whatever is at hand.

WE'RE WORKING TOWARD TRUSTING YOUR BODY MORE

The goal is always to practice listening your body, and learn to trust it.

In the beginning, or in times of stress, you'll need to use more guidelines. A combination of trusting your body and using guidelines is usually ideal for most people.

If you're just starting to work on these skills, you may find you aren't sure when you're hungry or full. You may need to wait longer to feel it. In this case, you may not notice you're full *during* the meal, and may need to plate healthy portions, and then check back with your stomach in an hour or two. You can self-check, and notice if you feel you had the right amount of food, if you had too much, or if you had too little.

That between-meals self-check is a cool way to practice internal focus…*before you get good at it*.

That practice of checking in with your stomach will help you get better at noticing your hunger and fullness cues. Eventually, you'll be able to use them mid-meal. This could take a year!

Even when you're really good at noticing your internal cues, you may find in times of intense stress, tiredness, or emotions, it's much harder to notice them.

When that happens, default back to an external focus. You'll use internal focus most of the time and external focus once in a while when things are hard.

TROUBLESHOOTING THREE COMMON ISSUES

1. *Reverting to dieting, and failing*
   Essentially, this is about not using guidelines or skills.

2. *Practicing trusting your body skills, but not losing weight*
   You get somewhat in touch with your body, but don't yet have enough skill or have too much stress and tiredness and need to use guidelines.

3. *Using guidelines to lose weight, but not using skills*
   This runs the risk of turning into a pseudo-diet, and you'll miss the longevity and wellbeing benefits of listening to your body. This means it's time to start practicing the skills again. Use the guides to help with skill learning, but start to experiment with trusting your body sometimes instead of only using guidelines.

GUIDELINES VERSUS LISTEN TO YOUR BODY—EASY VERSUS HARD

Guidelines are much simpler to practice. It's easy to tell when you have your plate set up properly. It's easy to know when you have a snack between meals.

Trusting your body skills are harder. These are trial-and-error skills that can take months or sometimes even a couple years to master. Essentially, the more time you've spent ignoring hunger and fullness—both ignoring hunger trying to diet and then ignoring fullness on "cheat days"—the more practice you've had teaching yourself to ignore those internal cues. Give yourself time to relearn them.

The really cool thing is, both trusting your body and using guidelines for food can co-exist. In fact, they help each other.

It's easier to eat just enough if you've plated healthy portion sizes. You might end up only needing a little more or a little less, but it's easier to figure that out if you start pretty close.

Like unit bias, which we talked about in the plating skill section, we're more likely to feel like something is the right amount if it's what's on our plate. That means if we pay attention, eat slowly, and plate our meals appropriately, when we do feel hungry, there's a pretty good chance we actually are. It's a way to set ourselves up to win.

At the same time, if a person has snacked or grazed throughout life, it can be really hard to distinguish hunger versus boredom or stress between meals. Having a guideline like "Eat every four to six hours" can help a person think through the craving that shows up two hours after breakfast.

PROBLEMS WITH ONE OR THE OTHER

The *listen-to-your-body skills* and using guidelines really do work together. This is probably a stark contrast to what you may have heard elsewhere in the nutrition world.

Most people in the weight loss field only teach dieting, which sucks. The people who are better at this usually only teach guidelines. Their clients never actually get in touch with their own bodies. They spend their entire life feeling like their hunger and fullness is an adversary, like they have to fight their bodies every day to lose weight. Even with the best intentions, this pretty quickly devolves into diet rules and a perceived deprivation experience.

Then, most people who teach trusting the body or intuitive eating tend to bristle against the mention of guidelines. This is usually the extreme anti-diet crowd. I may lean this way philosophically, but I'm also a realist. Trusting your body takes a long time to learn. It's worth starting with a fair amount of external cues, and then relying on them less and less over time. Also, in times of intense stress, many people don't "hear" their internal cues. In that case, relying on external cues is super helpful.

It's really awesome to have those cues inform your guidelines as you're practicing trusting your body. For example, if you're practicing eating just enough, you can self-check by eating every four to six hours. If you eat a meal and stop when you think you might be full, you can then see if it was the right amount. If you get truly hungry in three hours—not a craving or stress eating—you know it was too little. If you're still full at six hours, you know it was too much.

In this way, you can use an external cue of four to six hours between meals to help you learn the internal cue of stopping when full.

MULTIPLE SKILLS AT ONCE IS USUALLY BETTER THAN ONE AT A TIME

We talked earlier about using two skills together, like a *listen-to-your-body skill* and a guideline, both focused on the same thing. Let's look at using three skills to triangulate:

1. **Guideline**: Eat every four to six hours, without snacking in between.

2. **Listen to your body**: Note hunger 30 minutes before eating.

3. **Listen to your body**: Make sure to eat enough *OR* stop before eating too much.

Here you're using a guideline like *four to six hours between meals* to nail down not snacking between meals. Then, you're using *make sure to eat enough* OR *stop before eating too much* to work on eating the right amount at meals.

Triangulation/self-check: Here is where it gets really cool: Noting hunger 30 minutes before eating triangulates the two skills—if you eat the right amount at the meals, you should get hungry 30 minutes before your next meal, and that's four to six hours later.

Another example of using three skills to triangulate:

1. **Guideline**: Eat every four to six hours, without snacking in between.

2. **Listen to your body**: Distinguish hunger versus cravings, boredom, tiredness, emotions, or thoughts.

3. **Listen to your body**: Note hunger 30 minutes before eating.

You're using a guideline like *three or four meals per day* to nail down not snacking between meals. Then, you're using *distinguish hunger from boredom, cravings, and stress* to handle not snacking between those meals.

Triangulation/self-check: *Noting hunger 30 minutes before eating* triangulates the two skills—if you notice the cravings and stress and boredom snacking between meals, you're also recognizing true hunger.

You can tell when you're actually hungry, and after being hungry for 30 minutes, you can eat an actual balanced and satisfying meal.

EATING WHILE ON VACATION

When eating on vacation, one of the skills that travels best is to put the fork down between bites. This is usually the only skill people should practice while they're on vacation. If you're in Italy, you should:

1. Eat all of the amazing food.

2. Eat slowly enough to enjoy all of it.

If you're on vacation, eat like you're wine tasting. Enjoy every bite. Find each flavor; pick out the different seasonings. Look at your food while you're eating it. Look at your surroundings. Smell the food. Listen to the sounds particular to the place where you are—be there.

Many clients have had "weight neutral" vacations simply by putting the fork down between bites. They enjoyed their food more and noticed when they got full… and stopped eating.

Some clients have mentioned that on previous vacations to places with amazing food, they found themselves eating too much at meals and feeling sluggish. The sluggishness actually had a negative impact on their sightseeing later in the day.

Put the fork down between bites (or the pizza, taco, gyro, or baguette), and enjoy your food. Then, stop when you're full. Go and have a great time sightseeing.

SOCIAL EATING

Again, *putting the fork down between bites* can be a simple and magical way to regulate food while being social. It doesn't matter the content of the food that shows up, you can always put the fork down between bites.

Plating healthy portions works well more often than people think. If you're at a bar-b-que, you can probably balance your plate without too much effort. You can get some protein (steak, hamburger, chicken, hot-dog, pulled pork), get some carbohydrates (a bun, or chips, or beans, or potato salad), and people usually have some sort of vegetables (a salad, coleslaw, or a veggie plate).

The same goes for other places people typically assume they can't eat a balanced meal, like an Italian restaurant. You could get protein (chicken parmesan), carbohydrates (*one portion* of spaghetti), and a salad. They may serve you five portions of spaghetti, but you eat just the one. Some clients even draw a line in the portions with their fork.

But the point is, you get to eat out—to do something social. You aren't restricted. Once in a while you can eat anywhere. There's nothing terrible about spaghetti—just have one portion of spaghetti instead of five. It's portions two to five that get people in trouble, not portion one.

PHASES OF MORE GUIDELINES AND PHASES OF MORE *LISTEN- TO-YOUR-BODY SKILLS*

Clients often note that when things have been going well for a while, it's easier to rely on the *listen-to-your-body skills.* The body falls into a rhythm, and the regularity of normal life makes it fairly simple to eat every four to six hours, stop when full, not snack between meals, and so on.

On the flip side, when people come back from a vacation where they ate more treats, had bigger meals, and drank more alcohol than normal, they might find themselves craving far bigger meals and craving snacks more often than normal. They keep checking in and feeling like they "really want it," but simultaneously, they know it's just because they've recently gotten in the habit of eating more.

This is when it's totally normal to shut off the *listen-to-your-body skill* practice for a week, focus on eating guidelines, and just get back to normal. Often, after a week of guidelines, you'll feel reset, and it will be much easier to go back to *listen-to-your-body skills.*

It's okay to intervene. It's okay to say, "It fit my values to eat more food on vacation in Italy. And now, it fits my values to eat less food," then implement some guidelines.

If I value reasonableness: "It was reasonable to eat all the great food in Italy. It isn't reasonable to continue eating like I'm in Italy now that I'm home. It's unbalanced."

Similarly, if we're practicing saying "yes" to treats sometimes and "no" to treats other times, some weeks we may have more and other weeks we might have less.

That's normal and fine. But, if you find you've had treats every day for a week, you might notice that doesn't fit your values. You could implement a guideline for a couple days to end that streak of treats every day. Once you've done a mini reset, you can go back to checking in and choosing.

Eating guidelines are awesome for any time that checking in and trusting your body has gotten harder, like when you've fallen into a habit of eating in a way that doesn't fit your values. Guidelines are good for pattern-smashing.

IS IT POSSIBLE MY *LISTEN TO MY BODY SKILLS* ARE OUT OF WHACK?

Of course it is!

Usually, this is caused by stress, boredom, or emotions, but sometimes it's just habit.

If you're relying mostly on *listen-to-your-body skills* and you aren't losing weight, it's probably time to practice more guidelines. I've had dozens of clients with seasonally stressful jobs who found their *listen-to-your-body skills* worked really well in the less stressful times, and worked really poorly in the more stressful times. In the more stressful times, they totally used guidelines instead.

Sometimes, we're just used to eating more. Many people find, that after a couple weeks of using guidelines, they're happy and satisfied with less food than they thought they needed. They'd literally just gotten in the habit of eating more. There isn't any big thing to coach—there isn't anything complicated. It's just a habit. That's okay—that happens too.

WRAPPING UP EATING SKILLS AND GUIDELINES

Just remember, in terms of eating skills, there are only four things you ever need to work on:

	DURING MEALS	BETWEEN MEALS
LISTEN TO YOUR BODY	Notice when getting full, and stop	Distinguish true hunger versus cravings, boredom, tiredness, emotions, or thoughts
USE A GUIDELINE	Plate healthy and balanced portions	Eat a balanced meal every four to six hours, without snacking in between

You can work on any of the sub-skills related to these four elements, but these are the only four big things.

Remember, eating skills—just like learning to play a clarinet—take practice. Whoever practices the most frequently will get better the fastest. In the coming chapters, we'll take a look at what Meta-skills and Turning Points will set you up to be the most successful in your food skill practice.

SAMPLE TWELVE-WEEK FOOD TRACKER

WEEK ONE	DAY:	M	T	W	TH	F	S	SU
	DATE:							
DURING MEALS	Plating: Increase protein							
BETWEEN MEALS	Eat a meal every four to six hours, without snacking in between							

WEEK TWO	DAY:	M	T	W	TH	F	S	SU
	DATE:							
DURING MEALS	Plating: Increase Vegetables							
BETWEEN MEALS	Distinguish hunger from stress, boredom tiredness, or emotions							
	Eat a meal every four to six hours, without snacking in between							
PLANNING	If: Then:							

WEEK THREE	DAY:	M	T	W	TH	F	S	SU
	DATE:							
DURING MEALS	Plate balanced meals							
BETWEEN MEALS	Eat a meal every four to six hours, without snacking in between							
	Distinguish hunger from stress, boredom tiredness, or emotions							
PLANNING	If: Then:							
TURNING POINT	Practice excellence and self-compassion							

WEEK FOUR	DAY:	M	T	W	TH	F	S	SU
	DATE:							
DURING MEALS	Plate balanced meals							
	Put the fork down between bites							
BETWEEN MEALS	Eat a meal every four to six hours, without snacking in between							
	Distinguish hunger from stress, boredom tiredness, or emotions							
PLANNING	If: Then:							
TURNING POINT	Practice excellence and self-compassion							
WISE FIVE	Values (list three)							

WEEK FIVE	DAY:	M	T	W	TH	F	S	SU
	DATE:							
DURING MEALS	Wait ten minutes before having seconds							
BETWEEN MEALS	Defusion from unwanted thoughts, uncomfortable feelings, or cravings							

WEEK SIX	DAY: DATE:	M	T	W	TH	F	S	SU
DURING MEALS	Plate healthy portion sizes							
	Wait ten minutes before having seconds							
BETWEEN MEALS	Eat a meal every four to six hours, without snacking in between							
	Wait ten minutes before having snacks or treats							
PLANNING	If: Then:							

WEEK SEVEN	DAY: DATE:	M	T	W	TH	F	S	SU
DURING MEALS	Put the fork down between bites							
	Wait ten minutes before having seconds							
BETWEEN MEALS	Defusion from unwanted thoughts, uncomfortable feelings, or cravings							
	Wait ten minutes before having snacks or treats							
PLANNING	If: Then:							
TURNING POINT	Engagement/flow/goldilocksing							

WEEK EIGHT	DAY:	M	T	W	TH	F	S	SU
	DATE:							
DURING MEALS	Plate balanced meals							
	Put the fork down between bites							
BETWEEN MEALS	Wait ten minutes before having snacks or treats							
	Distinguish hunger from stress, boredom tiredness, or emotions							
PLANNING	If: Then:							
TURNING POINT	Engagement/flow/goldilocksing							
WISE FIVE	Values (list three)							

WEEK NINE	DAY:	M	T	W	TH	F	S	SU
	DATE:							
DURING MEALS	Notice when getting full, and stop							
	Five senses mindfulness during eating							
BETWEEN MEALS	Distinguish hunger from stress, boredom tiredness, or emotions							
	Deliberate self-care instead of snacking							

WEEK TEN	DAY:	M	T	W	TH	F	S	SU
	DATE:							
DURING MEALS	Plate healthy portion sizes							
	Five senses mindfulness during eating							
BETWEEN MEALS	Distinguish hunger from stress, boredom tiredness, or emotions							
	Defusion from unwanted thoughts, uncomfortable feelings, or cravings							
PLANNING	If: Then:							

WEEK ELEVEN	DAY:	M	T	W	TH	F	S	SU
	DATE:							
DURING MEALS	Notice when getting full, and stop							
	Five senses mindfulness during eating							
BETWEEN MEALS	Eat a meal every four to six hours, without snacking in between							
	Deliberate self-care instead of snacking							
PLANNING	If: Then:							
TURNING POINT	Weight loss comes from self-care							

WEEK TWELVE	DAY: DATE:	M	T	W	TH	F	S	SU
DURING MEALS	Plate balanced meals							
	Notice when getting full, and stop							
BETWEEN MEALS	Distinguish hunger from stress, boredom tiredness, or emotions							
	Defusion from unwanted thoughts, uncomfortable feelings, or cravings							
PLANNING	If: Then:							
TURNING POINT	Weight loss comes from self-care							
WISE FIVE	Values (list three)							

This sample 12 weeks has a fair amount of variety in the skills presented. You'll rotate through most of them. If you find this to be too much variety or it moves too quickly—as many people do—you can simply repeat the sample skills tracker in first chapter, *Your First Month*, page 29. I've had dozens of clients get awesome results just repeating the work on those four skills for months. For some clients, those were the only four skills they ever needed to practice.

You may notice this program is designed such that the first week you only focus on skill practice. The second week you have skill practice, plus If/Then planning. The third week, you include a turning point. The last week you include skills, If/Then planning, a turning point, and values reflection.

This is designed to keep refocusing on the simplest and most important thing: the skill practice. At the same time, you get to practice the higher order work for part of each month. It's okay if during the first month managing all of it feels like too much; the next month you'll start again with just skills. You'll cycle through the whole system, from the most basic to the most advanced every month.

You can find blank skill trackers at the back of the book beginning on page 251. After 12 weeks, you should be familiar with the system and your individual needs, and you can fill in the four skills and guidelines that make the biggest difference for you.

In Appendix 1, you'll find a longer skills program and skills programs designed to meet specific needs.

CHAPTER FOUR
WORKOUT SKILLS

WHAT IS GETTING STRONG? HOW DOES IT WORK?

Workouts are good for five things:

1. Making you lean;

2. Making you strong;

3. Reducing stress;

4. Increasing self-efficacy;

5. Being one component of changing your relationship to your body.

One thing workouts *are not* great for:

1. Weight loss.

Whatever your scale weight, the volume of strength training work you do plus your protein intake is the biggest determinate of leanness (read: ratio of muscle to fat).

Scale weight, on the other hand, is almost all about food skill practice.

Strength is a super cool adaptation to strength training. The body does this amazing thing called "supercompensation." Supercompensation means that when you repeatedly put your body under the same stress (like deadlifting every week for a month), your body *super*compensates—it makes you stronger than the stress you put it under. It doesn't

just adapt to the workout stress you gave it, it actually adapts extra to prepare you to do more.

We're going to use a few different principles to get you as strong as possible:

1. Mostly big movements: push, pull, squat, and hip hinge;

2. Mobility work and corrective exercise is done as "active rest" between strength exercises;

3. Pay attention to how each movement feels;

4. Treat workouts like skill practice;

5. We use short, medium, and long-term workout planning.

WORKOUT PROGRAM PLANNING (PERIODIZATION)

1. Monthly strength program planning: cycling through weeks of doing the right amount, doing a little too much, and then recovering and doing too little;

2. Quarterly strength planning: cycling through different adaptations of strength, leanness, and endurance;

3. Multi-year strength planning: average monthly volume of work increases over the first three years; third-year programs have almost twice as many total sets as first-year programs.

We're going to focus mostly on big, full-body movements in the following programs. I'm not against smaller isolation movements for bodybuilding purposes, but they won't show up much in this program. If you want to add some curls or triceps press-downs at the end of your workouts, that's totally fine, but the meat of this program is pushing, pulling, hip hinging, and squatting.

This is mostly a time thing. While we're going to have multiple *Lean and Strong* programs with different workloads, they're all three-day-per-week programs. If you want to do more of a bodybuilding split and strength train five or six days per week, that's awesome (and I've had some clients who have done that), but it isn't this book.

The majority of my clients have gotten great strength results lifting three days per week. Some of my clients have added or mixed in conditioning workouts, and that will be discussed on page 151. Suffice to say, the meat-and-potatoes of the program is three days of strength training.

HOW WORKING OUT MAKES YOU LEAN

Leanness is the ratio of muscle to fat at a given scale weight. More muscle means more leanness. Less fat means more leanness. When people say they want to get "toned," what they mean is "lean." And getting leaner is simply a matter of gaining muscle and losing fat.

Remember: Scale weight is always just calories. The amount of working out required to hit a weight loss goal without changing what you eat requires more time than most people have. Sure, when I was in Brazil training in Brazilian jiu-jitsu 35 hours per week, everyone there lost weight. Most people don't have that kind of time, so we handle scale weight with eating skills.

From a workout standpoint, leanness is about gaining muscle. There are two different things we need to look at for that:

1. Amount of weight lifted;
2. Total volume of work.

The amount of weight lifted is pretty simple. All things being equal, the person lifting more weight will be leaner than the person lifting less weight. Over months and years, the weight you lift should be going up.

Now, I'm sure I'm going to get email from folks who've been lifting 20, 30, 40 years who are going to tell me about the upper limits of lifting more weight. This is legit; there's absolutely a reasonable upper limit on the weights going up. At some point, we get to "enough." But, the majority of people reading this aren't at their upper limit of strength.

Total volume of work is usually calculated as *total sets per week x total reps per set*. It's actually simpler and more useful to forget the reps and just track how many hard workout sets you do in a week.

Let's take an example of a woman I worked with:

*Squat three sets of 20 repetitions
with a 35-pound kettlebell*

*Squat three sets of 3 repetitions
with a 155-pound barbell*

Both of those workouts included three sets of squats. For her, both workouts were appropriately hard. They're very different workouts, but if we just look at "three hard sets," it makes it easier to think about the volume of a workout.

WHY POWERLIFTING ISN'T REQUIRED FOR BEING STRONG

In this day and age, it's a little weird to have a book about getting strong that doesn't focus on the three powerlifts: bench press, deadlift, and back squat, or even Olympic weightlifting—the clean and jerk and the snatch.

But wait, should a book on being strong be filled with gymnastics movements? Should it be gymnastic ring work? Or handstand pushups? Working toward a planche?

Should it be strongman workouts? Heck, strongman even has "strong" in the name.

We start to see there are a lot of different ways in which to express strength. Right now, there are a million strength gurus all telling you the "right way" to be strong. Not surprisingly, each swears their favorite way to work on strength is the best.

Lean and Strong is for regular folks to get strong in basic movement patterns. It isn't about gymnastics or powerlifting or any other specialized strength sports. Those are all awesome, but they don't have a lot to do with what most people want. If you're looking for general strength and leanness, *Lean and Strong* is a program tailored toward your goals.

I'm going to tell you a secret about strength training programs: If you do them, you should get stronger at *what you're doing.*

- If someone is getting stronger at barbell back squats, that's cool.

- If someone is getting stronger at kettlebell front squats, that's cool.

- If someone is getting stronger at rear-foot-elevated split-squats, that's cool too.

Those are all legitimate strength movements.

Strength is about getting stronger in the movements you want to do. I think powerlifting is really cool and if you want to compete in powerlifting, you should do a program designed for that. *Unapologetically Powerful* by Jen Sinkler and Jennifer Vogelgesang Blake is awesome. If you just want to be strong in your life, *Lean and Strong* will be perfect.

WORKOUT GUIDELINES AND SKILLS

Workouts also have guidelines and skills. Workout guidelines have to do with weight selection and exercise selection. Workout skills have to do with mindfulness and focus during movement.

WORKOUT GUIDELINES	WORKOUT SKILLS
Exercise selection Weight selection	Internal focus during movement External focus during movement Specific form cues Tension skill Relaxation skill

WORKOUT GUIDELINES

Guideline: Exercise Selection, The Strength Moves We're Going to Use

The moves fall into five main categories:

PUSH

PULL

SQUAT

HIP HINGE

CORE

Using these movements is the most efficient way to get strong at the basics of human movement.

THE BIG "X" OF BALANCING WORKOUTS	
UPPER BODY PUSH	UPPER BODY PULL
LOWER BODY SQUAT	LOWER BODY HIP HINGE

It works out to be pretty close to a front-to-back "X"—balancing your pushing movements with pulls and balancing your squatting movements with deadlifts.

Then, for supersets we combine a front upper-body movement (push) with a back lower-body movement (deadlift) or a back upper-body movement (pull) with a front lower-body movement (squat). It also has the benefit of putting movements that fatigue your grip—like pullups and deadlifts—in different supersets.

Example superset combinations:

- Pushups and barbell deadlifts

- Dumbbell bent-over rows and lunges

- Dumbbell bench presses and kettlebell swings

- Pullups and double-kettlebell front squats

- Dumbbell incline bench presses and staggered-stance deadlifts

- Cable rows and goblet squats

VARIATIONS VERSUS PROGRESSIONS

In *Fat Loss Happens on Monday*, we grouped these categories of movements into progressions—as in, you'd progress from one to the next. For some movements, especially bodyweight exercises, progression is the way to make a movement harder. Going from a pushup to a one-arm pushup is a huge progression, with lots of steps in between.

In *Lean and Strong,* all of the categories are variations. There isn't a start or an end; they're just variations on the same patterns. There's really cool research on how humans learn, showing that multiple variations of the same principles leads to better learning than hammering the same variation all the time.[158] There are limits to this, which is why we aren't doing random movements. That being said, we're going to repeatedly vary the same basic patterns.

Two-leg Hip Hinge

- Romanian Deadlift
- Standard Deadlift
- Trap Bar Deadlift
- Split-stance Deadlift
- Cossack Deadlift
- Single-leg Deadlift
- One-arm Kettlebell Swing
- Dumbbell Single-leg Hip Bridge on Bench

Horizontal Push

- Double-Dumbbell Bench Press
- Single-kettlebell Floor Press
- Pushup

Vertical Push

- 45° Incline Double-Dumbbell Bench Press
- 75° Incline Single-Dumbbell Bench Press
- Single Kettlebell Military Press

Horizontal Pull

- Single-cable Split-stance Row
- Double-cable Row
- Bent-over Row

Vertical Pull

- Assisted Chin-up
- Chin-up
- Single-arm Lat Pulldown

Squat

- Double-kettlebell Squat
- Barbell Squat
- Walking Lunge
- Split Squats
- Rear-foot-elevated Split Squats

Core

- Band Dead Bug
- Kettlebell Dead Bug
- Ball Body Saw
- Pallof Press
- Horizontal Cable Rotation
- Low to High Cable Rotations
- High to Low Cable Rotation

You may notice that's significantly more variation than we used in *Fat Loss Happens on Monday. Fat Loss Happens on Monday* was a deliberately minimalist program. This program has an optimal amount of variation. For my clients who have access to a gym, this is the preferable program, and that's true for you too.

Research into motor learning shows that if people can learn multiple variations of a skill, they more robustly learn that skill.[159] For example—a person who learns how the hinge in a Romanian deadlift, the hinge in a staggered-stance deadlift, and the hinge in a kettlebell swing are all the same hinge really gets the feeling for "hinge."

That's a person to whom I could then expose other hinge variations, and who would pick them up very quickly.

The trick is to practice a version of the movement for a specified period of time—like a month—and then move on.

We're doing variety according to a plan. Randomness isn't the goal. We'll work with a couple variations on each movement for a month, and then change.

BARBELLS VERSUS DUMBBELLS VERSUS KETTLEBELLS—WHICH IS BETTER?

The short answer is whichever you have access to and whichever feels best for your body.

Here are different ways of looking at this:

Barbells

Pros: Barbells are the easiest to load, and we can typically do the most work with a barbell.

Cons: Not every move feels awesome with a barbell for everyone. Not everyone has access to barbells at their gym or at busy times at their gym.

Dumbbells

Pros: Dumbbells are probably available at every gym—can be used for almost every move in the book.

Cons: You'll never be able to use as much load with a dumbbell as with a barbell.

Cables

Pros: Cables are probably found at every gym and can be used for almost every move in the book. These are like dumbbells you can point in any direction.

Cons: You'll never be able to use as much load with a cable as with a barbell.

Suspension Trainer

Pros: A suspension trainer is good for home use, and can be used for most things that cables are used for with some creativity.

Cons: Some cable moves are easier to load with a cable or a band than a suspension trainer.

Bands

Pros: Bands are good for home use, and can be used for most things that cables are used for if you buy heavy enough bands.

Cons: Some core moves are easier to load with a band than cables or a suspension trainer. Most people don't buy heavy enough bands to do any real work.

Kettlebells

Pros: These can be used for almost every move in the book, although they're the only implements you can do kettlebell swings with. They're really solid for holding front squats.

Cons: You'll never be able to use as much load with a kettlebell as with a barbell.

The implement you use doesn't matter a whole lot. While I've listed specific implements with each exercise in the book, they're almost interchangeable. The only exception is swings since you need a kettlebell for those.

But if you're doing Romanian deadlifts with a barbell, two dumbbells, or two kettlebells, it doesn't matter. It changes the movement in an odd way, but you could even do Romanian deadlifts with two cables in a pinch.

Don't get too hung up on the tools; use whatever you have access to.

The workouts in this book are written to be done in a gym, but you could do every workout with kettlebells, bands, and a TRX, if that's the route you want to go.

NORMAL STANCE VERSUS SPLIT-STANCE VERSUS SINGLE-LEG—WHICH IS BETTER?

Do whichever stance feels best today.

We're going to do our best to work through all of them. There's a lot of benefit to this "same but different" variety. Again, we aren't doing random movements; we're working through different variations of the same movements.

Looking at hip hinges:

Normal-stance Romanian Deadlift—You can use a fair amount of weight on this deadlift with both legs under you splitting the workload.

Staggered-stance Deadlift—You really get to put a lot of the work onto one leg, while also using the other leg to help with balance.

Single-leg Deadlift—Here, all of the work is on one leg, but we sacrifice the amount of load we could use because of the balance challenge.

A CASE FOR SPLIT-STANCE AND SINGLE-LEG STRENGTH

The best case for split-stance and single-leg strength work is it works for just about everyone. I've had plenty of clients who at first couldn't do a barbell back squat without pain, but could do painless split-squats or step-downs. Similarly, I've never had a client who couldn't do staggered-stance deadlifts. These feel good for everyone.

Mike Boyle has made the case that past a certain age, most people are better off switching to rear-foot-elevated split-squats than barbell back squats. His basic argument is that there's a lower chance of injury with single-leg movements, and balance becomes a more important attribute as we age. It makes sense.

Ultimately, I want everyone to have the mobility to do whatever they want, and we will work toward that. In the meantime, staggered-stance and split-stance moves are solid choices for getting stronger. And people can get really, really strong in those moves. Of course, if barbell moves feel good, do them. They're awesome.

If they don't feel good in your body, either because you haven't done enough mobility work (yet) or because you've got a high-mileage body that they bug sometimes, it's okay to do something else.

Similarly, even if they feel great most of the time, if you have a night when you slept funny and they don't feel good that day, it's okay to switch to a split-stance or staggered-stance version for a day.

MOBILITY WORK

Mobility work plays three parts:

1. Most people need some mobility work.

2. It's active rest between sets of strength work.

3. It sets you up to move better in your workout, and creates an upward spiral of better movement.

We're going to do the most basic mobility work between sets—the stuff that seems to make a difference for everyone and that everyone needs. If you sit at a desk all day, it's good to be able to move into opposite positions to open up everything that's closed all day.

The cool thing about doing mobility work immediately paired with strength training is we can create mobility at a joint and then immediately load that movement and practice better movement with that new mobility. It could be argued that the loaded practice of the better movement has a bigger impact on being able to hold onto mobility than the mobility work itself.

Here is an example of what it might look like:

1. Deadlift
2. Pushup
3. *Hip flexor stretch*

The hip flexor stretch is mobility work that opens up the hip joint to be able to do a better deadlift.

By cycling through these three exercises, you do the mobility work so the move is better, and then you do the move to solidify that new mobility. The mobility work will be in italics in the tables throughout the book.

Mobility work also acts as a brake—it forces people to rest enough between strength sets and not turn every workout into a circuit.

MOBILITY WORK

- Quad T-spine Rotations

- Hip Flexor Stretch with Rotation

- Rear-foot-elevated Hip Flexor Stretch

- 360° Breathing

- Band Clamshells

- Bretzel

- Band/Wall Hamstring Stretch

PUSHUP VARIATIONS

This book isn't going to give you a catalog of pushup variations. The basics go like this:

- If you want an easier pushup variation, elevate your hands.

- If you want a harder pushup variation, elevate your feet.

If you're advanced, you could just keep elevating your feet until you're doing handstand pushups. And, handstand pushups are awesome.

That being said, if you're looking for more variety, that's totally fine. Any pushup variation you like that fits the rep range of the workout is fine. If you want to do suspension trainer pushups, spiderman pushups, archer pushups, pike pushups, one-arm pushups, or pushups with a band or weighted vest…all of those options are good. If you want a bigger variety of pushup variations, see my first book, *Fat Loss Happens on Monday*.

For most people, simply elevating your hands to make it easier is a good option. I like to use the Smith machine. And, at least for intermediate folks, elevating the feet will be enough to sufficiently challenge you. If you're advanced, I assume you already have some favorite variations.

WHY NO BARBELL HIP THRUSTS?

As of this writing, barbell hip thrusts are the new trendy movement. I think they're cool too, and you could totally substitute them into this program.

However, in many gyms, they're a pain to set up. I have clients who work out in gyms with great setups, and they do them all the time. Most of my clients, though, just do single-leg and high-rep dumbbell versions instead, which seems to work just as well.

Barbell hip thrusts are basically a glute bodybuilding movement and work well at high reps. I've never seen any need for the average client who wants to get lean and strong to do low-rep barbell hip thrusts. We still have plenty of low-rep deadlifts in the program, so that end of the spectrum is covered. High-rep single-leg, staggered-stance, and dumbbell hip bridges definitely do the trick of teaching people how to drive from their glutes, work the opposite end of the strength curve from deadlifts, and seem to make people better at all things lower body. I think they're rad. They're also portable and easy to set up.

Part of these decisions is just preference and style. If you like barbell hip thrusts and have a good setup to do them at your gym, you can totally substitute them for any of the glute bridges in this program.

GYM LOGISTICS AND PAIRING MOVEMENTS

When possible, I try to pair moves with equipment that's hard to move around, like assisted pullups, with moves that are easy to move around, like kettlebell front squats.

Some of my favorite pairs:

- Assisted Pullups, either band or machine (hard to move around)

- Kettlebell Front Squats

- Barbell Deadlifts (hard to move around)

- Pushups

- Dumbbell Bench Press (hard to move around)

- Staggered-stance Deadlifts

- Cable Rows (hard to move around)

- Walking Lunges

- Barbell Squats (hard to move around)

- Dumbbell Bent-over Rows

Whenever possible, try to put things together in a way that will work at the gym where you work out. It doesn't make sense to pair assisted pullups with deadlifts if the barbells and plates are on one side of the gym and the assisted pull-up machine is on the other side. Instead, deadlifts are almost always paired with pushups, which can be done anywhere.

I'll often put single-kettlebell floor presses in a program for a multitude of reasons. Folks with sensitive shoulders often find that floor presses feel great. Beginners gain control by learning to just barely touch their elbows on the ground each rep. Advanced trainees often like how safe a single-kettlebell floor press is for both setting up and finishing with a heavy kettlebell; you can use two

hands and a body roll to get in and out of position, just like you would for a Turkish getup.

In this program, floor presses are mostly used for logistical concerns: You can do a floor press anywhere, like next to the barbell you're deadlifting with or next to a cable machine you're using. If you're in a situation where you can and would prefer to use a bench instead of the floor for presses, you can switch those. For many people, though, the floor presses will work really well because they're easy to move around.

The workouts are set up in a way that should work for most people at most gyms. That being said, if your gym is set up in such a way that it makes sense to do the movements in that workout in a different order, feel free to change the order so it works for you.

GUIDELINE: WEIGHT SELECTION

The Two Mistakes

People usually make one of two mistakes:

1. They always push the weight higher, even at the expense of form.

2. They never push the weight higher.

How Much Weight to Lift Explained in 100 Email Messages

After *Fat Loss Happens on Monday* came out, I started getting email messages about the workouts. In fact, I still get messages every week that fall into one of two camps:

1. These workouts are brutal!

2. These workouts are way too easy!

"These workouts are brutal! I passed out in my car for the whole rest of the night afterward." I responded, "Tell me about the workouts; what weights are you lifting… how does it feel?"

The response: "I'm on the 3x12 phase. I used two 70-pound kettlebells for the squats, and did the pullups with a 60-pound weight vest. I did one-arm pushups for my pushup variation, and then two 53-pound kettlebells for the single-leg deadlifts. Then I passed out in my car for two hours."

Digging further, I usually find out the person is really strong and has been lifting heavy for low reps for the last few years. I'm all about going heavy, so that's cool. That being said, if passing out in your car for two hours is cutting into your family time, you might want to adjust the weights. It's probably cool to get in a good workout *and* be able to hang out with the fam.

On the other hand, I get messages like this:

"I'm on the 3x12 phase. I did the whole workout in ten minutes and it was super easy. I don't get why you're wasting my time." I responded back, "Tell me about the workouts; what weights are you lifting…how does it feel?"

The response: "I used two five-pound weights for the squats. For the assisted pullups, I assisted 95% of my body-weight. For the pushup variation, I did knee pushups, and I used two five-pound weights for the single-leg deadlifts."

The response: "I used two five-pound weights for the squats. For the assisted pullups, I assisted 95% of my body-weight. For the pushup variation, I did knee pushups, and I used two five-pound weights for the single-leg deadlifts."

Digging deeper still, I discover this person is used to doing cardio strength classes doing 30 to 40 sets of 20 reps, all with five-pound weights. If you're going to do 800 reps per workout, that makes sense.

But if you're doing a total of 36 reps (3x12), increase the weight. If you don't *have to* rest a minute between each group of exercises, it's way too light. Increase the weight.

The people who were emailing me saying it was "way too hard" were always strong people who hadn't lifted above five reps per set, in anything, for years. They were trying to use the same weights for 12- or even 20-rep sets, and getting crushed. My suggestion to them is, "Try using less weight." After two or three responses, we'd settle on the appropriate weights for each rep range.

The people who were saying it was "way too easy" were the opposite—they had never gone up in weight. They were used to doing group exercise classes with eight-pound dumbbells, for literally hundreds of reps per workout.

When they went to a lower volume, fewer sets and reps program, it didn't occur to them to use a heavier weight. The correspondence back and forth with them, sometimes six messages in a row, would be, "Try using more weight." Then again later, "Try using more weight." Often after bumping up the weights five or six times, they'd find they got a great workout.

Both ends of the spectrum surprised me. It never came up in in-person training because if something looked right form-wise and didn't look challenging, I'd always ask, "How do you feel about increasing the weight?" and if form started coming apart, I'd ask, "How about we drop the weight a little and clean up your form?"

Usually, we'll have a series of email exchanges adjusting the weight until everyone ends up with the right amount of weight for them for that workout…for that phase. For some people, it will be less weight; for others, it will be more.

For anyone who's reading this and rolling their eyes, I wouldn't have thought I'd have to explain it, but I've now received hundreds of messages like this.

A similar email I get often goes like this: "The lunges are really hard, but the bent-over rows are super easy."

We want to get as close as possible to equalizing the difficulty across exercises. With some exercises, you may need to increase the weight…others you may need to decrease the weight. You should be able to get them all pretty close to even.

REP RANGES
AND WHEN TO INCREASE OR DECREASE

This book doesn't list actual rep ranges, but you can assume that every set and rep scheme listed can be treated as "plus or minus two reps, ish." If you can't do within two reps fewer than the suggested rep range, you should probably drop the weight. If you can do more than two reps more, increase the weight.

If you're ever doing one of these workouts and thinking, "This is way too easy," try doing as many of that move as possible with the weight you're using. If you get five or eight more reps than the rep range, that's a good indicator to move up in weight. If you get 10 or 20 more reps than the rep range, that's a good indicator you should have moved up the weight years ago.

For example:

If the rep range is 12, and you get to 17 reps, you should move up in weight.

CYCLES OF INCREASING WEIGHT
AND CLEANING UP FORM

I'm not going to give a structure for this because this cycle can exist independently of the rest of the cycles in the program. And there are already plenty of cycles in the program.

You want to go through cycles of:

- Pushing to increase the weight and/or reps lifted;

- Digging deep on form and cleaning up your movement.

WORKOUT SKILLS

WORKOUT SKILLS
Internal focus during movement
External focus during movement
Specific form cues
Tension skill
Relaxation skill

At its most basic, *internal focus* is focusing on the feeling in the muscle during a movement. Which muscles are doing the work? It could also be noticing if you feel the movement in your muscles or your joints. Lastly, it could be where you feel the weight balanced below your feet (like in a squat) or if you feel a balanced amount of weight in both hands (like in a bench press).

External focus is about moving something external such as a kettlebell toward or away from something else. In a deadlift, that could be "pushing the ground away." In a military press, that could be "pushing the kettlebell toward the ceiling." External focus is moving a weight toward or away from something.

Specific form cues are what we typically think of with workout skills—discovering if things are lined up right… if we're in the right position.

Tension skills are about generating more tension. With heavy low-rep work, more tension in the right places creates more strength and more safety.

Relaxation skills are about being able to relax the right things in the right amount. In endurance-based workouts, relaxation is a big part of getting to higher repetitions. Even in low-rep strength work, you probably want to relax your jaw and neck. Power, speed, and gracefulness all involve the right amount of relaxation at the right time.

Workout skills are all about awareness. Internal and external focus are the first two kinds of awareness we'll cover.

INTERNAL FOCUS	EXTERNAL FOCUS
Where do I feel this working?	What am I moving the weight toward or away from?

For example, on a deadlift, you could ask yourself:

Internal

Do I feel that in my butt and hamstrings?

Or do I feel it in my low back?

External

Did I focus on pushing the ground away?

In this example, internal focus is often a good way to check in and see if things are going well. If you feel the deadlift in your low back instead of your butt and hamstrings, you know something is wrong.

External focus could then be used to fix the issue: Instead of thinking about pulling the weight up (which often causes people to use the low back), you're going to focus on pushing the ground away (which usually fixes that).

You may even use a combination of the two: Focus on flexing your butt really hard (internal) and focus on pushing the ground away (external).

These questions are the most basic, but for fun, you could ask yourself different questions at different times.

External focus has been found to be most effective for movement efficiency, gaining strength, and for movement learning.[160] On the flip side, internal focus has been found to be most effective for muscle growth.[161] Someone who most wants to get stronger would more often use external focus; someone wanting to get lean would most often use internal focus, and someone who wants to be lean *and* strong would use both at different times.

MINDFULNESS IS NOT A "100% OF THE TIME" THING

I don't expect you to become a workout monk, with every rep of every workout being 100% present and mindful. That isn't realistic or necessary.

It's normal to have some workouts where you just clock in, do the moves, and leave. Sometimes, just making it in to the gym is a win.

Also, it's normal to have your attention and mindfulness vary throughout your practice. If you can be mindful of a few reps in each set or one set of each exercise, it will make a difference. Pick a set or two each workout and really focus. Or, pick a few reps—like the last few reps of each set—and really be there.

You may notice other things—like how heavy low-rep sets require more mindfulness than high-rep sets. In heavy, low-rep sets, your ability to be mindful has a direct impact on how much weight you can lift. Similarly, in heavy low-rep sets, that mindfulness is required to lift the weights safely. That's another reason heavy low-rep sets can be more draining—they require more attentional focus.

The awareness you bring to some parts of your workouts some of the time will pay big dividends in all your workouts.

In terms of your connection with your body, the mindfulness you bring to your workouts is everything. We'll dig in on this more later in the book.

20 QUESTIONS FOR INTERNAL AND EXTERNAL MINDFUL MOVEMENT

INTERNAL MINDFULNESS	EXTERNAL MINDFULNESS
Is this easy, medium, or hard?	What are you focused on moving?
Is this hard in an endurance way or a strength way?	Where is the target—what are you moving it toward?
Where did you feel that working?	Does the movement feel smooth or jerky?
How do your joints feel?	What one form detail are you focused on this set?
How do your muscles feel?	How did the exercise look when you videoed it with your phone?
Do you feel too tight? (in high-rep phases)	
Too loose? (low-rep phases)	
Just right?	
How loose and efficient can you be? (high rep)	
How tight and solid can you be? (low rep)	
How's your posture in this movement?	
Do your face, jaw, and neck feel relaxed?	
Does this exercise feel safe?	
Does this exercise feel strong?	
How was your breathing in that exercise?	

If you really want to dig in and develop your body awareness over a lifetime, asking yourself a few of those questions each workout can have a huge impact.

The basics of mindfulness in exercise are:

- When you notice your mind wandering, bring it back to how you feel in your body (high-rep sets), or;
- When you notice your mind wandering, bring it back to a specific cue or intention for the set you're focusing on (low-rep sets).

In high-rep sets, it can be really effective to bring your attention back internally to how it feels in a certain muscle group. For low-rep sets, it will bring your attention back externally, like how you're pushing the dumbbell toward the ceiling. Of course, this isn't rigid—you could bring your attention back to either internal or external awareness with either high- or low-rep exercises. This is just a useful and intuitive place to start.

It's normal for your mind to wander. Mindfulness in this case is simply bringing it back to something you feel in your body or the target—the direction or a literal target— you have for the weight you're moving.

The mindfulness you bring to your workouts will dramatically change your execution of each exercise. It will bring a depth to your practice that will make your workouts more fun, more challenging, and more engaging. It will reduce injury and make you stronger.

EXERCISE FORM-SPECIFIC MINDFULNESS

EXERCISE	INTERNAL	EXTERNAL
DEADLIFT	Is your back neutral or slightly arched? Can you feel it in your butt?	Are your back pockets moving toward the back wall? Are your feet pushing the floor away?
PUSHUP	Do you feel it working in your chest and back of your arms? Do you feel your weight equally in both hands?	Are you pushing the ground away?
SQUAT	Do you feel this in your quads? Do you feel the weight equally in both feet?	Are you pushing the ground away?
SPLIT SQUAT	Do you feel most of your weight in the front foot?	Are you pushing the ground away?

EXERCISE FORM-SPECIFIC MINDFULNESS		
EXERCISE	**INTERNAL**	**EXTERNAL**
STAGGERED-STANCE DEADLIFT	Do you feel like your butt is doing most of the work? Do you feel most of the weight in your front foot?	Are your back pockets moving toward the back wall? Are your feet pushing the floor away?
CABLE ROW	Do you feel this in your lats?	Are you pulling your shirt sleeve back and down at the top of each rep?
PLANK	Is your back neutral or slightly rounded? Do you feel like you're doing a static crunch?	Are you pushing the ground away? Are you getting taller from your ponytail?
PULL-UP	Do you feel this in your lats?	Are you pulling the bar to your shirt?
DUMBBELL BENCH PRESS	Do you feel this in your chest and triceps?	Are you pressing the dumbbells up to the ceiling?
CABLE ROTATION	Are you bracing your butt and abs?	Are you turning your belt buckle to the wall in front of you? Are you turning your back shoe around?

GOING DEEP IN FORM AS A LIFETIME PRACTICE

More people need to think about lifting like martial arts. It's normal to start out at a white belt in a martial art and spend a decade or two working up to a black belt. Then they spend the rest of their lives deepening their skills as a black belt.

Everyone starts lifting as a white belt; over years, you should spend time deepening your skill practice of each movement. Go deep into how it feels, the cues that help you lift the most weight, and dialing in your form.

The most engaging part of strength training is the skill practice. Deep skill practice over years is the part that can have the biggest impact on the way we know our bodies and in our relationships to our bodies.

Over the years, these increases in form should come with increases in strength. But the longer you go, the more skill refinement may be required for incremental increases in strength.

If we live long enough, we'll even see our strength decline. But the skill practice can still be worthwhile and engaging while we maintain as much strength as possible.

TENSION AS A SKILL VERSUS RELAXATION AS A SKILL

Adding the appropriate amount of tension can be the most important skill for safely lifting heavy weights. Tension also significantly increases strength.

Essentially, we're practicing deliberately tightening ourselves up. It usually looks like:

- Flexing your butt;

- Bracing your abs;

- Squeezing the bar;

- Gripping the ground with your feet.

During low-rep workouts, usually in the three- to five-rep range, you to want to get really tight. You're going to practice adding tension *before* the first rep.

In a dumbbell bench press, you could pop the weight up over your shoulders, then go through the mental checklist: Brace your abs, flex your butt, squeeze the dumbbells—then start.

In a barbell deadlift, you can go through a similar checklist: Brace your abs, flex your butt, squeeze the bar as hard as you can, grip the ground with your feet—then push the ground away.

As this skill develops, people feel both safer and stronger with heavier weights. In your strength-phase workouts (sets of five reps), you should be practicing getting tighter. This is a skill you can get better at over months and years, and it will make a huge difference in your strength.

Note about what not to tighten: Regardless of how tight you get below the neck, you don't want to add tension above the neck. Your neck should be relatively relaxed. Your face should be relaxed. You don't want to hike your shoulders up when you're tightening up. You don't want to clench your jaw. If you're getting sore in your neck or shoulders, video yourself doing the movements to double check that you aren't adding tension at your neck and face.

This is a short but solid primer on tension techniques, and is what I work on with most of my clients. That being said, you can go deeper if you'd like. If you want to really dig in, I recommend *Power to the People* and *The Naked Warrior* by Pavel Tsatsouline.

Relaxation techniques are on the other end of the spectrum—your ability to do high-rep sets (15–20 reps) is about how much you can relax while still maintaining proper form. Endurance is primarily about efficiency.

The thing about the high-tension techniques is that these are exhausting after more than five reps. High tension is a power tool that's effective for one job—lifting heavy. It's terrible for other things like endurance.

In higher-rep sets, try to relax as much as possible. You might still brace your core and flex your butt, but maybe only at 50%. You might instead focus more on getting long and tall through your spine.

Relaxation, like tension, is also a skill. In high-rep sets, ask yourself—is this harder because I'm tightening up too much? Can I relax a little and still keep my form? Be aware of when you're adding tension at times when it's costing you reps.

HIGH-REP WORKOUTS VERSUS LOW-REP WORKOUTS

We're going to do workouts in three different rep ranges. We'll talk more about when to use each of those rep ranges in the next section, Meta-skills. For now, just know there are three basic rep ranges, and we'll be looking at them differently.

Different Workouts, Different Skills

Strong (low rep range):

- Get as tight as possible to build a strong base to move from.

- Really focus on external cues (move this to that).

- Workouts are hard because the weight is heavy, and your focus on form is so intense.

Fit (medium rep range):

- Get as relaxed as possible while you can still maintain form so you can do as many reps as possible.

- Really focus on internal cues (what you feel working).

- Workouts are hard in a sweaty and muscle-burning kind of way.

Lean (medium rep range):

- Have a balanced amount of tension and relaxation.

- Balance focus between internal and external cues.

- Workouts are hard in a sweaty and muscle-burning kind of way and in a "the weight is heavy kind of way."

SHOULD I LIFT TO FAILURE?

A couple rules of thumb:

You can lift closer to failure on movements like pushups.

And you want to stay away from failure on movements like barbell deadlifts.

You can lift closer to failure on high-rep workouts.

And you want to stay away from failure on low-rep workouts.

The big barbell lifts like the deadlift are intense enough that you don't need to lift to failure to get a benefit from them. If you're doing heavy deadlifts, you run a risk of hurting yourself if you go to the absolute limit. In general, keep a rep or two in the bank. If you feel like you can do six reps, do five. If you feel like you can do five reps, do four.

With simpler exercises that have less chance of hurting you, you can often go closer to failure…or even to failure. There isn't a lot at risk doing pushups to failure. With dumbbell bench press, you can get pretty close to failure; just make sure you save enough strength to safely drop the dumbbells.

Three things to consider:

— **Don't hurt yourself.** On complex, heavy lifts, keeping a rep or two in the bank is helpful for safety.

— **For strength**, going to failure often isn't required. As long as you're increasing in strength (lifting more weight), I don't care if you ever go to failure. If the goal is to lift more, the goal is to lift more. If you're making solid progress, increasing the weight on the bar, and you never lift to failure, that's fine. Training to failure isn't required to increase strength.[162,163,164]

— **For leanness**, there's a benefit to going to failure on moderate- or high-rep exercises. Besides weight and volume, metabolic stress makes a difference in increasing muscle.[165]

If you want to go to failure on simple, medium- and high-rep exercises, don't go to failure on every set—usually just the last set. Some people can go to failure in three workouts per week, and make progress and increase strength. Other people may find they get stronger faster when going to failure less often. It's individual, and it's worth experimenting with this.

POST-WORKOUT REFLECTION

The fastest route to get better at any important practice:

1. Plan the practice

2. Practice (mindfully)

3. Reflect on the practice

Similarly, Dan John, discussing strength training, often quotes J. Stanton's book, *The Gnoll Credo*, "Plan the hunt, hunt, discuss the hunt."

There are questions you can ask yourself to reflect on your workouts. Just pick one or two that jump out at you on a given day. You can do it in less than a minute.

INTERNAL POST WORKOUT	EXTERNAL PORT WORKOUT
What was your favorite part of that workout?	How many sets are in the program each day this week?
How did you express your values in this workout?	How many sets will there be each day next week?
What did you learn during this workout?	Are you stronger in this move than when you started this program?
What did you notice about your body this workout?	Is it time to move up the weight in any exercises?
How hard was that set on a scale of one to ten?	Is it more appropriate to stay the same or even lift less in any exercises?

WORKOUT SKILLS RECAP

You have a couple guidelines to work on and five different skills to focus on:

WORKOUT GUIDELINES	WORKOUT SKILLS
Exercise selection	Internal focus during movement
Weight selection	External focus during movement
	Specific form cues
	Tension skill
	Relaxation skill

Just like eating skills, workout skills get better over time. It's a matter of practice.

Often, the difference between getting stronger and leaner over time hinges on whether you work out mindlessly or if you build skills over time.

For sure, the most engagement equates to the most enjoyment. And the most flow you can get in a workout requires spending time practicing workout skills. The kind of confidence and mastery that changes a person's relationship to the body and to fitness is a direct result of developing workout skills.

CHAPTER FIVE
META-SKILLS—
FOOD AND WORKOUT

Don't Diet	The first step is to stop doing things that don't work
Eating Skills and Workout Skills	What skills to practice to get lean and strong
Meta-skills	How to practice the skills so your practice is successful each week
The Ten Turning Points	How to think about your skills practice so you don't sabotage your results every eight weeks
The Wise Five	Understanding intrinsic motivation and how it works

Let's review the eating skills:

	DURING MEALS	BETWEEN MEALS
LISTEN TO YOUR BODY	Notice when getting full, and stop when full	Distinguish hunger versus cravings, boredom, tiredness, emotions, or thoughts
USE A GUIDELINE	Plate healthy and balanced portions	Eat a balanced meal every four to six hours, without snacking in between

The eating skills are **what** you're practicing:

- *What* I'm practicing is putting my fork down between bites.
- *What* I'm practicing is noticing when I'm full.

The Meta-skills are **how** and **why** you're doing it:

- *Why* I'm practicing putting my fork down between bites is because I value health.
- *Why* I'm practicing noticing when I'm full is because I value energy.
- *How* I'm practicing noticing when I am full: I'm planning that *if* I have pizza for dinner, it's harder to tell when I am full in the moment. I know I always want another slice in the moment. So, if I have pizza, *then* I'll have to wait 20 minutes after eating my first serving before being able to notice if I'm full.
- *How* I'm moderating eating treats is I'm practicing eating flexibility: I practice saying "yes" to treats sometimes, and I practice saying "no" to treats other times.
- *How* I'm moderating eating treats is I'm practicing psychological flexibility: I know sometimes it's normal to feel sad, and I don't have to try to fix that *with food*.

The Meta-skills are the context that encompass the eating skills.

FOOD META-SKILLS

If/Then Planning

Flexibility

Decision making
from personal values

PLANNING FOR FOOD: IF/THEN PLANNING

The most important Meta-skill for behavior change is If/Then Planning. If/Then planning is simply a matter of planning for:

3.   IF obstacle _____ shows up,

4.   THEN I'm going to do _____ to overcome that obstacle.

It's been shown goal setting is usually not enough, and *obstacle planning* is an important and often missing piece of the puzzle.[166] People take more consistent action and have more consistent practice if they expect and plan to overcome obstacles. In research, this is called *implementation intention*. It means your plans to overcome the obstacles that always come up are what make the difference in success.

Most people fail in behavior change because they repeatedly assume no obstacles will come up. They don't think things through and they end up with a horrible If/Then plan: "IF everything goes perfectly in my life today, THEN I'll practice my skills." Unless you have a charmed life, that's a recipe for failure.

Research on If/Then Planning

A meta-analysis of 94 individual studies found If/Then planning to be an extremely consistent and robust predictor of goal achievement.[167] In every case, people who created If/Then plans to overcome obstacles were more successful in their actions, habit change, and goal achievement than people who didn't.

The first thing to know is planning for healthy eating has been shown to be incredibly effective...but that planning not to eat unhealthy food has been found to be incredibly ineffective.[168] This is often the biggest mistake people make—they say, "If I see some chocolate I want, then I won't eat it." Planning not to do something or not eat the thing just doesn't work. You have to make your "then" plan be something you *will* do, like accept that cravings are normal, or eat a carrot, or go for a walk. It has to be a "doing" thing, not a "not doing" thing.

Another thing to keep in mind: If/Then plans have been shown to be effective when the person focuses on the action (in our case, skills and guidelines or workouts) and not to be effective when a person focuses on the outcome, such as weight loss or strength.[169] Build your planning around the actions you want to take.

Interestingly, If/Then plans have shown to be effective for working on hard habit changes, but not easy ones.[170]

You actually won't need them for things that come easily to you; they'll be the most useful for the skills and guidelines you struggle with the most.

Similarly, If/Then plans are effective when you're tired, irritable, anxious, or in a bad mood. One study manipulated people into good or bad states of mind, and then had them complete hard tasks. For people in happy, positive states of mind, task completion was high with or without If/Then planning. Of the people who were irritable and tired, If/Then planning made a huge difference in task completion, such that they were *equally as effective* as the people who were in great moods.[171]

EFFECTIVE	NOT EFFECTIVE
Using If/Then plans to eat healthy food	Using If/Then plans not to eat unhealthy food
Using If/Then plans focusing on skills, guidelines, and workouts	Using If/Then plans focusing weight loss and strength gain
Using If/Then plans to work on hard skills, guidelines, and workouts	Using If/Then plans are unnecessary when working on easy things
Using If/Then plans is most effective when you are tired, irritable, anxious, or in a bad mood	Using If/Then plans are unnecessary when you are stoked about everything

IF/THEN PLANNING WITH CLIENTS

Clients really like If/Then planning for two reasons: First, they get to see, when they mess up, it isn't a personal failing; it's a failure to plan. Second, they get to make specific plans each week for how to overcome the obstacles that come up most often in their lives. Most of those coaching calls are simply reflecting on what did and didn't work, and creating If/Then plans for the things that were hard.

THINKING THINGS THROUGH

Again, *thinking through obstacles* is the most important element of behavior change.

There are two things people typically don't consider:

- Obstacles are part of life; we need to accept these are part of life and expect them.
- Successful food skill practice isn't a matter of not having obstacles; it's a matter of expecting obstacles and planning for them.

There are two kinds of obstacles we face:

External obstacles: *People bringing pizza into the office or having a really stressful and draining workday*

Internal obstacles: *Not wanting to feel sad, tired, have cravings, be angry, or have unwanted thoughts*

Most clients find one of these two obstacles is tougher for them.

Sometimes If/Then planning may revolve all around external obstacles:

Obstacle: *Eating fast food for dinner when tired*

> **IF** I have a 12-hour workday every Wednesday,
> **THEN** I know I need to cook Wednesday's dinner on Tuesday.

Obstacle: *Eating too much at restaurants*

> **IF** I get served too much food at the restaurant,
> **THEN** I need to box some up and take it home.

Obstacle: *Starving at dinner, then eating too fast and overeating*

> **IF** I have eight hours of work on my schedule between lunch and dinner,
> **THEN** I'm going to need a snack halfway in between.

Obstacle: *Eating mid-morning when bored at work*

> **IF** I crave a snack at 10:00 a.m.,
> **THEN** I'm going to check to see if it's been four to six hours since breakfast.

For other people, it's all internal obstacles:

Obstacle: *Eating too much candy at work*

> **IF** I have a craving for candy in the middle of the afternoon,
> **THEN** I'm going to check to see if I'm hungry for a balanced meal.

Obstacle: *Late-night stress eating*

> **IF** I have a stressful day at work,
> **THEN** I'm going to veg out on TV after I put the kids to bed.

Obstacle: *Emotional eating*

> **IF** I feel sad,
> **THEN** I'm going to go for a walk.

Obstacle: *Boredom eating*

> **IF** I feel bored,
> **THEN** I'm going to work on a craft.

Or we can look at internal obstacles from acceptance:

Obstacle: *Eating too much candy at work*

> **IF** I have a craving for candy in the middle of the afternoon,
> **THEN** I'm going to remember it's normal to crave candy.

Obstacle: *Late-night stress eating*

> **IF** I have a stressful day at work,
> **THEN** I'm going to remember it's normal and okay that work is stressful sometimes.

Obstacle: *Emotional eating*

> **IF** I feel sad,
> **THEN** I'm going to remember it's normal and human to feel sad sometimes.

Obstacle: *Boredom eating*

> **IF** I feel bored,
> **THEN** I'm going to remember it's normal and human to feel bored sometimes.

Most people find if they do just a little reflection about the previous week, they can anticipate what obstacles they might find in the upcoming week.

Reflection is a useful tool in your tool box, and it's necessary for your If/Then planning. Consider all the skills and Meta-skills and take some time each week to reflect on how things are going. Sometimes, my clients will give themselves multiple options:

IF I have a stressful day at work,
THEN I'm going to do one of the following:

- Remember it's okay if work is stressful sometimes.
- Go for a ten-minute walk.
- Do five minutes of yoga.
- Watch funny cat videos on YouTube.
- Drink some tea.

It can be nice to have choices. But there's a huge difference between having mapped out your choices ahead of time—before you're stressed out—versus trying to figure things out in the moment. Having a plan ahead of time is what makes the biggest difference.

And, your plan can have multiple options.

IF/THEN PLANNING ON YOUR SKILLS TRACKER

It can really work well to add an If/Then plan to your tracker. Plan to overcome an obstacle each week:

		DAY:	M	T	W	TH	F	S	SU
		DATE:	7	8	9	10	11	12	13
EATING SKILLS	Check in with my stomach mid meal								
	Check in with my stomach one hour after eating								
FOOD GUIDES	Put the fork down between bites								
	Eat a meal every four to six hours								
VALUES (LIST THREE)	Persistence, compassion, connectedness								
IF/THEN PLANNING	If: I get stressed out at work Then: I'm going to walk a lap around the building								

Research indicates that If/Then planning is personal—it works better if you come up with your own plan.

If/Then planning for the following week is one of the biggest things I do with my coaching clients. You should have a coaching session for yourself every week in your skill tracker. If it helps, you can journal about the previous week before your internal coaching session.

Really though, it's just as simple as identifying one obstacle you had, and then creating a plan for how to overcome it the following week.

YOUR IF/THEN PLANS FOR ONE OBSTACLE MIGHT WORK FOR MULTIPLE OBSTACLES

In the beginning, most obstacles will feel like they're separate. It will seem like each time you hit an obstacle, it was a completely new problem you've never encountered.

A funny thing happens over time—

- As you reflect on the obstacles you've encountered, you'll start to see many of the obstacles that seemed completely different are actually the same two or three obstacles, just in slightly different situations.

- The more If/Then plans you create, you start to see there are certain If/Then plans that overcome multiple obstacles.

This is the highest level of skill practice—when you can take skills and If/Then plans and apply them to multiple situations. This only comes with practice and reflection and planning. But if you're doing that practice and reflection and planning, over time you will see this start to generalize. You'll even find yourself using skills or If/Then plans in situations that are totally new.

Ultimately, what looked like a million obstacles will probably only be two or three. And where skills might seem really different in different situations, like on weekdays versus weekends, they will all start to become the same skill.

For now, just do your practice, but have in the back of your mind to be looking for how to generalize your practice to multiple situations over time.

PLANNING FOR WORKOUTS: PERIODIZATION

There are five things we currently know about workout programming:

1. People get stronger over time with almost any consistent strength program.

2. People get stronger faster with some sort of structured plan—this is called "periodization."

3. Most people get stronger faster when they use a variety of rep ranges—on a monthly basis, that's called block periodization.

4. People get stronger faster when they cycle the volume of work in some way—volume periodization.

5. Advanced people get stronger the fastest when they use multiple rep ranges within a week—advanced programs should use undulating periodization.

There's been really cool progress in strength training research over the last ten years. People are doing better research that more closely resembles how people actually work out in a gym. Brad Schoenfeld, for example, has really pushed for more strength training research using people who aren't new to training, and using program variables people actually use in real life.

What they have found is that people get better results with a structured program. Which kind of structured program is definitively best is harder to pin down, but here's what the evidence points to:

- If you're a beginner, anything works.

- If you're intermediate, you want some sort of structured program, like block or linear.

- If you're advanced, you'll likely get the best results by doing undulating periodization.

PERIODIZATION RESEARCH

A meta-analysis of 11 studies found that having a periodized program was more effective for gaining strength, regardless of age, gender, or length of time training. In all conditions, people got stronger with a periodized workout program than without.[172]

One study compared three different four-month workout programs. The first group lifted 5x10 (five sets of ten reps) for the whole four months. The second group lifted 6x8 for four months. The third group, the closest to what we are doing in *Lean and Strong,* changed rep ranges every month: month one was 5x10; month two was 6x8; month three, 3x6; and month four, 3x4. That third group got significantly stronger than the first or second groups.[173]

A study with collegiate women tennis players compared periodized versus non-periodized programming, and found that the athletes in the periodized training group got significantly stronger and leaner. What's cool about this study is that the participants were high-level athletes, both very strong and very lean. The nine-month program rotated weekly between 6–8 reps per set, 12–15 reps per set, and 8–12 reps per set. The athletes had no change in bodyweight, but went from an already lean and athletic 22.9% bodyfat to a very lean 19.1% bodyfat. They also had significant increases in maximum strength, anaerobic power (think high intensity interval training), and tennis serve velocity.[174] They replicated the study a

few years later and found similar increases in leanness, strength, and sport-specific power.[175]

On the other hand, a systematic review looked at periodized versus non-periodized training for adults who had never worked out. They found if you're an adult new to working out, it doesn't make a big difference—everything works.[176] If you're in your first three months of working out, you could do literally any program and get stronger and leaner. The longer you've been working out, the more difference periodization makes.

One study on young untrained women and strength training was interesting in that it found different results for leanness and strength with two types of periodization. The two kinds of periodization included linear, where the reps changed every month (like the intermediate *Lean and Strong* program) and undulating periodization, where there were three set-and-rep ranges each week (like the *Lean and Strong* advanced program).

In both groups, the young women studied got leaner and stronger. In the linear periodization group with sets and reps change monthly, the women got much leaner. With undulating periodization where the sets and reps rotate daily, the women got significantly stronger. Again, both groups got leaner and stronger, but the results suggest that you choose your program based on the primary goal.[177]

In terms of rep ranges, in the short term, high reps create more muscular endurance, and medium and low reps create more maximum strength.[178,179,180] That being said, low reps, medium reps, and high reps, all increase strength and leanness.[181,182]

Lastly, one study looked at rugby players' strength training with different rep ranges, and tested the strength gains each individual athlete had in each rep range. Some got better results at 3x5 reps, heavy; some got better results at 3x10, medium heavy; some got the best results at 5x15 with light weights, and some got the best results at 4x5, light weight.[183]

As a whole, the results don't fit any of ways we normally look at strength training. The big takeaway is that different athletes responded to drastically different things. It's a good reason to work with different set and rep ranges: You don't know your best fit, but if you do them all in a systematic way, you're definitely going to spend some time in the range that's best for you.

To wrap this up, a bunch of studies have found that any periodization is better than none.[184,185] Other studies have shown that undulating periodization (the *Lean and Strong* advanced program) beats other forms of periodization for recreationally trained women.[186] Similar results found undulating periodization won for recreationally trained men.[187]

On the other hand, a study of both male and female track athletes found block periodization, which is the *Lean and Strong* intermediate program, to be more effective for strength.[188]

PERIODIZATION WITH CLIENTS

My clients often note they just enjoy periodized workout programming. They like knowing there's a plan; they like understanding the cycles the program goes through. They enjoy having something consistent enough that they can see progress, but also changing often enough that it stays interesting. They find it both engaging as an activity and effective in that they get stronger and leaner.

Linear Periodization

Linear periodization is where we start with higher reps and work our way down to lower reps. As the reps get lower, we increase the weight. We start with endurance, and work our way, linearly, to strength. It's a straightforward way to structure a program, and that's why we're going to have the beginner program be linear periodization.

The beginner six-month linear periodization program looks like:

1. Fit: 3x20

2. Lean and fit: 3x15

3. Lean: 3x12

4. Lean: 3x10

5. Strong and lean: 3x8

6. Strong: 3x5

A note about the names: Naming these ranges is always weird.

"Strong," the lower-rep range, is generally the best for practicing the skills of getting strong.

"Fit," the high-rep range, is usually the best for practicing the skills of creating endurance. Honestly, if it matched the other two ranges, I would have called this rep range "endurance" or "conditioning."

"Lean," the medium-rep range, is right in the middle. Sometimes it's called the "hypertrophy" range—the muscle-building range—and sometimes people say it's best for "toning." It's still funny to think of muscle building and toning as the same thing, usually marketed to different genders. Basically, the quality of having more muscle and less fat is "leanness," and this is the phase that's probably best for that.

Here's what we know:

* People get stronger in all three rep ranges. They just best express their strength in the rep range they've been practicing.

* All three rep ranges make people leaner.

* Spending some time in each of the three is probably the most effective.

- Volume —the total number of hard sets—also has a big impact on strength and leanness.

In most cases and for most people, the sum is more than the parts. We get more of all three if we do the work of cyclically practicing all three.

Block Periodization

Block periodization simply means working through different "blocks" of rep ranges. We'll cycle through blocks of leanness, strength, and endurance, but not in a linear order as shown earlier. In addition to the fact that it works really well, people like feeling as if each block of the program has a definitive thing to work on.

When you're working on endurance, you know you're working on endurance, and then that block ends. When you're working on strength, you work on strength, and then that block ends. The blocks change like seasons, and it's engaging and fun. People find that each time they cycle through, they're a little stronger in that block than they were the time before.

The intermediate six-month block periodization program looks like this:

1. Lean: 3x10
2. Fit: 3x20
3. Lean and strong: 3x8
4. Lean: 3x12
5. Lean and fit: 3x15
6. Strong: 3x5

Undulating Periodization

(We really need a different name for this)

Undulating periodization is where you have one day per week to work on strength, one day to work on endurance, and one to work on leanness. The body responds to this

extremely well—some of the research cited in the previous section suggests this might have an edge on strength building for advanced workout folks.

For a beginner trainee, or even intermediate, this can be unwieldy. Beginners often find there aren't enough differences between their days for it to make an impact. People who are intermediate may find it's more to keep track of than they'd like.

For people who are advanced, as long as they track the workouts, it's manageable and effective.

This is similar to how a skill changes over time—for someone who's intermediate, it's overwhelming; for someone advanced, it's engaging.

In the advanced undulating periodization program, each week looks like:

- Monday—Strong: 3x5
- Wednesday—Fit: 3x15
- Friday—Lean: 3x10

WHY NOT JUST DO STRONG BLOCKS IF I WANT TO GET STRONG?

Here you could ask the questions:

- Why not just do the strong block over and over if I just want to get strong?
- Why not just do the lean block if I want to get lean?

Per the research mentioned, general fitness folks get both the strongest and leanest faster when they work through different rep ranges, like lean, strong, and fit.

Next, we'll take a look at the subject of practice.

DIFFERENT WORKOUTS, DIFFERENT SKILLS

"Strong" rep range:

- Get as tight as possible to build a strong base to move from.

- Really focus on external cues—move this to that.

- Workouts are hard because the weight is heavy, and your focus on form is so intense.

"Fit" rep range:

- Get as relaxed as possible while you can still maintain form so you can do as many reps as possible.

- Really focus on internal cues—what you feel working.

- Workouts are hard in a sweaty and muscle burning kind of way.

"Lean" rep range:

- Have a balanced amount of tension and relaxation.

- Balance focus between internal and external cues.

- Workouts are hard in a sweaty and muscle burning kind of way, and in a "the weights are heavy kind of way."

Volume: Low, Medium, and High

The other way we periodize workouts is with total volume. Volume is simply the number of hard sets in each workout.

In *Lean and Strong,* we have three intermediate and three advanced workouts. Excluding the core exercises and conditioning, here's the volume (including all exercises) for each phase:

Intermediate, low volume
120 sets per month

Intermediate, medium volume
152 sets per month

Intermediate, high volume
180 sets per month

Advanced, low volume
132 sets per month

Advanced, medium volume
160 sets per month

Advanced, high volume
190 sets per month

All things being equal, the person who does the most volume will get the leanest and strongest. Oh, if only life were that simple.

Considerations for volume:

- The volume should increase the longer you've been working out. Someone new to training cannot lift heavy with high volume. It can take a few years of consistent lifting to work up to high-volume workouts.

- Your stress level will impact how much volume you can recover from. If your life is super stressful, you often won't be able to recover from and make progress with a high-volume program. And if your relationships, career, food, and sleep are all awesome, you should go ahead and rock out on a high-volume program.

- Not everyone has time in their lives to do a high-volume program. It's better to do a program that actually fits into your life.

- The volume of work you do should cycle over time. Within each month, it should cycle from low to high. Over the course of a year, it can also cycle from low to high. If it works for your life, it makes sense to do a low-, medium-, and high-volume program, and then start the cycle all over again.

A meta-analysis of nine studies found that medium- and high-volume workouts produced better strength results than low-volume workouts.[189] Another meta-analysis and review looking at 15 studies found a dose-response relationship with muscle gain—every added set per week had a significant effect on results.[190]

A study on untrained adult men found that people in low-volume, medium-volume, and-high volume strength training programs all got leaner and increased strength, but the men in the high-volume group got the best results.[191] A program comparing low-volume and high-volume strength training for women found that the women in both groups got leaner and stronger, but the women in the high-volume group got significantly leaner and stronger.[192] The study was a little weird in that the low-volume group did circuits and the high-volume group did a periodized strength training program, like *Lean and Strong*. Regardless, the higher-volume group got better results.

An absolutely giant meta-analysis in *The Journal of Strength and Conditioning* looking at a whopping 177 studies found different results for people who were untrained, recreationally trained, or athletes. Of people who were untrained or recreationally trained, medium volume was the most effective. For people who were athletes, high volume was the most effective.[193]

WHERE TO START

Beginner Low		
Intermediate Low	**Intermediate Medium**	Intermediate High
Advanced Low	Advanced Medium	Advanced High

Ninety percent of the people reading *Lean and Strong* should start with the intermediate medium-volume program. Try that for three months and adjust from there.

If you haven't followed a structured program for at least six months, do the beginner program. If you've been lifting consistently for more than three years, try the advanced medium-volume program.

CARDIO AND ADDING MORE

When my clients want to do more, my favorite thing is to have them *walk* on their off days. The program literally looks like:

- Strength training three days per week

- Walk three days per week

The biggest benefit of walking is chilling out. It's one of the most effective and positive coping strategies for stress or unwanted emotions. It's good to relax, look at the birds and the sky and the trees and the houses, and get away from electronics.

Research shows that moderately intense walking reduces the stress hormone cortisol.[194] If you walk outdoors[195] and notice the birds and trees on your walk, [196] it increases emotional wellbeing.

You could just as easily do some gentle yoga, deep breathing exercises, qigong, or meditation. I like walking because it's simple and accessible.

People expect to hear about crushing themselves with punishing cardio to burn more calories. Honestly, most people will get better results by using walking to cope with stress and *doing less stress eating.*

You can ramp this up to cycling or elliptical or jogging or rowing or whatever you like. But most people will get a better result from treating this addition as relaxation. Use it to wind yourself down. Down-regulate yourself for a change.

Most people are better off doing some chill cardio to manage stress. Listen to music or a fun podcast. Or listen to nothing and just be with your thoughts. Move your body and sweat a little, but don't do a crushing, punishing cardio workout. Save your effort for the strength workouts.

Useful things you can do on your walks:

- Practice mindfulness by noticing what you see, hear, and smell;

- Let your mind wander;

- Reflect on your values;

- Think through If/Then planning for your skill practice;

- Listen to a podcast;

- Relax and de-stress.

Walking has been shown to reduce cravings for sweets and chocolate. One study looking at 47 people who were overweight and self-described sugary snack eaters found that a 15-minute walk reduced their stress response and had a significant impact on chocolate consumption.[197]

If you are already fit, these walks could become jogs or bike rides or time on a rowing machine or elliptical. You can do moderate intensity of whatever you enjoy. The point is, these workouts are more about chilling out than they are about crushing it.

Moderate cardiovascular exercise like brisk walking or easy jogging has been shown to short-circuit the chronic stress response and re-set the HPA axis.[198,199] If you do easy-to-moderate cardio on your off days, the reduced stress and subsequently reduced snack intake might be the most important aspect of working out for leanness.

The other option for adding a fourth workout is to add a strength-conditioning day. Sometimes people call these met-cons—metabolic conditioning…but whatever. It's basically interval training. It could look like battling ropes, rowing intervals, bear crawls, kettlebell swings, sled pushing, maybe some higher rep TRX strength moves—that kind of stuff.

If that's your jam, go ahead and throw in a day like that. Just keep it to about 30 minutes and go have fun.

This would now look like:

- Strength training three days per week

- Strength-conditioning one day per week

Lots of people really like how this feels. If you totally love doing it, do it. It can be fun to push yourself in an endurance kind of way. Keep it short, rock out, and have fun.

Can you add more conditioning days or high intensity interval training? Maybe.

If your life is super low stress, you might be able to crush it six days per week and still get stronger. Everyone has had a time in life when everything is going their way and they have tons of free time and you really can kill it six days per week. For me, it was a few years in my 20s.

However, if you're partner at a law firm, have a high-stress job and can't seem to de-stress at night without using food or alcohol, you might get more from going for a walk and letting your mind wander for a half-hour.

That half-hour of no deadlines or stimulus or anything to do, with no email or text messages might be what you really need to handle to hit your weight-loss goals—walking to relax instead of using food or alcohol.

If the goal is to get strong, save your energy, focus, and recovery for the strength workouts. Keep the main goal the main goal.

One benefit of doing chill cardio is it doesn't compete with the strength work.

WEEKLY WORKOUT OPTIONS

MAIN LEAN AND STRONG PROGRAM		
STRENGTH TRAINING	HARD CONDITIONING/ INTERVAL TRAINING	WALKING OR MODERATE CARDIO
Three days per week	None	Whenever you have time or need stress relief

ALTERNATE LEAN AND STRONG PROGRAMS		
STRENGTH TRAINING	HARD CONDITIONING/ INTERVAL TRAINING	WALKING OR MODERATE CARDIO
Two days per week	Two days per week	Whenever you have time or need stress relief
Two days per week	One day per week	Whenever you have time or need stress relief
Two days per week	None	Whenever you have time or need stress relief

EXAMPLE OF CONDITIONING WORKOUTS

EXAMPLE CONDITIONING DAY A		
DURATION	MOVEMENT	INTERVAL
5–10 minutes	Bear crawl Original Strength style	30 seconds work 30 seconds rest
5–10 minutes	Battling ropes	15–30 seconds work 30–45 seconds rest
5–10 minutes	Sled push	Up and back as many times in 5–10 minutes

EXAMPLE CONDITIONING DAY B

DURATION	MOVEMENT	INTERVAL
4, 6, 8, or 10 minutes	One-arm kettlebell swings	30 seconds work 30 seconds rest
5–10 minutes	Bear crawl Original Strength style	30 seconds work 30 seconds rest
5–10 minutes	Battling ropes	15–30 seconds work 30–45 seconds rest

EXAMPLE CONDITIONING DAY C

DURATION	MOVEMENT	INTERVAL
4, 6, 8, or 10 minutes	One-arm kettlebell swings	30 seconds work 30 seconds rest
5–10 minutes	Bear crawl Original Strength style	30 seconds work 30 seconds rest
5–10 minutes	Assault AirBike or Spin bike	30 seconds work 30 seconds rest

EXAMPLE CONDITIONING DAY D

DURATION	MOVEMENT	INTERVAL
4, 6, 8, or 10 minutes	One-arm kettlebell swings	30 seconds work 30 seconds rest
5–10 minutes	Battling ropes	15–30 seconds work 30–45 seconds rest
5–10 minutes	Elliptical	30 seconds work 30 seconds rest

EXAMPLE CONDITIONING DAY E

DURATION	MOVEMENT	INTERVAL
5–10 minutes	Bear crawl	30 seconds work 30 seconds rest
5–10 minutes	Rowing Machine	30 seconds work 30 seconds rest
5–10 minutes	Battling ropes	15–30 seconds work 30–45 seconds rest

Again, this is just bonus stuff to do if you like it. Feel free to mix up the rest intervals. If you get bored, you could try:

- Harder/faster/heavier intervals at 15 seconds work with 45 seconds rest
- Easier/slower/lighter intervals at 45 seconds work with 15 seconds rest

There really isn't a lot of magic to the conditioning days. Just rock out.

The one thing you will notice about conditioning days is this: All of the movements are self-limiting. We aren't doing high-repetition barbell snatches, which have a high degree of technical skill and can come apart under pronounced fatigue. Instead, we use something like battling ropes, in which typically under fatigue, people just stop.

Even kettlebell swings, which people sometimes totally massacre with two hands, are pretty self-limiting with one hand. With two hands, often people's heads jut forward and their shoulders elevate, back arch, hips pike that come from trying to pull the weight up with the arms—all horrible, horrible form for kettlebell swings. Those are much rarer with one-arm swings. With one-arm swings, unless the weight is waaay too light, you have to use your hips to do the work.

MAKING DECISIONS FROM VALUES

Clients who put their values first in making decisions about food skill practice and workout programs hit their goals fairly easily. Values-based practice is the foundation of making smart decisions about fitness.

You'll notice values show up multiple times in *Lean and Strong*. They show up here in the Meta-skills; they show up in The Ten Turning Points (the paradox of values and goals), and really extensive values reflections show up in The Wise Five.

What you need to know right now: *Goals = destination and Values = direction.*

"Life is a journey, not a destination," is about the most cliché thing you can say, so I'm not going to say it—even though it's true.

What I'm going to say is this: People who get the direction right and move in that direction have no trouble hitting their goals. In weight-loss terms, people who get their values about food right and practice appropriate skills get leaner and stronger.

The more people obsess about their weight-loss goals, the more they do flat-out dumb things. They do stupid cleanses. They try to force weight loss with starvation. *They do things that go against all their values.* They essentially try to cheat the system and cut corners; they think the rules don't apply to them.

Another way to look at values versus goals:

Goals = specific achievements

Values = character strengths

Think about the *values* you want teach your kids: hard work, doing what's right, being reasonable, being diligent, being kind. Now, apply those to weight loss. When people approach their food from those values, things go amazingly well. And they go fast.

But when people obsess about weight-loss goals, they *throw out everything that works* and try to cheat. They try completely silly things like cleanses and elimination diets. Is some magic food group really the answer?

Do you remember reading the news about Enron, the energy company that went from the darling of Wall Street to massive scandals around fraudulent accounting? They went from making smart moves to trying to cut corners and hide their mistakes in pursuit of their goal to keep the stock price up. As often happens when you throw out your values in pursuit of goals, everything fell apart.

It's a really good metaphor for how people throw out their values when they diet.

If your goals take you in the opposite direction of your values, you either have the wrong goals, or you aren't mature enough to have goals at all. Either way, you need to work on your values, and true up your skill practice to your values.

WHY GOALS USUALLY AREN'T EFFECTIVE FOR WEIGHT LOSS

To set a goal, you need to have two things:

1. Clearly defined milestones that occur at regular intervals;

2. A strong track record of success.

Almost everyone in weight loss fails at number two. If your weight-loss history is mostly failure, you don't have any business setting goals about weight loss. If you've consistently failed at weight loss, setting a goal just means you're going to push yourself to fail faster. What you did in the past *did not work*. Doing more of what doesn't work is just failure that takes more effort. Don't take dumb things and do more of them.

Let's say you set a weight-loss goal of losing 60 pounds. Then, you do something dumb (diet). You fail a few times, and fall behind schedule. Since you're behind schedule on your goal, you decide to do something dumber (a cleanse, remove an entire food group, or fast) and fail even more spectacularly.

The answer to doing dumb things isn't to do dumb things faster. The answer is also not to do dumber things. The answer is to do smarter things.

Smarter things always are congruent with your values.

THE COLLEGE METAPHOR
Clear Milestones plus a History of Success

Let's say Sally is a junior in college. Sally is getting Bs in all of her classes and is taking 12 credits per semester.

Sally can easily set a goal for when she is going to graduate. For the last two years, she's done 12 credits per semester and has been successful. She set a goal to graduate in three years, based on continuing at that pace. She has a strong track record of success, so it makes sense to set a goal.

Stephanie has been getting Ds and Fs in college for the last two years. Though she has taken 12 units per semester, she's only completed three to six units. She has a track record of failure. This is where most people are in weight loss. In weight loss, most people *do more…badly.* The way most people set weight-loss goals would be like if Stephanie decided to take 30 or 40 credits per semester so she can "catch up" or "because she's really motivated." Setting a goal for her is crazy. She needs to return to basic values like consistency, reasonableness, and patience.

In that metaphor, a values-based approach would be to work on study skills, not take more units. In fact, taking fewer units would probably be smart. It would be better to get six units of As than to get 12 units of Fs.

Six units of As actually moves her in the *direction* of her goals, where 12 units of Fs moves her in the *opposite direction*. If she's obsessed with her goal, she'll keep taking more and more, because she "has to hit her goal."

Doesn't that sound like how much people approach weight-loss goals?

THE HUMAN BODY NEVER MAKES LINEAR PROGRESS

To make it even worse, not only do most people have a track record of failure—which would preclude us from goal setting—weight loss doesn't have perfect milestones. Where college can be measured in units that happen each semester with regularity, nothing in the human body is that neat and tidy. The human body is messy.

Everything in the human body is nonlinear. Recovery from injury isn't linear; people often get better for a couple weeks, then worse, then better again. Learning isn't linear;

people practice and get better, then they practice and still stay plateaued, and then one day it clicks.

Similarly, weight loss is rarely linear: People lose weight, then plateau, then lose weight, then plateau. If you get freaked out by getting behind on your goals every time you plateau, you're guaranteed to fail.

Think back to the example of a kid learning to play a clarinet. There are long stretches of bad notes when it looks like nothing is getting better. Then all of a sudden, things click. These stretches of no progress followed by explosions of progress go on for years. Over time, the trend is strongly upward.

Over weeks and months, goal orientation is really frustrating, as things might not go forward, or might even go backward. But the value-driven approach—knowing practice is the right direction—drives the trend line in the right direction over time.

VALUES, MOTIVATION, AND WEIGHT LOSS RESEARCH

Longitudinal data—observing long-term results—has shown that people who pursue actions related to their values are more likely to hit their goals, and they derive more wellbeing from the results.[200]

A review and conceptual model of goal achievement, personality, and values, looked at studies showing that 1) value-directed action increases performance, 2) the personality trait of conscientiousness increases performance, and 3) the combination of value-directed action and consciousness increase performance.[201]

Self Determination Theory, the preeminent theory of intrinsic motivation, explains that we want to move from external motivation (reward and punishment, guilt and contingent self-esteem) to more internal motivation (fully integrated personal values).

Goal contents matter, goals that are external don't always meet our basic psychological needs, and getting those basic psychological needs met is the foundation of motivation and wellbeing. As we move from less self-determined (reward and punishment) to more self-determined (values), we increase motivation, increase performance, and increase wellbeing.[202]

SELF DETERMINATION THEORY'S FOUR KINDS OF MOTIVATION			
MORE EXTERNAL		MORE INTERNAL	
I work out so I can have a cookie afterward or If I miss my workout, no carbohydrates tomorrow	I work out to meet a societal standard of beauty. or I work out so I don't feel guilty.	I work out because I have a goal that aligns with my value of strength.	It's deeply important to me to be strong. Working out is an expression of being the kind of person I want to be.

A review of Self Determination Theory and health behavior looked at research where intrinsic motivation increased goal achievement. They found intrinsic motivation to drive results in multiple health domains, including weight loss, smoking cessation, and health screening. Increased intrinsic motivation not only increased goal achievement, but also increased people's ability to maintain their results as well. They gave the example of extrinsic motivation being losing weight to win a prize versus intrinsic motivation of losing weight because it matches your personal values.[203]

Complete behavioral weight loss studies, including values work, have been extraordinarily successful. It should be noted that besides values work, all of these studies included acceptance skills, defusion skills, and other specific eating skills. They also all had a huge values component similar to the values work in this book.[204,205,206,207,208]

One of these studies, "The Mind Your Health Project," has a publically available treatment manual, *Effective Weight Loss*. In *Effective Weight Loss*, values are distinguished as the reason a person would engage in hard behavior change. We're willing to deal with the discomfort of taking these actions and practicing skills because it's consistent with the kind of people we want to be.[209]

In the textbook *The Art and Science of Valuing in Psychotherapy*, the authors outline that values work helps 1) define what matters to you, 2) create meaning and purpose, 3) have a framework for choosing goals, 4) have a reason to experience and work through difficult thoughts and emotions, and 5) be aware of why you're taking certain actions, and how they relate to being the kind of person you want to be.[210]

Lastly, an article, *Motivating the unmotivated: how can health behavior be changed in those unwilling to change?* in the journal *Frontiers in Psychology* noted "values exploration" as an effective tool for increasing intrinsic motivation with health behaviors.[211]

The big takeaway is that values work is your access to getting to be the kind of person you want to be and do the things that matter to you. It's the context from which you'll overcome your hardest obstacles.

BRINGING A VALUE-BASED APPROACH TO SKILL PRACTICE

Value-based approaches usually include values like reasonableness, kindness, intelligence, diligence, and practice. These are things everyone knows always lead to the best results in every area of their lives…yet almost no one thinks to use them with their weight, food, and workouts.

VALUES REFLECTIONS

There are 12 weeks of values reflections in The Wise Five section, and many comparisons of values versus goals. For now, we'll just start by picking your values from a menu.

Now, you don't have to pick your values from the menu. You can write out your own, and just use the menu to get some ideas. Just remember: A value is a *direction*, not a *destination*.

Pick three values; each week you'll spend some time with your eating skills tracker, reflecting on how your values do or don't match your skill practice.

Again, in The Wise Five section of the book you'll find beginning on page 199, you'll have eight weeks of journaling exercises to clarify your values around food and fitness, and to connect your skill practice to those values. For now, just identify them and put them on your eating skills tracker each week.

EXAMPLE VALUES

YOU CAN CIRCLE YOUR TOP ONE TO THREE VALUES, OR COME UP WITH YOUR OWN

Acceptance	Flexibility	Play
Adventure	Freedom	Reciprocity
Assertiveness	Friendship	Respect
Authenticity	Forgiveness	Resourcefulness
Balance	Fun	Responsibility
Beauty	Generosity	Romance
Caring	Gratitude	Safety
Challenge	Home	Self-awareness
Collaboration	Honesty	Self-care
Community	Humor	Self-discipline
Compassion	Humility	Self-expression
Connection	Industriousness	Self-respect
Contribution	Independence	Service
Cooperation	Intimacy	Skillfulness
Courage	Joy	Spirituality
Creativity	Justice	Stewardship
Curiosity	Kindness	Strength
Design	Knowledge	Supportiveness
Dignity	Leadership	Teamwork
Diversity	Learning	Tradition
Encouragement	Love	Trustworthiness
Ethics	Loyalty	Understanding
Equality	Mindfulness	Uniqueness
Excitement	Order	Usefulness
Exploration	Open-mindedness	Vision
Fairness	Optimism	Vulnerability
Faith	Patience	Wellbeing
Family	Persistence	Wholeheartedness
Fitness	Personal Development	Wisdom

BALANCED VALUES

Most people naturally tend to approach their fitness from one extreme end of the spectrum or the other. They either set up their values as all "go, go, go," or they set them up as "chill, chill, chill." Obviously, it's more effective to pick values that balance each other.

Examples of balanced values:

- Excellence and Compassion

- Passion and Mindfulness

- Conscientiousness and Reasonableness

- Adventure and Intelligence

- Strength and Vulnerability

- Powerful and Connected

Values that have that kind of balance between action and humanity work really well in pursuit of fitness goals.

Think about movies: We love seeing vulnerable, flawed people doing amazing things. That's a hit for our own pursuits of goals and taking actions in line with our values—we're allowed to be vulnerable at the same time we're building strength. We're allowed to have self-compassion at the same time we're pursuing excellence.

This isn't a compromise; this is significantly more effective. People who pursue excellence without self-compassion tend to hit the wall and break…over and over again. They miss the times when the smarter and more effective play is rest or self-care or acceptance. We aren't robots; we can't go all-out all the time. We need to deliberately add values like self-compassion.

If you want to really go for it, you could add a third value related to connecting with others.

Examples of those third values:

- Connectedness

- Family

- Community

- Being an example

- Mentoring

- Generosity

- Making a difference

- Charity

- Contribution

A person might finish with three values like Excellence and Compassion and Community. That's one way to look at crafting a very cool and well-rounded life.

Whatever you select, choose what's important to *you*, in your life…right now. Choose meaningful things. Choose things that represent the kind of person you want to be. You get to choose.

MAKING DECISIONS FROM VALUES

Once you have a sense of your values, you can integrate those into how you make decisions with your food every week.

When you do your weekly planning and reflection session, you can reflect on how your food skill practice did or didn't reflect your values. Then you can consider how you could more clearly express your values in your skill practice the following week.

On the following page, you'll find a simple prompt for values reflection each week.

	VALUE	RATE YOUR SKILL PRACTICE IN RELATIONSHIP TO THAT VALUE	HOW DO YOU WANT TO EXPRESS THIS VALUE IN YOUR SKILL PRACTICE NEXT WEEK?
ONE		1 2 3 4 5	
TWO		1 2 3 4 5	
THREE		1 2 3 4 5	

First, write down three values in the first column, again remembering values are not goals. Values are the kind of person you want to be.

In the middle column, circle how close you got to expressing that particular value in your food skill practice the previous week. This isn't a way to punish yourself or compare yourself to an ideal. It's just a way to look at your value as a target to point toward, and see how close your skill practice was in pointing to the target. Again, skill practice is about actions. It's not what you thought or how you felt; it's what you *did*. Over time, we want to slowly bring your skill practice closer in the direction of your values.

Finally, make a quick note of how you'd like to express your values in your skill practice the following week. It's okay if it's the same as the previous week, especially if the previous week went well.

VALUES FOR EATING SKILLS— VALUES FOR WORKOUT PROGRAMS

With food, you might have a value of longevity or intelligence, and that leads you to practice eating skills instead of doing a stupid crash diet or an idiotic cleanse. You're playing a longer, smarter game, and you don't get caught up in quick diets that are destined to fail and hurt you.

Similarly, with workouts, those same values—longevity and intelligence—might have a similar effect. They may cause you to take it easy on a workout day when you feel bad. You know you're playing a long game, and it's okay to have an off day, to go through the motions, and not get hurt.

And, you're fine with that because you know you have other days that feel awesome when you can crank up the weight and rock out. Because you value longevity and intelligence, you're willing to listen to your body, not get hurt, and build serious strength over time.

VALUES IN AREAS OF YOUR LIFE WHERE YOU'RE REALLY SUCCESSFUL

Often, my clients are really successful in multiple areas of their lives—their families, their careers, or their hobbies. They often find they've been successful in those areas because they took a values-based approach. In those areas of their lives, they never tried to cut corners.

The way people tend to approach dieting and workouts—through looking for magic fixes and trying to find shortcuts—is generally the opposite of how they approach everything else in their lives. It's the opposite of what they teach their kids. It's the opposite of how they are at work. It's the opposite of advice they'd give to a friend.

The whole diet world has taught us to try to cheat the system. Marketing is always based on magic diets and secret fixes. We've been sold an entire field based on cheating, forcing an outcome, or buying magic beans. Let's recognize all of the fitness and diet advertising for what it is—the opposite of our personal values.

If you start to approach eating skills like anything else you've ever been successful at, you'll do really well. If you approach mastery of your workouts like anything else you've ever learned, you'll do really well. Treat food skill practice and workout programs like other things you've done well at. Make decisions from your personal values. Use your own history of success as a template for how to do well.

FLEXIBILITY

Rigid Diet Rules Predict Failure

We looked at *The Diet Cycle of Failure* in the first section "Don't Diet." On pages 47, we looked at 14 different studies that outlined how rigid dietary restraint often leads to rebound eating and weight gain, and how flexible regulation of eating is effective for weight loss, weight maintenance, and wellbeing. In this section, we're going to look at ways to apply that kind of flexibility to your skill practice.

Importantly, I want to point out that eating skills are not diet rules. When most people start using a skill-based approach, what they're really doing is turning the skills into rules. They apply the same rigid perfectionist attitude, which leads to failure and quitting.

Look, I get it—we've been taught the rule perspective for decades. You may have done a half-dozen or more diets in your life. Rules are all you know. It can be hard not to pretend these skills are rules.

So remember, *rules and perfectionism are the path to quitting and failure.*

Skills and practice are the path to excellence.

Flexibility is the Goal

Flexibility gets a bad rap, mostly because people don't know how to teach it. They go from rigid rules to free-for-all, with nothing in between.

The thing about skills is they are always flexible. Let's take a look at a gym example:

Skill: The Hip Hinge

The hip hinge is a skill that shows up in multiple movements: kettlebell swings, deadlifts, Romanian deadlifts, trap bar deadlifts, single-leg deadlifts, Cossack deadlifts, side-lunge deadlifts. It can show up when we pick up a box when moving. It can show up when we lean in to listen to a friend tell a good story.

One skill, many applications.

At the same time, because it's a skill and not a rule, you aren't forced to use it at all times. You may find that when picking up a pencil off the floor, you don't need to use a perfect hip hinge. You might pick up a baby out of crib with a rounded back. It turns out, there are just as many situations where it's appropriate not to use the skill as there are situations where it is.

PLAYING BASS LIKE FLEA

I have a client who's a musician. He once told me he wants to be able to use eating skills like Flea, the bassist of the Red Hot Chili Peppers, plays bass. Flea clearly has the skills to hit the right notes and play a tune, but he also has the flexibility to go off the pattern. He can solo. He can add extra notes. He can skip notes. He flows. Part of his artistry is knowing when to play on beat and when to play behind the beat.

Flea has flexibility. And flexibility is hard.

By hard, I mean it takes more skill practice. Often when we learn a new skill, we learn it in one specific scenario, like putting the fork down between bites…at lunch… at work. As we get better, we can generalize that skill to multiple scenarios. We can put the fork down between bites at lunch at work; we can put the fork down between bites at lunch on the weekend with our kids; we can put the fork down between bites on date night; we can put the fork down between bites at the backyard Bar-B-Que.

With practice, we're able to first build the skill and then to generalize it to different situations.

With a lot of practice, we know when we can even not pay attention to the skill at all. It's like Flea knowing if he hits a certain number of notes, we get the song. Sometimes he can drop the notes, and it sounds cool and we still get it.

The height of flexibility isn't just knowing how to use a skill in multiple situations, but to be okay with *not* using the skill at times, with no fear of "blowing it" or worrying if you're capable. Flexibility means knowing you have the skill, and are able to choose to use it when you want.

This hinges on your personal values. You may clarify your values, and find you want to use skills most of the time. But there are other times when you don't want to use the skills, like at your grandma's 100th birthday party with relatives you haven't seen in decades. You can forget about all of the skills, be with your family, and nothing changes in your skill practice the following week.

Most people agree, the kind of people they really want to be have that flexibility, and still eat in line with their values.

You only need to fear flexibility if you haven't clarified your values, and have no skills you've practiced. If you've practiced skills, you can always rely on them.

If you've clarified your values and found values like family and longevity and socializing and joy, you prob- ably want to be able *not* to focus on skill practice every minute of your life.

If you've clarified your values, and found values like health and fitness and vitality and self-care, you probably want to use your skills most of the time. If you've found some combination of those values, you see a healthy and complete life includes all of those at different times, in the amount you get to determine.

People who are flexible and know their values don't have free-for-alls very often. That's not Flea playing a song; that's like smashing your bass onstage. In reality, you want to play a million songs in your life. Some will be fast and some will be slow and some will be more and some will be less.

Similarly, you'll eat a million meals in your life, and some will be more and some will be less and some will be social and some will be goal oriented, and all of those will show up on a continuum—that's flexibility. Make sure those experiences of the eating skills showing up differently in different contexts fit your values.

Rules don't work because a chocolate chip cookie at your favorite bakery with your friends really *is* different from a chocolate chip cookie when you are bored in the middle of the afternoon. Splitting a bottle of wine on date night really *is* different than having a couple of glasses of wine because you had a bad day. Having a plate of spaghetti for dinner on your first-ever trip to Rome really *is* different from having a plate of spaghetti for dinner because you don't feel like cooking.

The thing that's really amazing about Flea playing bass is he's paying attention to the song, the other musicians, and the audience, and plays what fits the best right then. Flexibility in eating skills more than anything is about paying attention to the food, the situation, and the people you're with, and applying the skills as they make sense right then.

SAYING YES SOMETIMES AND NO OTHER TIMES

People really complicate flexibility. It's really as simple as saying "yes" sometimes and saying "no" other times.

The rigid diet person thinks:
I have to say 'no' all the time!"

Meanwhile, the stress eater thinks:
"I have to say 'yes' all the time!"

The answer for both is in the middle. The way to gain flexibility is simply to practice—sometimes—the opposite of what you mostly do now.

People fail at diets over and over again because they truly believe it's about saying "no" all the time. Then, when they break down and say "yes" to a treat, they have a free-for-all and eat like it's their last-ever shot at food.

People who stress eat are equally rigid. They believe the only fix for stress or negative emotions is to eat a treat. Because they only have one response to a situation, they have no control.

FLIP THE SCRIPT

It should be obvious by this point that rigidness (aka failure) is a practice. On the inverse, flexibility (aka success) is also a practice. Possible situations might include:

THE PERFECTIONIST/DIETER NEEDS TO PRACTICE SAYING "YES"	THE STRESS EATER/SWEET TOOTH NEEDS TO PRACTICE SAYING "NO"
Is it my grandma's 100th birthday? Maybe I should try saying "yes" to birthday cake.	Is it the 17th office birthday cake this month? Maybe I'll say "no."
Is it date night? Maybe I'll try saying "yes" to a glass of wine.	Am I stressed out from a long day at work? Maybe I'll say "no" to a glass of wine and go for a walk instead.
I'm at my favorite bakery in the world, with literally the best cake ever. Maybe I should try saying "yes."	I walked by the break room at work and there are some crappy baked goods. Maybe I'll say "no."

DIETING AND THE LOSS OF CONTROL

For the chronic dieter, saying yes might be scary. You may have a feeling you'll lose control if you ever say yes. Keep in mind, the primary reason you lost control in the past was because you set things up in a no-win situation. Every time you had a treat, it meant total failure…so you went all-in. After all, it would be the last time, and you'd never have that treat again.

Doesn't it sound a little silly?

If you can say yes to a treat when you really want it, it takes away that horrible, constantly building fear of missing out. You can evaluate when it really matters and you really want it—like when it's date night—versus when you don't really care.

The hard work is in thinking things through.

Hint: Don't think about if it's "worth it;" think about *if it fits your values*. Look at your personal values.

When people tell me they skipped the birthday cake at their grandma's birthday, I know that's a choice that doesn't fit anyone's values. That's such terribly sad diet rule-making, and has nothing to do with the kind of person anyone really wants to be.

THE STRESS EATER OR SEE-FOOD EATER HAS TO EAT

For the stress eater, saying yes is the only way to fix feeling bad. Or, seeing a food you like means you have to eat it. The practice to fix this revolves around noticing you're using food to fix non-food problems. You've practiced using food as the only solution for so long, you can't imagine there's anything else.

Turning it all around is mostly a matter of practicing trying other things. You'll start distinguishing cravings and stress from hunger. It requires eating a real meal when you're really hungry. Another part of turning it around is adding coping skills and real-life treats. Sometimes, it might be just as simple as going for a walk when you're sad.

Fixing this is a matter of practicing saying no to food sometimes and saying yes to something else, be that self-care or acceptance. For more on acceptance, see The Wise Five section, pages 199–244.

RIGID EXTREMES VERSUS FLEXIBLE CHOICES

The least successful people in weight control tend to only make choices from rigid extremes. They pretend there are always only two options: the absolute most diet-y choice there is or just have whatever they want.

For example, people tend to act like they can have full-sugar soda or water, with no choices in between.

WHAT TO DRINK				
RIGID	Full sugar soda	Pretends there is nothing in between		Water
FLEXIBLE	Full sugar soda	Diet soda	Flavored carbonated water	Unsweetened tea	Water

The most successful people know any choice in the middle is better for their goals than full-sugar soda.

Sometimes they might still have full-sugar soda. Other times they might have diet soda. Sometimes they'll have tea. They have options. On balance, all of their middle options add up to better results than of the people who took an all-or-nothing approach.

EATING OUT		
RIGID	Burrito with rice, beans, cheese, tortilla, guacamole, sour cream	Pretends there is nothing in between	Bowl with chicken, lettuce, and rice

EATING OUT					
FLEXIBLE	Burrito with chicken, rice, beans, cheese, a tortilla, guacamole, sour cream, and salsa (no vegetables)	Burrito with chicken, rice, beans, cheese, a tortilla, guacamole, and salsa (no vegetables)	Bowl with chicken, fajita veggies, rice, beans, cheese, and salsa	Bowl with chicken, fajita veggies, lettuce, rice, and salsa	Bowl with chicken, lettuce, and rice

It works the same with eating out. Some of my most successful clients eat at fast-casual restaurants all the time. They know that wherever they go, there's always a continuum of options. They can sort out a healthy meal by what they choose.

They know anything in the middle has fewer calories, and can still be a filling and healthy meal they enjoy. They can always have one portion of carbohydrates, instead of the three that's normally served. They can always add vegetables. If it's a place that normally serves five servings of guacamole, they might skip the guacamole.

Over time, those middle options add up to better results. The people who take a black-or-white approach almost always fail in the end.

DIET SODA WILL NOT KILL YOU

A guy is 40 pounds overweight and drinks two or three full sugar sodas every day.

I say, "How about switching to diet soda? You could probably lose ten pounds just doing that."

He says, "No way; diet soda will kill you!"

That kind of black-and-white thinking is crazy. Of course, water is better than diet soda. But also, of course, diet soda is better than full-sugar soda. I've seen clients lose 15 pounds just switching from full-sugar soda to diet options. It's a better step along a continuum.

The more you can think in the world of *continuums*, the better you'll do.

I love that in *Original Strength*, Tim Anderson talks about "good, better, best." For most of us, doing something "good," is, well, good. We get so caught up in doing what's "best" that we miss out on opportunities to take useful, effective, and meaningful steps. Spend some time starting with good, and work your way up to better.

Don't get caught up on the idea that pure water would be best if you aren't ready to switch from full-sugar soda to water. Instead, take a step to good…maybe diet soda. Maybe better might be that fancy new flavored carbonated water. Or maybe better is lemon water or unsweetened tea.

Rigidness is thinking it's the best or nothing, which is pretty silly. Try to avoid rigid rules about what you "have to do." All of the perfectionism, the rigidness, the rules, the adherence to "best or nothing" are just excuses not to do the real work—doing a little better.

THINKING IS REQUIRED IN SAYING YES OR NO

It takes effort and thought to consider your values and make a decision about what actions fit the kind of person you want to be.

Only robots say no to dessert all the time. That's NOT the kind of person you or I want to be. I want to be the kind of person who says no when something sucks, and says yes when it's awesome.

You might want to say yes to a glass or two of wine on date night. You might want to say no to a glass of wine every night while you're making dinner. Or maybe you want to flip that. The cool thing is, you get to say.

The big thing with doing the thinking: Give yourself time to think. Wait for a couple minutes and actually think things over. Most people fail in these choices simply because they don't slow down and give themselves time to think.

YOU GET TO SAY

You get to pick and clarify your own values. You get to use your values to figure out what kind of person you want to be. You get to sort out what balance of "yeses" and "nos" fit the kind of person you want to be.

You get to say. Not me. Not the diet police. Not your parents. Not your spouse. Not your friend who's always failing at diets. Not your friend who's a personal trainer who has never struggled with food. Not the people in a magazine or on TV.

You get to decide what your values are.

Flexibility is simply practicing your values.

And the practice based on your values looks like figuring out when it fits to say yes and when it fits to say no. That practice looks like trying out saying no to see how it goes, then figuring out if you would do things the same or differently in the future.

Most people do well by starting with saying yes half the time and saying no half the time.

For the people who always say no, this gives them a lot of practice saying yes. For the people who always say yes, that's a lot of practice saying no.

Start with 50/50. Pay attention to how you evaluate situations and if you consider all of your personal values. Over time, you can change the ratio. But start with 50/50.

FLEXIBILITY AND WORKOUTS

Workouts are a little simpler. We're actually confronted with significantly fewer decisions in our workouts. We don't have people coming up to us during our workouts and offering us other workouts. We don't have to make workout decisions multiple times per day. Workouts are simpler.

But workout decisions still require flexibility.

FLEXIBILITY AND NOT GETTING HURT IN WORKOUTS

Usually when someone gets hurt in the gym, it's simply a lack of flexibility, but not physical flexibility such as tight hamstrings. Here we're talking about psychological flexibility—being able to adapt.

I've known trainees who've gone into the gym, knew their backs hurt that day and deadlifted anyway because it was in the program. They ended up hurting their backs more and having to take a couple weeks off or even to see a physical therapist. This kind of inflexibility always ends badly.

If your back hurts, flexibility might look like skipping deadlifts or switching from barbell deadlifts to single-leg or staggered-stance deadlifts if those feel good that day. It could be doing glute bridges instead. Flexibility is realizing there are multiple options for working around those little tweaks when you woke up feeling bad.

Flexibility with exercise includes knowing, even if a movement doesn't feel good one day, you can modify or work around it. That same movement might feel great the following week.

FLEXIBILITY AND YOUR SCHEDULE AND STRESS

It's cool to be real about your schedule and stress levels, and actually do fewer or shorter workouts. That's part of why we have three levels of volume. Regardless of the program you're on, it's okay to dial things back when you're getting crushed with work or family stuff.

Getting in part of a workout is always better than doing none. Some people fail because they adhere to a rigid standard of what a workout has to look like or feel like. They think it has to be the full workout as written or it isn't worth going to the gym at all. That's silly.

RIGID WORKOUT BELIEFS	FLEXIBLE, SELF-AWARE WORKOUT BELIEFS
My workout has to be at least an hour, or it's not worth doing.	Any amount I can get of my workout is cool. If I can only get 15 minutes today, that's much better than none.
I have to work out three times per week, or there's no point.	If my schedule is tough right now, it's better to get one or two workouts per week than none.
With young kids, I never have time to get a full workout. If I can't do it all, it just doesn't feel like a real workout.	Having young kids is tough. If I can get in a set or two of an exercise whenever I can, I know it all adds up.
I know I'm sick, but I have to get my workout, or I'm off schedule.	I really need to focus on getting better and taking care of myself. My workout program will be there when I'm not sick.
My shoulder hurts, but I really want to hit this pressing goal, so I'm going to work out anyway.	I know if my goal really matters to me, I need to take care of my body. Today, I'm going to skip pressing and just do everything else. If it doesn't feel better by next week, I'll go see a physical therapist.

FLEXIBILITY AND GRIT

Sometimes this comes down to doing what you said you would do, even if it doesn't sound fun. It can mean finishing the program you're on, even when you're bored with it, or doing the sets in the program because it's in the program.

If this seems like it's in contrast to the previous section, it isn't. Flexibility and not getting hurt means listening to your body, noticing when you're truly exhausted or when something hurts in a joint.

The flip side is having thoughts about not wanting to finish the program, or wanting to do different things, or feeling like things are not working, or whatever judgments you have in the moment. One is about listening to your body. If your body hurts, listen to it…trust it, stop. Change the exercises or call it done for the day. Listen to your body.

The other is about not taking every thought so seriously. Do the program as it's written because that's the program, not letting your feelings and thoughts make your choices for you—fickle as they are, like the weather.

"Grit" is doing something even after the excitement that started you on the program has run out.

I want you to listen to your body tell you how it's doing. Do the warmup and one set of each of the exercises and see how it feels. Do you feel weak or strong today? Are you moving well? Do you feel extra tight or loose in the mobility section?

Listen to your body.

- If your body feels awesome, trust it. Rock out on your program that day.
- If your body feels terrible, trust it. Chill back on the weight or the number of sets in your program.

Where grit comes in is in accepting it's normal not to want to do everything all the time, and doing what's called for anyway. I want you to expect your mind to give you thoughts that are sometimes helpful and sometimes totally unhelpful…and doing what matters to you regardless of your thoughts.

- If you have thoughts telling you to follow the program, and do the work, cool. Follow the program, and do the work.
- If you have thoughts telling you not to follow a program, sometimes that's to be expected. Acknowledge it's normal to have those thoughts. Follow the program, and do the work anyway.

People make the mistake of flipping this: When they feel motivated, they ignore their bodies and work out. But when they don't feel motivated, they listen to their thoughts and skip the training.

- Flexibility is about listening to your body and adjusting your workouts accordingly.
- Grit is about knowing it's normal not to feel motivated or want to do the work all the time, and doing the work anyway.

One is physical and the other is mental.

Flexibility means paying attention to your body and what it needs. An example might be doing one set of everything and seeing how it feels—including being willing to call it right there and go home if you feel terrible.

When you have grit, you'll take action regardless of whether or not you feel motivated. Grit is going to the gym even when you don't feel like it, so you can do that one set of everything to check in and see how you feel. You'll find that the days when you do or don't feel motivated often don't correlate with the days you feel strong after getting to the gym and doing a couple sets.

FLEXIBILITY WITHIN STRUCTURE

Flexibility is inherent *within the skills of the program.* You have options about how many skills to practice, which skills to practice, and how often.

But flexibility does not mean "do whatever you want." People often assume if they aren't dieting, there are no guidelines and nothing to track, and they'll just see what happens. This is chaos. If it works, it works by accident and not by design. If getting lean and strong just worked for you by accident, it's likely you wouldn't be reading this book.

That's why we have a program structure. You're setting up the boundaries of the game in such a way that they move you toward your goals and what matters to you. Within those boundaries, you have flexibility.

- On vacation, you might only practice the skill of putting the fork down between bites. When you get home, you might work on four skills. That's flexibility.

- When life is really stressful (see "green light, yellow light, and red light" life stress on page 235), you might only practice one or two skills. When things are going really well, you might practice four or five skills. That's flexibility.

- When things are stressful, you might use more guidelines. When things are chill, you could use more listen-to-your-body skills. That's flexibility.

In all of those cases, you have a ton of flexibility to make the program work with the normal ebbs and flows of life. But you still have enough structure that you'll make progress. You still have a plan—you're still working a plan.

RIGID VERSUS FLEXIBLE WORKOUT THOUGHTS

RIGID WORKOUT BELIEFS	FLEXIBLE, SELF-AWARE WORKOUT BELIEFS
If my form isn't perfect, there's no point in doing it.	The best way to get better is to practice. If something feels awkward and weird now, I can practice more, read more about it, and get better over time.
I really want to hit this deadlift goal. I have to deadlift heavy this session, even though I slept poorly, and my back hurts today.	I really want to hit this deadlift goal so I'm going to make sure not to hurt myself. Today my back hurts so I'll try staggered-stance deadlifts, or maybe single-leg hip thrusts. I'll do whatever feels good. I know next week I'll probably feel fine again and deadlift heavy then.

RIGID WORKOUT BELIEFS	FLEXIBLE, SELF-AWARE WORKOUT BELIEFS
Only circuit training "feels" like working out so I'm going to change the program and do all of the sets back to back.	I know this is a strength program, and I'll get stronger following the program.
I'm bored with this program. I'm going to change some of the exercises so it's more fun.	It's normal to get bored sometimes, but I'm going to follow the program. It changes every four weeks anyway.
I wasn't sore after the last workout so I'm going to change everything.	Soreness isn't a gauge of progress. I know I'll be sore sometimes and not others. Any time I'm not sure if the workout is hard enough, I'll re-evaluate and see if I'm lifting enough weight in each exercise.

You'll see that rigid thoughts can come up around both ignoring your body and thoughts about not following a program. It's normal to have those thoughts; most people have rigid responses to those thoughts. Notice when you're having rigid thoughts, but take action that's flexible anyway.

META-SKILLS RECAP

The three Meta-skills are about how to be successful at the eating skills and workout programs.

META-SKILLS		
IF/THEN PLANNING	VALUES	FLEXIBILITY

If/Then planning is the *most effective* way to change behavior.

Your values are *why* you change behavior.

Flexibility is the key that makes all of this *work in real life*.

You now have three of the pieces of the *Lean and Strong* system: You know what not to do; you know what to do, and you know how to make that happen.

In the next two sections, we're going to go deeper into the psychology required to be lean and strong for life.

CHAPTER SIX
THE TEN TURNING POINTS

Don't Diet	
	The first step is to stop doing things that don't work
Eating Skills and Workout Skills	
	What skills to practice to get lean and strong
Meta-skills	
	How to practice the skills so your practice is successful each week
The Ten Turning Points	
	How to think about your skills practice so you don't sabotage your results every eight weeks
The Wise Five	
	Understanding intrinsic motivation and how it works

We've discussed the small picture (skills) and the medium picture (Meta-skills). Now it's time to get big picture into mindset.

THE TEN TURNING POINTS

My most successful clients figure out The Ten Turning Points after about a year of practicing the skills. When they discover these turning points, *nothing is ever the same for them.* They reach a new level of food skill and strength practices.

Each of these turning points is a complete shift in context. You could call it a paradigm shift. You could call it a change of mindset. These are the things people understand that help them lose weight faster, and never regain it.

For lifetime results, these turning points are mandatory.

*"One's mind, once stretched by a new idea,
never regains its original dimensions."*
—*Oliver Wendell Holmes Sr.*

From contextual behavioral science, we learn the context—the meaning and the reason—you have when taking an action can change the quality of that action and the amount of wellbeing you derive from it. These ten points are the context that encompass your skill practice. While your skill practice doesn't change, these turning points mark a paradigm shift in how you approach your practice.

A couple years ago, I got this genius idea (sarcasm) that if these are the turning points everyone figures out after a year, why don't I just tell people ahead of time? It's a little silly I didn't figure it out sooner. Then, it took me a year to catalog all of them from my client notes. After that, I began telling my clients about them during coaching calls, and having them deliberately practice them. I know this is a shock: People made the turning points much, much faster when they knew about them ahead of time.

The way you're going to approach these is to pick one each month and write it on your tracker. Just reflect on it for ten seconds each time you fill out your skill tracker. Think about it from time to time as you practice your skills during the day.

That's all—that's all it takes.

THE TEN TURNING POINTS

1. The difference between unsustainable and unrealistic practices versus personal failure

2. Engagement—flow—goldilocksing versus doing too much all of the time

3. Perfectionism versus excellence and self-compassion

4. I do it because it feels good versus meeting a societal standard

5. This is what practice looks like in real life versus an idealized fantasy

6. Intuitive eating versus objectification

7. Feel your feelings versus fake optimism and forced positivity

8. Weight loss comes from self-care versus punishment

9. The paradox of values versus goals

10. Leanness and strength as a part of life versus the fix for all of my life

THE TEN TURNING POINTS UNDERSTANDING WHAT WORKS VERSUS WHAT CAUSES FAILURE	
WHAT WORKS	**WHAT FAILS**
Understanding unsustainable practices	Assuming personal failure
Practicing excellence and self-compassion	Practicing perfectionism
Engagement, flow, goldilocksing	Too much all of the time
I do it because I feel good	I do it to meet a societal standard
What practice actually looks like	Idealized fantasy of what dieting and workouts look like
Intuitive eating	Objectification
Feel your feelings, and be a human	Good-vibes-only trap causes emotional eating
Weight loss comes from self-care	Weight loss comes from punishment
Value based practice	Excessive focus on goal achievement
Leanness and strength are an important part of my life	Leanness and strength will fix all of my problems

UNSUSTAINABLE PRACTICES VERSUS PERSONAL FAILURE

Most people have had so many diet failures, they've started to think the problem is them. They might decide they don't have enough willpower, or they have a broken metabolism, or any other reason to explain why they can't be successful at getting lean or strong.

I'm not saying there aren't differences. There really are genetic differences, differences in your previous relationship to food, and definitely differences in habit and skill proficiency. These affect both getting lean and getting strong. It isn't that everyone is the same…but everyone can get lean and strong. If it takes you a little longer than someone else, that's okay as long as you're doing the things that are effective, and your results are moving in the right direction.

That's the thing: Most people aren't doing things that are effective. As we covered in the first section, *Don't Diet,* diets just don't work for the majority of people. They're too much; they're too rigid, and they're unnecessarily strict. They're unsustainable for nearly everyone.

The problem is, we've been told over and over, if we failed at a diet, it's a personal failing—that it's some sort of lack of character. That totally sucks.

The truth is, we need a better plan. We need eating skills and eating guidelines. We need The Meta-skills to be successful at the skills. We need to know The Ten Turning Points and we need The Wise Five. We need better than what the diet world has given us.

Most people fail because dieting is unsustainable.

When people fail with skills, it's usually because they turned the skills into diet rules. They're forgetting all the turning points and all The Meta-skills and all The Wise Five. Then they feel like a personal failure again.

Diet thoughts include thoughts about this being a personal failing. It's normal to continue to have diet thoughts, especially for the first few years you practice skills. You'll be having thoughts about this being personal failure for years after you've already gotten good at the skills, and hit all your goals. These diet thoughts fade *very slowly.*

When you have thoughts about weight being a personal failure, notice those as diet thoughts. Go back to your Meta-skills, especially If/Then planning and flexibility. Take a look at which turning points you're ignoring, particularly goldilocksing.

It's never a failure of who you are. It's always a failure of your plan. So…adjust your plan.

Stop trying to turn the skills into diet rules. Stop trying to turn the skills into diet rules. Stop trying to turn the skills into diet rules.

I know I'm beating a dead horse, but it happens with every client…every time. The first three months are always spent practicing skills, doing well, then turning the skills into diet rules and hitting a wall. When people hit a wall, they feel like a failure.

Look, always remember section one, *Don't Diet.* When you feel like a failure, it's usually that you're trying to diet again. It's not that you're a failure; it's that dieting is unsustainable for most people. When you make mistakes, that's okay; learn from them and plan.

Do things that are sustainable, like Skills, Meta-skills, The Ten Turning Points, and The Wise Five.

PRACTICING PERFECTIONISM VERSUS PRACTICING EXCELLENCE AND SELF-COMPASSION

Sarah Campbell, one of the most amazing eating skills coaches I know, puts it best:

> *"Part of perfectionism is about unrealistic self-expectations.*
>
> *This produces self-generated internal pressure.*
>
> *What happens when something is squeezed too much?*
>
> *It is immobilized.*
>
> *This is how perfectionism leads to feeling stuck."*

Perfectionism is fantasizing that we're perfect robots. When we can't measure up to robot perfection, we quit. There's a deep unwillingness to *do work* in spite of our own humanity and imperfections.

If you practice perfectionism, you're setting yourself up for failure. On some level, you already know that. You can look back at every time you've ever said, "I blew my diet," and know that was the point you decided to just eat whatever you wanted. But that's not what we tell ourselves about perfectionism.

There's an interesting lie about perfectionism—that it's about having a high standard. Unfortunately, nothing could be further from the truth.

1. **Perfectionism is about fear of failure.** In research, perfectionism is defined by people quitting something when it's hard. Perfectionism in nutrition simply means "I quit my diet a lot." People who practice perfectionism are practicing quitting when they hit an obstacle or when they make a mistake. Perfectionism is the actual practice of quitting. [212,213]

2. **Pursuit of excellence is about wanting to increase skills.** Pursuit of excellence is defined by how much someone practices. It simply means "I get in lots of food skill practice." When people practicing excellence make a mistake, they know making mistakes is part of the process of learning. They just practice again at the next meal. The pursuit of excellence is a philosophy of repeated practice.

RESEARCH ON PERFECTIONISM

A meta-analysis looked at 57 studies on perfectionism in multiple domains, including work, school, and sport. Perfectionism was found to be strongly related to burnout, whereas the pursuit of excellence was related to lower risk of burnout. Perfectionism led to burnout, as noted by emotional exhaustion, disconnection, and eventually a reduction in skill level. [214]

Multiple studies have found that perfectionism is a driver of binge eating and that perfectionism predicts four different binge triggers. [215]

It's also been found that a continuum of perfectionism predicts a continuum of disordered eating from normal to disordered eating symptoms, to a full-blown eating disorder. Essentially, the greater the perfectionism, the worse the disordered eating symptoms. [216] It's even been found that perfectionism is a predictor of disordered eating in athletes. [217]

A review, *Disordered Eating in Women: Implications for the Obesity Pandemic*, cited the "Perfectionism Model of Binge Eating." The model is fairly large and complex, with multiple factors, but the most simplified version is this: Perfectionism predicts body dissatisfaction, and body dissatisfaction predicts binge eating. [218]

One really interesting study looked at binge eating, perfectionism, and basic psychological needs. You might not be familiar with the term "psychological needs," but you will be after reading the last section of this book, The Wise Five. Researchers found, first, binge eating was predicted by not having psychological needs met—and they looked at the first three needs of The Wise Five. Then, they found perfectionism predicted binge eating, which we already know. They found the two were related—perfectionism actually thwarts people's ability to get their basic psychological needs met. It fits all of the other perfectionism research that perfectionism lowers wellbeing, but this was particularly cool because it studied the three psychological needs we'll look at later in the book. [219]

The big takeaway is perfectionism with food and body is related to both restrictive dieting, followed by snapping and over-eating (the Diet Cycle of Failure). Also, when people were perfectionists about their bodies, they'd eat to cope with the dissatisfaction. Either way, perfectionism is bad for getting lean and strong.

Perfectionism Research Covered Earlier in *Lean and Strong*

All of the research in the first section of the book (page 23) on perfectionism and how it's related to worse performance and worse wellbeing still applies. Perfectionism does not mean pursuing excellence—it's more like avoiding shame and guilt.

Also, *all* of the research presented in the "Don't Diet" section of the book on black-and-white food rules and how they're the number one psychological predictor of weight-loss failure apply to food perfectionism. Essentially, having to maintain perfect diet rules is an extremely robust predictor of failure.

The big takeaway on all of the previous research is, if you relate to your food in perfectionist ways—labeling some good and some bad and rigidly adhering to only eating what's good—you're going to snap and overeat. On top of that, your relationship to your body and your wellbeing will go down after every cycle of restricting and failing.

PERFECTIONISM AS A PRACTICE

No one is born a perfectionist. Perfectionism is a practice. The more you practice perfectionism in food, the more practice you get quitting a diet.

Remember: *"Perfectionism" is just practicing quitting a lot.*

If you've been a perfectionist in the past, don't worry—you can practice something new!

Practicing excellence is simply a matter of practicing your eating skills. When you mess up—and everyone messes up—just practice again at the next meal. When you hit an obstacle, you can strategize how to overcome that same obstacle in the future. Then, you can practice that strategy. When your life situation gets stressful, you can step back your practice because you know that any practice is more effective than no practice.

The pursuit of excellence is just practicing your eating skills. Regardless of what comes up, just practice at your next meal.

IT'S NOT THE "GOOD" WEEKS THAT PREDICT SUCCESS; IT'S THE "BAD" WEEKS

Success isn't about how "perfect" the good weeks are. Trying to have perfect weeks is a complete waste of your time. I hate to break it to you—you're a human. Humans aren't perfect—none of us.

The game worth playing—the game that will make the biggest difference in your results—is how good the "bad" weeks are. You want to look at how much practice you get *after you mess up.* What's important is how much practice you get at starting back on your skills the next meal, no matter what happened at the previous meal.

The person who has perfect weeks always has complete quitting weeks.

The person who continues to practice during the tough weeks is the person who never has to worry about gaining weight ever again. This is the person who gets better faster. This is the person who is in pursuit of excellence.

PURSUIT OF EXCELLENCE

The pursuit of excellence is simply practicing and studying. Someone who pursues excellence knows anything worth doing is going to include messing up. That's how practice works.

When people practicing perfectionism make a mistake, they quit. They fail.

When people practicing excellence make a mistake, they keep practicing. They reread parts of this book. They do a new If/Then plan to sort out how they can improve their practice in the future.

Excellence is about practice. Excellence requires making mistakes. Excellence is about learning from mistakes and practicing again.

Practicing perfectionism is a three-step process:

1. Practice
2. Make a mistake
3. Quit, fail

Practicing excellence is at least a seven-step process:

1. Practice
2. Make a mistake and learn
3. Practice
4. Make a mistake and learn
5. Practice
6. Make a mistake and learn
7. Become excellent at that skill!

Excellence comes from making mistakes and learning. Learning research shows very clearly that people learn the best from repeated practice where they're allowed to make mistakes and learn from them.

PERFECTIONISM VERSUS SELF-COMPASSION

It turns out, self-compassion is the primary difference between perfectionism and pursuit of excellence.[220] Self-compassion is a healthy way of relating to ourselves and can be cultivated with practice.[221]

People are often afraid self-compassion will lead to not taking action, but this isn't the case. Instead, the self-care involved in self-compassion can drive us to practice our eating skills and workouts.

Self-compassion allows us to be human, without beating ourselves up about it. We allow ourselves to make mistakes without excessively dwelling on them. In practice, self-compassion means having all of these things show up, feeling the feelings that come with them, and then moving on.

SELF-COMPASSION	LACK OF SELF-COMPASSION
Allowing ourselves to make mistakes, and moving on	Dwelling on or beating ourselves up about mistakes, stopping the action
Allowing ourselves to be human, and practicing anyway	Intense pressure to be a perfect robot that stops us from taking action
Allowing ourselves to have feelings like sadness, frustration, and guilt that come and go in their own time, and practicing anyway	Suppressing feelings like sadness, frustration, and guilt because robots don't have feelings, then exploding, and eating our feelings

Perfectionism is an unwillingness to *do work when confronted with our own humanity*, abdicating responsibility every time we see evidence of being human.

Self-compassion is acknowledging it's normal to make mistakes. It's normal to have all kinds of emotions, like happiness and sadness. It's normal to have cravings. It's normal to make mistakes. It's normal to feel guilty about making mistakes.

When we have self-compassion, we notice all of our judgments about ourselves are just thoughts. We've had judgmental thoughts—maybe for decades—and we know it's a habit. We don't need to debate them; we don't need to figure out if they're true or false; we don't need to fight or change them; we don't need repeat them over and over and beat ourselves up. We can notice that these are just thoughts, and forgive ourselves when they show up.

The game we are playing is continuing to practice our food skills and workouts, simply because they're self-care.

Remind yourself that no matter how together everyone else looks on the outside, everyone has human issues. People have different easy and hard things in their lives, but everyone has hard things. Everyone makes mistakes. We're all human.

There are three ways to approach self-compassion:

1. My thoughts are just passing events (defusion, described on page 91).

2. I can respond to those thoughts with kindness.

3. Imperfection and mistakes are a normal part of everyone's lives.[222]

SELF-COMPASSION	PERFECTIONISM
My thoughts are just passing events.	My thoughts are always true.
I can respond to my thoughts with kindness.	I must beat myself up about my thoughts.
Making mistakes is normal and human. Everyone makes mistakes.	Making mistakes means I suck at this. I'm terrible. Everyone else has it all together.

IT'S OKAY TO HAVE PERFECTIONIST THOUGHTS

We live in a world that gives us consistent perfectionist messages about diet. The entire diet world is about perfection. That's why it always fails.

Here's where you need to make an important distinction: Just because you have perfectionist thoughts doesn't mean you need to act on them. You don't need to quit and fail because you had a perfectionist thought.

Thoughts and actions are completely unrelated:
- You can have a perfectionist thought and quit.
- You have a perfectionist thought, but practice excellence in spite of it.

The path to failure is having a perfectionist thought and then *practicing* quitting. It's not the thought that's the problem; it's taking actions like restricting, then taking actions like quitting.

The path to excellence is having a perfectionist thought, and then practicing your skills anyway. It's messing up and not being perfect, and simply returning to your practice. You can keep practicing excellence even when you have perfectionist thoughts.

This probably flies in the face of everything you've ever heard. Your favorite diet guru probably preaches that you need to "change your thoughts!" I'm here to tell you that you don't need to change your thoughts. In our diet-obsessed world, it's weird not to have perfectionist thoughts, so don't be surprised if you keep having them.

If you've practiced perfectionism for years or decades, you're going to keep having perfectionist thoughts for a few years.

The goal is to practice excellence—to keep practicing your skills even after mistakes, even when you have perfectionist thoughts.

PERFECTIONISM IN WORKOUTS

In workouts, perfectionism usually shows up like this: "I didn't have time to do a full workout, so I didn't do anything."

Each workout does not have to be a perfect masterpiece. Life doesn't always allow for the full workouts we plan—sometimes we get off work late; sometimes kids have a surprise project they need help with; sometimes there's an important errand we have to run. That's life. We don't always have time to do everything exactly the way we plan.

Doing one set of everything is fine. If you have time to go to the gym, do one set of everything and go home. That's the pursuit of excellence. Most of the time, do the whole workout, but sometimes just get in whatever you can.

Doing a modified version of the workout at home is fine. If you have home gym equipment, but you prefer to work out at a gym, that's good too. You can do most of the workouts at the gym, but once in a while do a home workout. Get as close as you can with the weights and the bands you have and a pullup bar. If you have to change the rep range a bit, that's okay. Once in a while, get in whatever you can.

Doing one or two workouts a week is fine. I've seen people quit a program because they didn't get a third workout in a week. That's absurd. I've had dozens of clients who never worked out more than twice per week. I've had clients who worked out once per week when life got stressful. Something is always better than nothing.

Doing the workout split up over the day is fine. I've had many clients who were moms with kids under four do these workouts split up over the course of a day. Of course, you have to have kettlebells and bands and equipment at home. It's okay to do a couple sets literally whenever you get a spare minute. They don't have to be back to back and they don't have to be in one continuous session. You can split them up over the course of the week or over the course of a day, however it fits into your life.

A workout doesn't have to be perfect. You can do what you can with what you've got. It all adds up. Excellence is doing what you can, whenever you can.

PRACTICE COMPARING YOUR CURRENT SELF TO SIX MONTHS AGO

Humans usually spend too much time looking at the ideal of perfection and not enough time looking at progress from the start. This isn't even a glass half-full thing; this is a "paying attention to all of reality" thing.

Regularly compare your skills practice to six months ago, a year ago, or before you started your skills practice. Look at the real progress you've made—look at the actual increase in frequency of your skill practice.

If you've been keeping your skill and workout trackers, you can look back and see how far you have progressed. This is real, objective data about the progress you've made, and it's smart to reflect on it every couple weeks. It's a good way to remind yourself that—even though you were never perfect—you've been making real, measurable progress in your eating skills and strength.

ENGAGEMENT—FLOW

Skills, Challenge, and Growth Engagement—Flow

The coolest thing about a skills-based approach is that increasing skills is naturally engaging. Humans thrive on playing games at the edge of our skill level.

One reason people tend to fail at diets is because the diet presents a win or lose scenario that's unnecessarily above their skill level. While the game itself is above their skill level, they can hold on with hustle and sheer force of will for a short period of time—usually 8–12 weeks. Then they crash and burn; it all feels overwhelming, and is no longer engaging.

From game theory, we know three things:

- A game that's too easy is boring.

- A game that's too hard is crushing.

- A game that's just right is engaging.

That's why we goldilocks our skills—so we can have just the right practice, right at the edge of our skill level, where it's challenging, engaging, and we learn and grow.

The right level is somewhere around 85% success.

If you're practicing your skills and hitting what you set out to do eight or nine out of ten times, that's probably perfect. If you're getting ten out of ten every time, it might be too easy. If you're getting five out of ten, it's too hard. Optimal learning happens somewhere between eight or nine out of ten.

But that's what's so cool about skills. Skills are goldilocks-able!

Here are some examples:

Increasing Protein

- **Good:** Try to have a source of protein at every meal.

- **Better:** Have one serving of protein at every meal.

- **Best:** Check protein guidelines for strength on page 77. Have that many servings of protein per day.

Moderating Carbohydrates

- **Good:** Have one source of carbohydrates per meal, instead of multiple sources of carbohydrates.

- **Better:** Limit to two servings of carbohydrates per meal.

- **Best:** Limit to one serving of carbohydrates per meal.

Moderating Fat Intake

- **Good:** Have one source of fat per meal instead of multiple sources of fat.

- **Better:** Limit to two tablespoons of fat per meal.

- **Best:** Limit to one tablespoon of fat per meal.

Plating Balanced Meals

- **Good:** Plate one balanced meal per day.

- **Better:** Plate two balanced meals per day.

- **Best:** Plate three balanced meals per day.

Eating a Meal Every Four to Six Hours

- **Good:** Notice when having snacks between meals. Limit having snacks to only 50% of the times you feel a craving for them.

- **Better:** No snacks between meals during the hardest time of the day for you (between breakfast and lunch, lunch and dinner, or between dinner and going to sleep).

- **Best:** No snacks between meals. Eat a meal every four to six hours.

Feeling True Hunger 30 minutes before eating

- **Good:** Notice hunger before eating sometimes.

- **Better:** Notice hunger before eating at lunch and dinner.

- **Best:** Notice hunger and wait 30 minutes before eating, at lunch and dinner.

Distinguish Between True Hunger versus Stress, Boredom, Cravings, and Tiredness

- **Good:** Use the three questions to determine if it's hunger or not.

- **Better:** Use the three questions to determine if it's hunger or not. Fifty percent of the time, if it's not hunger, don't eat a snack or treat. Instead, accept it's normal to feel that way, or put in some self-care to address the issue.

- **Best:** Use the three questions to determine if it's hunger. If it's not hunger, either accept it as normal, or do self-care to address the issue.

Plating Balanced Meals

- **Good:** Put the fork down between bites for a few bites, for one meal per day.

- **Better:** Put the fork down between bites most of the bites, one or two meals per day.

- **Best:** Put the fork down between bites most of the bites, two or three meals per day.

Defusion from Unwanted Thoughts, Feelings, and Cravings

- **Good:** Notice thoughts as thoughts and emotions as emotions.

- **Better:** Journal about thoughts, use the feelings wheel, or use the weather metaphor, or think about the movie *Inside Out* to get distance from thoughts. Fifty percent of the time, practice your eating skills even in the presence of thoughts.

- **Best:** Journal about thoughts, use the feelings wheel, or use the weather metaphor, or think about the movie *Inside Out* to get distance from thoughts. Practice your eating skills even in the presence of thoughts.

Waiting Ten Minutes before Having a Snack

- **Good:** Wait ten minutes before having a snack.

- **Better:** Wait ten minutes, think about what you really want, and choose to have the snack 50% of the time, and not have the snack 50% of the time.

- **Best:** Wait ten minutes, think about what you really want, and choose to have the snack only when you truly feel hungry, or the snack is awesome, and you really want it.

Those are examples of how some of the skills and guidelines can be goldilocksed. Many people don't initially think what falls under "good" counts as practicing the skill, yet for many people, starting at "good" is what makes the whole system work. Building up a solid volume of practice at "good" allows us to progress to "better."

Most people will find they make solid progress toward their goals at the "good" and "better" levels. It doesn't require being at "best" to make progress; it just requires doing a step more than you used to do.

I definitely want to acknowledge some amazing people who had a huge impact on how the goldilocksing section looks. First, I love how Tim Anderson and Original Strength frame their system as good, better, and best.

Second, I love how Jennifer Campbell, Annie Brees, and Lauren Koski at Balance 365 frame their food habits with level targets. Thinking through the genius of both of their systems gave this section a much clearer framework for how to present goldilocksing.

There many variations you can do with each skill. You can practice at certain times of day. You can practice in certain situations. You can practice during one or two meals per day. You can practice more frequently during the week and less frequently on the weekend.

You get to set up the game—set it up so you're successful about 85% of the time, right at the edge of your ability level.

MOST PEOPLE DO TOO MUCH

The standard diet approach is that every meal must be perfect. This is, of course, far beyond most people's skill level. They struggle at a game that's far too hard… until they break.

It's silly.

If you grew up playing the Nintendo Entertainment System in the late '80s, you remember *Super Mario Brothers*. You were Mario, a plumber, fighting a turtle/dragon thing named King Koopa to save Princess Toadstool. Makes perfect sense.

Like most video games, it starts off fairly easy and gradually increases in difficulty at each level. People get to play through until they hit the edge of their skill level. Playing more often, people get better and can get further and further in the game. This is just like what we do with eating skills.

Most people don't know there was a sequel in Japan called *Super Mario 2* that was completely different from the *Super Mario 2* released in the USA (it was released in the US a few years ago as *Super Mario: The Lost Levels*). It was an expanded and much, much more difficult version of the first *Mario Brothers*. You had to time jumps perfectly; there were power-ups that powered you down, and even weather patterns that could blow you off cliffs.

It was so difficult that Nintendo of America thought it would kill their entire market. It started off too hard, and only got harder from there. It was too much, and it wasn't fun because it of that. People hated it, and quit playing almost immediately. Nintendo of America waited a couple years until a more playable game was created, and released that as *Super Mario 2*. The goldilocksed *Super Mario 2* was extremely popular, and they've been able to make a dozen more appropriately challenging games since.

That's where dieting is similar: It's too hard of a game. You're jumping into the hardest level right from go. In fact, you're jumping into a game that's harder than you *ever* need to play to hit your goals. It's needlessly, pointlessly difficult, and we want to stop playing. Because of that, most people don't stay engaged long enough to develop any skills.

WHY IT'S CALLED GOLDILOCKSING

In *Goldilocks and the Three Bears*:

- Papa Bear's porridge was too hot;
- Mama Bear's porridge was too cold;
- Baby Bear's porridge was just right.

We want to find the porridge that's just right.

If you've ever played tennis, you know it's the most fun to play with someone right at your skill level, where you don't know who's going to win and each player has to play their best. It's no fun if you play someone much better than you and you get crushed. Similarly, it's boring to crush someone much worse than you. Tennis is the most fun when it's goldilocksed just right.

Eating skills are like that. When you do too much, it's demoralizing. When you do too little, it's boring. When you goldilocks it just beyond your comfort zone, it's fun and engaging.

People love to grow. People love games that are appropriately challenging. Set up your food skill practice each week with a reasonable goal.

Sometimes that means practicing a skill one meal per day.

Sometimes that means practicing a skill two meals per day.

Sometimes that means practicing a skill three meals per day.

Sometimes that means practicing one skill at a time.

Sometimes that means practicing two or three skills at a time.

Sometimes that means practicing four skills at a time.

Set it up so it's challenging and fun.

GOLDILOCKSING WORKOUTS

We goldilocks workouts three ways:

1. Which program we choose;

2. Which movements we choose;

3. How much weight we use.

The Program Volume

The reason the workouts have different levels of volume (low, medium, and high) is so you can goldilocks the total amount of work. If you're new to working out, low is probably a good place to start. If you've been working out consistently for years, high is a good program to use.

Intermediate or Advanced

If you're new to working out, the advanced program will be needlessly complex. It'll be a lot to manage different weights for each exercise on different days. On top of that, you might not be strong enough and the weights aren't very different between the low-rep day and the high-rep day. If you're new, you'll get the best results on the beginning program.

If you've been working out for a while, the intermediate or advanced programs will be better for your results. On top of that, you'll enjoy the extra complexity of managing different weights on different days. You should be strong enough that the low-rep and high-rep days feel like entirely different workouts.

What Movements to Choose

If you're brand new, we might do all double-leg exercises. Just learning the basic movements, like squatting and deadlifting, is enough. Single-leg exercises and the balance required for them might be too much.

After a month or two, we want to start working in some staggered-stance and single-leg exercises. The balance challenge will be appropriate, and we can work on things like balancing left-to-right leg strength.

Similarly, a person might have a hard time learning kettlebell swings on their own if they've never done Romanian deadlifts. It might be smart to take out the speed and timing components of the swing and work slowly on the same hip-hinge pattern.

How Much Weight to Use

I've gotten many messages from people using inappropriate weights. On one hand, people tell me the programs are boring or easy, so they just need to increase the weight they're using. On the other hand, people tell me the workouts completely and totally destroy them; they need to decrease the weights.

Your workouts should all be appropriately challenging. Increase or decrease the weight accordingly.

Each exercise in each workout should feel like it's about the same level of difficulty as all of the others in the workout. Increase or decrease the weights as needed.

I DO IT BECAUSE IT FEELS GOOD VERSUS MEETING A SOCIETAL STANDARD

Most people initially start practicing the eating skills and doing the workout programs because they want to meet a societal standard of looking good.

That's okay. It's totally normal to want to look good. It's normal to want to feel good in your clothes.

The problem is when it becomes all about the status that comes from looking good and trying to look good for other people. As we'll cover in the last section, The Wise Five, you'll discover status and looking good for other people are some of the lowest and weakest forms of motivation. It's not that they don't work; it's that they don't work for very long.

However, if you practice your eating skills and workout programs simply because you feel good doing them, you'll do them forever. This is one of the most important turning points, because it's completely self-reinforcing.

When people start to practice their eating skills simply because they like the way their body feels eating like that, they'll eat like that for life.

When people practice the workouts simply because they like the way their body feels when they work out regularly, they'll work out for life.

Somewhere between three and six months of practicing the skills, everyone starts to love the way they feel. When they mess up and overeat, they don't like that overstuffed feeling and the sluggishness that comes with it. At this point, they're practicing the skills for their own sake.

This a profound shift as the practice becomes its own reward. It's self-reinforcing.

When you do the practice because it feels good, you want to keep practicing. When you keep practicing, you get all of the results you want.

The way to add this extra level of motivation is to start paying attention to how you feel.

After workouts, ask yourself how your body feels. After stopping when full, ask yourself how you feel. Pay attention to how these affect your mood and energy level over the course of each week. Notice when they make you feel better.

It's totally okay to have thoughts about status and looking good. It's sometimes even okay to be motivated by those. Just make sure to reflect on how the eating skills and workout programs make you feel.

THIS IS WHAT PRACTICE LOOKS LIKE IN REAL LIFE VERSUS IDEALIZED FANTASY

Often, people assume leaning up looks like dieting. Similarly, they assume getting stronger looks like boot camp workouts, powerlifting, or bodybuilding.

In reality, most of getting lean and strong looks like working on The Meta-skills, The Ten Turning Points, and The Wise Five.

This freaks people out because they think they're working on the wrong things. It doesn't look like the social media stories or the videos they've seen on TV. But the tools that work for the people for whom getting lean and strong is easy are different than what are needed for the people for whom getting lean and strong is hard.

- When leaning up is easy, dieting and counting calories really does work. That's nice for them, but that's not us.

- When leaning up is hard, people need the Skills, Guides, The Meta-skills, and The Wise Five.

- When getting strong is easy, they can do almost anything. That's nice for them, but that's not us.

- When getting strong is hard, people need to work on Skills, The Meta-skills, Programming, and The Wise Five.

Normal Obstacle:
It's Not Exciting Anymore

It's normal for people to stop doing the skills after two to three months. Some people stop because they're bored. Some people stop for no reason. Everyone who does the skills work gets results, so it's weird people stop while getting results…but they do.

I've seen it so many times, it no longer freaks me out. So, look, when you're one or two months in and you stop doing the skills for a week, nothing is wrong. There's a really easy fix—start doing the skills again.

Not being excited about the work is okay. Practicing the skills while not being excited is part of how this looks in real life.

Normal Obstacle:
Life Stress

Everyone freaks out when they start a diet, but then something in their lives changes. Either their work schedule ramps up or a community commitment starts demanding more time, or there's something they need to do for the family. Life stress increases, and they can't maintain their "diet." They're so used to diet rules, they think if they do less than the full rules of the program, they're "off." This program isn't like that.

Just do fewer of the skills and guides. Work out less. Goldilocks things down from "best" to "better" or "good."

The difference between none and two workouts per week is much bigger than the difference between two or three workouts. The difference between working on none and two eating skills is much bigger than the difference between working on two or eight skills.

Don't fall into the trap of doing nothing because you can't do everything.

The people who do something are those who are the most successful. Dial things back. Do one or two skills, and do a couple short workouts. That's it. Goldilockings is what practice looks like in real life.

The trick is to always do *some*.

Normal Obstacle:
Vacations

People also flip out about vacations. Usually, all I suggest is to eat slowly and stop when full. Eat whatever you want. But you don't have to eat to the point of feeling gross. Eat the great food; eat slowly, enjoy it, stop when full.

Going on vacation and working on some but not all of the skills is okay. Coming back and working on more is okay. That's what practice looks like in real life.

Normal Obstacle:
I'm Not Doing Enough

We've been programmed to think diets are about starving and suffering and workouts are about sweat and puke. We almost never feel like we're doing enough.

You might have a history of dieting such that these skills feel "too easy." I've had clients majorly disturbed because it didn't feel like suffering. And this is while those clients were getting results. They were losing weight and getting stronger, but were still concerned they weren't doing enough.

Stop romanticizing suffering. Just do the simple things that get results.

We think this work is doing heroic feats of suffering. Nothing could be further from the truth. The work is doing the skills three months from now when it's no longer exciting. The work is doing it when you don't want to. The work is simple skill practice over time. Do what's effective.

Having it not produce enormous amounts of suffering is okay. Just mundanely practicing the skills and getting results is enough. That's what this looks like in real life.

Normal Obstacle:
I'm Not Losing Weight Fast Enough

Shows like *The Biggest Loser* taught us we should be losing ten pounds per week. Gym challenges tell us we should be losing two or three pounds a week. Your friend who cut carbs lost eight pounds the first week… or whatever. We've all heard these things: lots of weight loss, really fast.

And, you've probably done those yourself. You've lost weight fast, and gained it back faster. Thus, again, we have the diet cycle of failure.

My weight-loss clients typically lose about two pounds per month. That's a half-pound per week, which sounds boring. No, it's losing 26 pounds per year, which is amazing.

They lose that half-pound per week, and they lose it for life.

They never have to worry about gaining that back. They could lose 30 pounds in a year. And they never have to worry about that weight again.

I used to have clients lose two pounds *per week* and it quickly became a real grind. It often set them up for the diet cycle of failure. Now, my clients are stoked to lose two pounds per month, and lose those two pounds for life. They never have to worry about those two pounds again. It's done. It ends up being faster in the long run. It's like the tortoise and the hare.

While all the people in challenges sprint really fast and lose, you can do steady food skill and workout practice, and always come out ahead. It's always faster to do it right and lose it once. Eating skills allow you to move forward, and get better results every year.

It's always slower to sprint and lose a lot, then fail and gain back more. The diet cycle of failure puts you backward every year. It's a fast way to fail, over and over again.

Losing a couple pounds per month is awesome. That's significantly faster than everyone in the diet cycle of failure who never actually lose anything from year to year. According to CDC data, the average American *gains* one or two pounds per year.[223] Being able to *lose 26 pounds per year* and actually keep it off puts you ahead of everyone who's dieting.

Losing weight slowly and keeping it off isn't what you normally see on social media. That's okay. This is what it looks like in real life.

INTUITIVE EATING
VERSUS OBJECTIFICATION

Objectification thwarts intuitive eating, and that's something that shows up in research repeatedly, but isn't something people normally think about. Put simply, the more people take an observer's perspective on their bodies (and assume that observer's perspective equates to their self-worth), the less success they have at noticing their own hunger and fullness cues. And, the more people accept and have self-compassion for their bodies, the more effective they are at noticing their hunger and fullness cues.[224,225,226,227]

We're taught to identify our value with how our body looks (objectification), and then we're taught to ignore our body's hunger and fullness cues so we can change our bodies. Objectifying yourself is a huge barrier to doing the *listen-to-your-body skills*.

To revisit intuitive eating, intuitive eating is:

- Unconditional permission to eat when hungry and what food is desired at the moment—by not ignoring hunger signals or classifying food into acceptable and non-acceptable categories;

- Eating to satisfy physical hunger rather than to cope with emotional fluctuations and/or distress;

- Reliance on—reflecting an awareness and trust of—internal hunger and satiety cues to determine when and how much to eat.

It should be clear that intuitive eating is similar to the *listen-to-your-body skills*. Intuitive eating, as shown in the above-referenced research, is connected to self-objectification. They're inversely related:

- When self-objectification goes up, intuitive eating goes down.

- When self-objectification goes down, intuitive eating goes up.

This is the part where most trainers and fitness gurus tell you to start loving your body more. I think that's ridiculous. If you could flip a switch and love your body, you'd already have done that. And, if you had already done that, you'd likely already have a handle on intuitive eating skills and not need this book at all.

Nope. We're going the opposite direction. I don't want you to love your body; I want you to *have compassion* for your body. I want you to accept that our society is constantly giving us messages that we should hate our bodies. And because of that, I want you to accept that it's normal not to love your body every minute of the day. Have compassion for your body, and have compassion for yourself for having those thoughts programmed by the diet world.

With the amount of media messages telling us our bodies aren't good enough, it would actually be weird for you only to have shiny happy thoughts about your body. In our society, it's much more normal to have thoughts about hating it.

Now, I don't want you to hate your body either. I just want you to notice that thoughts about body dissatisfaction are normal. You don't have to fight them. You don't need to make them go away (good luck with that one!). You don't need to change them.

- Have compassion for your body.

- Accept that you're inundated with messages from the diet world about hating your body.

- Accept that it's normal to have thoughts emanating from the diet world.

- Give yourself compassion about having those thoughts.

THESE AREN'T THE ABSOLUTE TRUTH

These ideas of body dissatisfaction aren't true or false. They're just thoughts. We all have a million thoughts; some are useful and some aren't. We can work with the useful thoughts and can use them for planning and taking actions in line with our values.

The thoughts that aren't useful—those we can just let be. We don't need to fight or stop them or make them something else. We don't need to feed them or spin them over and over either. We can just let them be and go back to practicing our skills.

It's enough to notice these aren't your thoughts. They're thoughts from other people, and they aren't necessarily true. They for sure aren't helpful. Notice unhelpful thoughts as simply being unhelpful thoughts. Recognize it's normal to sometimes have unhelpful thoughts.

We have a million thoughts that come from diet world, completely objectifying us. They aren't our thoughts. They aren't true. But, because of the world we live in, your brain will remember those diet-world thoughts. Brains give us totally unhelpful diet world thoughts, and it doesn't mean anything at all. It's more a commentary on the books and magazines we've read, the things we've seen on TV, and the conversations we've heard. The thoughts *aren't from us*. They aren't true. They're just thoughts. Brains are just gonna be thinkin' thoughts.

Even when you have unhelpful thoughts, you can still take actions consistent with your values.

VALUED ACTION VERSUS LOVING YOUR BODY

What I like about taking actions that fit your values is it's something we can *do*. There's a contentment that comes from taking actions in line with our values.

Usually, the intuitive eating skills—the *listen-to-your-body skills*—match up really well with our values. And we can practice those skills whether we like our body today or not.

Tomorrow you may wake up and totally love your body.

1. Awesome. It's wonderful to feel like that— enjoy that feeling.

2. Practice the eating skills because they fit your values.

The day after, you may wake up and totally hate your body.

1. Bummer. That feels bad and it really sucks to feel that way. We all feel like that some days.

2. Have compassion for yourself for having objectifying diet-world thoughts show up in your brain. It's the world we live in.

3. Practice the eating skills because they fit your values.

Hating our bodies doesn't change anything. Loving our bodies may not change anything either. Practicing eating skills that fits our values does.

I don't have any skills up my sleeve that are going to make you love your body every minute of the day. But I do know practicing skills that fit your personal values will give contentment with your life and with who you are.

The contentment that comes from taking actions in line with your values will help you be more resilient so you can weather all of the ups and downs that come with body image. Self-compassion is a realistic and effective way to approach those ups and downs.

FEEL YOUR FEELINGS VERSUS FAKE OPTIMISM AND FORCED POSITIVITY

Fitness has a weird cult of optimism and positivity.

I've seen personal trainers and yoga teachers and boot camp instructors and social media celebrities all preaching things like "Be positive!" and "Good vibes only!"

I've seen them completely bulldoze a client's feelings when the client was legitimately having a bad day. At the absolute worst, I've seen trainers let other trainers get away with committing actual crimes because they "wanted to keep things positive."

Things aren't always great. People have real problems. Sometimes people get sick. Sometimes people die. Sometimes they get in car accidents. There are things that are legitimately terrible, and we need to let people know it's okay to feel bad when things are completely awful.

I know people usually have good intentions when they tell people they should be grateful, things will turn out great in the end, or they should look on the bright side. Well, my mom always said, "The road to Hell is paved with good intentions." And regardless of our intentions, forcing people to try to be happy and positive all the time is super unhealthy.

By telling them, almost explicitly, that they shouldn't feel their feelings, people start to think their feelings aren't normal. They might think other people really are happy every minute of the day.

TRYING TO BE ENDLESSLY HAPPY DRIVES EMOTIONAL EATING

Study after study has shown that if we try to suppress negative feelings, they rebound hard. We just end up with more of those feelings later. Let's take a look:

You may have heard of the study where they told people, "Don't think of a polar bear," and everyone, of course, thinks about a polar bear for the next five minutes.[228] More interestingly, they've tested the polar bear thought experiment with emotionally upsetting thoughts and found that the more emotionally upsetting something is, the bigger the rebound from thought suppression.[229]

One of the big sticking points, though, is that many people report they're initially successful with thought suppression. That's the thing—it's not that it doesn't work for a little while; it's that it works, and then you have a rebound where it's worse than before.[230] Suppressing thoughts or changing thoughts related to cravings can also work initially, and then cause a rebound where people eat more.[231,232,233]

Similarly, we find people who think they aren't supposed to feel sad are more likely to eat when they feel sad. They think their feelings are wrong, so they eat to numb them.

These same people—studies have shown over and over again—will then eat when they feel bad. Or, if they're able to suppress feeling bad and push their feelings away or bottle them up, they'll rebound and emotionally eat three times as much.

Optimism and Pessimism

New research in the world of positive psychology shows both optimism and pessimism can lead to worse life outcomes. Optimists tend to be terrible at planning and do stupid things...and they fail. Pessimists tend not to plan or try at all...and they fail.

Studies have shown that people who are too optimistic engage in fewer health behaviors,[234] are less likely to get more education about health behaviors,[235] and do less exercise when faced with a health issue that would be improved by exercise.[236] We've also seen that unrealistic optimists consistently underestimate the length of time or difficulty of completing tasks.[237]

On the following page, we'll look at optimism, pessimism, and reality.

OPTIMISM	PESSIMISM	OPENNESS
Everything will go well. This is not accurate.	Everything will go wrong. This is not accurate.	Sometimes things will go well. I should be present and grateful and enjoy that. Sometimes things will go wrong. I need to be able to accept that and cope with it in a healthy way.
I should be happy all the time. This is not possible.	I should be sad all the time. This is not balanced.	Sometimes I will be happy. I should be present and grateful and enjoy that. Sometimes I will be sad. I need to be able to accept that and cope with it in a healthy way.

With eating skill practice, optimists don't do If/Then planning very well—they say things like, "I'll just do better next time." That's not a plan; that's a wish.

When things don't go well and they fail, optimists get crushed. Since their optimism is tied to forced positivity, they end up trying to deny themselves normal human feelings of frustration. This usually leads to quitting or emotional eating.

Pessimists just don't ever try. Since action is the driver of results, they fail because they never actually start.

What's effective is simply realism:

It's normal to be happy sometimes,
and sad other times.

It's realistic to accept that things go well sometimes,
and go poorly other times.

If we expect to be happy sometimes and sad other times, we won't be completely caught off guard and emotionally eat every time we get sad. If we expect things to go well sometimes and poorly other times, we won't be shocked and crushed when we run into obstacles or even bad luck.

And…we get to really enjoy it when things are going well, and really be present and connected when we're happy.

The people who are the most successful are those who are able to weather all the normal human emotions. True empowerment is being able to take actions in line with your values, even when you have unwanted emotions.

Similarly, it's effective to expect that you won't actually be able to control everything. Expect things to go wrong sometimes, and you'll be able to keep taking actions in line with your values anyway.

When we can be open to the entire cornucopia of human experience, we're better able to cope with harder times, and we're better able to enjoy the better times. This openness to the positive and negative is considered a fundamental aspect of mental health.[238]

We're beginning to distinguish between things like positive growth versus positive thinking—these are massively different. Ironically, acceptance, openness, and coping strategies for both positive and negative experiences are a part of positive mental health.[239] The most effective path to positive growth is to embrace a balanced positive and negative thinking, optimism and pessimism, and to notice how often growth comes after hard, uncomfortable, and "negative" circumstances and emotions.[240]

We'll talk much more about this turning point in The Wise Five section on acceptance, pages 199–244.

WEIGHT LOSS COMES FROM SELF-CARE VERSUS PUNISHMENT

Another persistent myth in the fitness world is that we need to "punish" ourselves into losing weight. If we feel bad and suffer, we're doing it right.

It's ridiculous. Look, this is taking something that's supposed to be good for us and *deliberately* making it bad. People can only endure so much suffering. Eventually people get sick of punishing themselves and stop.

The only thing sadder than people who give up on punishing themselves are people who don't. There are people who are able to endure suffering for weight loss, sometimes for years. They derive no pleasure, no joy, and no satisfaction from hitting their goals. At best, they might—once in a while—get temporary relief. Constant punishment makes people exhausted and sad.

The irony is that self-care is the best thing we can do for weight loss. If we take care of ourselves by eating well and eating the right amount, we feel good. If we take care of ourselves by working out, we feel good.

This is a profound contextual shift:

— Some people might eat less because they hate their bodies; they count every calorie, thinking they need to punish themselves into losing weight.

— Others might eat less because they ate slowly, without distractions; they enjoyed their food more and noticed when they were full.

Two people can have the same result of eating less and losing weight, but have completely different experiences. One person is punishing his or herself, while the other is trusting and taking care of his or herself.

Similarly:

— Some people might do crushing workouts, always working to exhaustion and soreness, and think they need to punish themselves to lose weight.

— Others might do hard workouts because they enjoy a challenge; they like feeling strong, and feel like they have a better mood when they work out.

These people are both doing hard workouts, but they have completely different experiences. People whose context is punishment are more likely to hurt themselves because they're likely to ignore the body's warning signals. They're likely to work out when it's actually more appropriate to rest because they're afraid to stop the punishment.

The others will listen to their bodies because the whole point of a workout is to take care of themselves. These are two different contexts for the same action.

WORKOUTS AS THE MAGIC BULLET FOR STRESS

Let's get super nerdy for a second and talk about the stress system: the HPA Axis.

When your body senses a threat, the hypothalamus sends a hormone to the pituitary gland. The pituitary gland sends a hormone to the adrenal cortex. The adrenal cortex produces adrenaline (in the short term) and cortisol (in the long term). The system of the hypothalamus, pituitary gland, and the adrenal cortex is called the HPA Axis.

Cortisol is the hormone you've probably heard of causing multiple stress-related problems.

Exercise does this cool thing where beta-endorphins work on both the hypothalamus and the pituitary gland. The beta-endorphins effect both levels: Both the hypothalamus and the pituitary gland produce less of the stress-related hormones, causing a double drop in those hormones going to the adrenal cortex. It produces much less cortisol.

For the people whose eyes just glazed over, all you need to know is this: That's how the whole HPA Axis returns to normal. *Exercise is sort of like a reset for the stress response.*

Now, if there are any super-mega-nerds reading this, please forgive me for how much I simplified a very complex process. I just want to get the basic idea across.

If we're smart, we can use our workouts as self-care. We can use workouts to reset our stress response. It might be one of the most important pieces of our self-care puzzle.

IT'S NORMAL TO HAVE PUNISHMENT THOUGHTS

Like everything related to our diet culture, we've been given punishment thoughts so often—and we might have practiced them for years—that we're likely to keep having them for a while.

Like the previous turning points, just remember it's normal to have unhelpful thoughts—to think you need to punish yourself. You don't need to act on them. You can have those punishment thoughts, but still *practice self-care.*

Practice trusting your body. Practice self-compassion. Practice taking care of yourself.

Thoughts are just thoughts. You can notice you're having the thought that you need to do a workout to punish yourself for eating delicious food. Once you notice the thought, you can think about where it came from (the diet world), and you can move on. You can practice self-care in spite of unhelpful punishment thoughts.

SELF-CARE MAKES WEIGHT LOSS EASIER

People have an easier time losing weight when they go to sleep at the right time. That's self-care.

People have an easier time losing weight when they practice stopping when full—that's self-care too.

People feel better when they eat balanced meals; that's self-care.

People feel better when they work out—that's self-care.

MORE ABOUT SELF-CARE

There's much more about self-care in the skills section under the guideline of deliberate self-care on page 70. It will clear up some misconceptions about self-care; it'll describe the three kinds of self-care and you can figure out where you need more.

For now, just remember, the path to weight loss is self-care, not punishment. When you have punishment thoughts, passively disregard them and practice self-care anyway. When people listen to, trust, and take care of their bodies, weight loss is a natural result.

THE PARADOX OF VALUES VERSUS GOALS

There's a weird paradox between values and goals:

- People who focus mostly on values tend to hit their goals.

- People who focus exclusively on goals can sometimes sacrifice their values, or get discouraged by the slowness of progress, and fail to hit their goals.

I'm not anti-goal. Goals can be a fun, optional game to play if they're based on your values. And, they're affective if the way you play the game comes from your values.

Let's take a look at what values look like—values as compared to goals.

Values are always intrinsic. They're about being the kind of person you want to be, what you stand for, and what matters to you.

Goals are always extrinsic; they're about attaining something outside of yourself. They can become destructive when they're about symbols we think will make us look good to others. Goals can be healthy when they represent our core values.

We can divide each into three broad categories:

INTRINSIC META-VALUES	EXTERNAL META-GOALS
Contribution to community	Money and power
Skill building and growth	Physical attractiveness
Close relationships	Status-based popularity

Essentially, intrinsic meta values are all about meaning in life, about knowing what you stand for, and who you want to be. These are part of The Wise Five.

External meta goals are all about looking cool for other people. This is covered in the Failure Five.

Again, there's nothing wrong with having external goals. What's unhealthy is when you only have external goals with no connection to your intrinsic values.

What's *really unhealthy* is when your external goals actually take you the opposite direction from your intrinsic values.

This is a huge point in the diet and fitness world.

- If people say they value strength, but keep hurting themselves doing stupid challenge workouts

because they want to look cool on social media, their external goal is taking them away from what they value.

- If people say they value health, but starve themselves on stupid crash diets to meet a societal standard of beauty, their external goal is taking them away from what they value.

- If people say they value friendship, but can't go to social events because their elimination diet to get them abs by summertime is so restrictive they can't eat with other humans, their external goal is taking them away from what they value.

Let's take a look at possible intrinsic values people might have...and contrast those with extrinsic goals they might have.

INTERNAL VALUES	EXTERNAL GOALS
Health	Getting abs
Strength	Doing three pullups
Connectedness	Looking cool on social media
Family	Driving a luxury car
Contribution	Winning an award
Education	Getting a master's degree
Spirituality	Getting a promotion at work
Longevity	Deadlifting 275 pounds
Movement	Having a perfect butt
Loyalty	Having 10,000 social media friends
Adventure	Taking a tropical vacation
Mindfulness	Getting a perfect video of a cool trick
Courage	Winning a competition
Cooperation	Getting a title that denotes leadership
Patience	Completing a marathon
Authenticity	Getting thousands of likes on a picture

If you choose your goals before you understand your values, you've put the cart before the horse.

Your values are character strengths. If the character strength you want to express is wisdom, but you choose a goal that requires you do something stupid, like a crash diet or a cleanse, you have a terrible goal. And yet, this happens *all the time in fitness.*

Figure out your values first. Then, pick goals that would be the natural consequences of acting in line with your values.

Let's say you enroll in a master's degree program. An external goal would be to get the master's degree because it will look good for others. An internal value would be to pursue the master's degree because you value education.

In both cases, you're taking the same classes, but one motivation is external and one is internal.

Or consider deadlifting. On one hand, you could pursue a goal of deadlifting a certain amount of weight to look cool on social media. On the other hand, you could be consistent with your deadlift workouts because you value strength. Again, you might be doing the same workouts, but the motivation and the experience of doing the workouts is completely different.

GOALS NOT REQUIRED— GOALS CAN CHANGE

I've had clients who got awesome results, but never had goals. They just figured out their values and kept taking actions in line with them. Someone who values health, longevity, and mindfulness and who practices eating skills that match those values is going to settle at a healthy level of leanness and strength, even if that was never a goal.

It's the actions you take that matter. If your actions match your values, you're probably going to get everything you want anyway.

Sometimes the "goals versus values" concept throws people. But there are tons of examples of how we do really important actions without goals.

For example, an emergency room surgeon doesn't set a goal for the number of lives to save each day; that would silly. Instead, the docs value saving lives and they go in and do their best every day. Sometimes they save lives. Sometimes they fail. But neither result affects their commitment or their values. Their commitment to others is a character strength they want to do their best to express every day.

Or, consider being a parent. You don't set an age goal for your kids. You get up and be a parent every day because you value family and love. It's not about any desired outcome; you just do what matters to you.

It can take time and reflection for people to connect to their fitness this way, but that's all it takes. Interventions involving a simple weekly practice of reflecting on values and actions has been shown to be really effective.[241,242]

If you do set goals, make sure they match your values. And always make sure the value is more important than the goal.

If people value strength and do these workouts for six months with a goal of getting three pullups, that's awesome. If in six months, they decide a deadlift goal is a better expression of their value of strength than their previous pullup goal…that works too. Either goal—pullups or deadlifts—is an expression of strength. Either way, to match their value of strength, they're going to the gym three days per week. It really doesn't matter which of their strength goals they pursue because whatever the goal, they're working out. And working out is an action that matches their value of strength.

This is probably the opposite of everything you've ever heard about goals. I know, right? Sounds totally silly.

And yet, research on intrinsic motivation (specifically research based on Self Determination Theory) consistently backs up the power of things that are personally and internally meaningful for health and fitness motivation.[243]

1. Take actions related to your personal values.

2. If you set goals, derive them from your values.

3. Reflect weekly on your values and how your actions relate to them.

HEALTHY GOALS

Goals can be totally healthy and fun when based on your values, and when you stick to your values in the pursuit.

Most of my clients still set goals. And I'm getting paid to help them hit their goals so we make sure to do that.

The funny thing is, my clients who do food skill practice and workout programs consistent with their values always hit their goals.

There is a weird circularity to it:

— A healthy goal is a goal we'll certainly achieve if we're acting in line with our values.

— If we pursue a goal from our values, we get to become the kind of person we want to be.

— If we're being the kind of people we want to be, we hit our goals.

If your goals and your practice match your values, you hit your goals as a natural expression of being yourself. If you take actions in line with your values, you become the kind of person you want to be. People who do this make measurable progress toward their goals every week, simply by being themselves.

LEANNESS AND STRENGTH AS A PART OF LIFE VERSUS THE FIX FOR ALL OF MY LIFE

We're often marketed leanness and fitness as the ultimate fix for everything in our lives. Like, "If you just had abs, you'd be loved and adored by everyone!" After nearly 20 years of helping clients hit goals, I can tell you this: Fitness solves the problem of fitness…and nothing else.

Look, fitness is a really important part of life. It affects the things we can do for fun, like if we're capable of snowboarding or rock climbing or long hikes. Fitness effects how easy it is to shop for clothes, and how we feel in those clothes. Fitness can even affect how much energy we have throughout the day, and can reduce our stress level.

That's a lot of cool things fitness can do.

The issue is when people start to live as if "My life is going to be amazing once I have abs!" In truth, when you have abs, you'll have abs. It's cool, but it doesn't fix the existential hole many people feel. Having abs doesn't bring

meaning to our lives. Abs won't change the quality of our relationships. Abs don't make us better at doing things.

In reality, our lives have a mix of things that matter to us, like family, career, friends, hobbies, and communities we're involved in. Most of those will have a bigger impact on how we feel about our lives than will our fitness. If we clarify our personal values and take actions consistent with those values in multiple areas of our lives, that's a much bigger deal than having abs.

Another funny paradox is that people do better at getting lean and strong when they don't put leanness or strength on a pedestal. You'd think focusing your whole life around it would make sense, but in reality, the opposite is more effective. People do well when they fit their fitness into the patchwork of things in their lives that matter to them.

Getting lean and strong always comes back to skill practice. People practice their eating skills and do their workout programs more consistently when they're just one part of their lives. Ironically, when eating skills and workouts are just one of the things that matter to us, we end up being more consistent with our practice.

When people hold fitness up as the ultimate thing that's going to fix how they feel about themselves, the process gets emotional and puts their emotions on a rollercoaster. People get totally spun out if the scale doesn't change for a week. Often, people fall into perfectionist and punishment diet traps when they put too much value on fitness.

When people put fitness in perspective, as *one* of the things that matters to them, they usually practice *more often* and *more consistently*. If strength gains stall for a couple weeks, it's okay because they have other things in their lives that matter to them. What's more, they can easily see how continuing with their workouts reduces stress and makes them more effective at the other important things in their lives. Similarly, if their scale weight doesn't go down for a week, they don't freak out. They can see how practicing the eating skills gives them more energy and focus throughout the day and helps them be more connected to other things that matter to them.

When your eating skills and workouts support things that matter to you, you practice them a lot. And practicing a lot is where we get results.

THE TEN TURNING POINTS RECAP

The Ten Turning Points are the ten things you need to understand about getting lean and strong that will help you stop struggling, get results, and maintain those results for a lifetime.

THE TEN TURNING POINTS UNDERSTANDING WHAT WORKS VERSUS WHAT CAUSES FAILURE	
WHAT WORKS	**WHAT FAILS**
Understanding unsustainable practices	Assuming personal failure
Practicing excellence and self-compassion	Practicing perfectionism
Engagement, flow, goldilocksing	Too much all of the time
I do it because I feel good	I do it to meet a societal standard
What practice actually looks like	Idealized fantasy of what dieting and workouts look like
Intuitive eating	Objectification
Feel your feelings, and be a human	Good-vibes-only trap causes emotional eating
Weight loss comes from self-care	Weight loss comes from punishment
Value based practice	Excessive focus on goal achievement
Leanness and strength are an important part of my life	Leanness and strength will fix all of my problems

It's normal in our diet culture to notice yourself having thoughts that don't work. We've been programmed with them for years. We may even have practiced those thoughts for decades.

What surprises people the most is that we don't need to make those thoughts go away. We just notice ourselves having those thoughts, and remember they came from the diet world. Noticing the thoughts and knowing where they came from means we don't have to act on them.

We can have thoughts that don't work, but still take actions consistent with what does. Don't worry about changing your thoughts; just change your actions.

If there's a way to change your thoughts, it probably comes from first changing your actions. Change your actions for a few years, and your thoughts might change.

Most of my clients had been unsuccessful trying to change their thoughts in the past, and are usually really relieved to learn they don't have to. They can just let the diet thoughts be, while practicing taking action from The Ten Turning Points.

The Ten Turning Points remind us to:

1. Notice ineffective thoughts from the diet world. Accept them as simply being echoes from diet culture. Practice self-compassion when they show up. Let them come and go in their own time.

2. Take actions consistent with what works. You can take effective actions regardless of what thoughts show up.

CHAPTER SEVEN
THE WISE FIVE

Don't Diet	
	The first step is to stop doing things that don't work
Eating Skills and Workout Skills	
	What skills to practice to get lean and strong
Meta-skills	
	How to practice the skills so your practice is successful each week
The Ten Turning Points	
	How to think about your skills practice so you don't sabotage your results every eight weeks
The Wise Five	
	Understanding intrinsic motivation and how it works

In this section, we're going to dig deep into the psychology of intrinsic motivation. We're going to look at how research describes motivation. We'll cover what actually drives motivation—it's almost certainly the opposite of everything you've heard. Lastly, we're going to look at how to use that intrinsic motivation to rock your food skill practice, even when it's hard and uncomfortable.

If you've ever struggled with the motivation to do the things that fit your goals and values, this is the chapter you need to study.

DISCLAIMER

We're going to talk about psychology and motivation in this section. It all comes from research into health behaviors and behavioral weight loss based on Self Determination Theory and contextual behavioral science.

Of course, if you go to a clinical or counseling psychologist and are instructed to approach things in different ways from how they are presented here, always follow the advice of your mental health professional. These are just recommendations on what's most effective for changing health behaviors for people in the general population.

PRACTICING THE UNCOMFORTABLE

The major stumbling block most people run into with eating skills is being uncomfortable.

Maybe, even though you've failed at 15 diets, you feel *comfortable* doing another one. Another diet feels familiar and you like the idea of it. Even though you know another diet is going to fail, it's something you already have a lot of practice doing. You might find yourself wanting do the diet again just because it's what you know the best.

Eating skills, on the other hand, are super *uncomfortable!* It's all new. You don't feel good at it yet. Sometimes you're even unsure if you're doing it right. Plus, you keep reading about new diets, and they all sound magical.

To get good at eating skills, you're going to need to spend some time doing them while they are uncomfortable.

You'll have to lean on your personal values. You're likely to find the eating skills fit your values. Dieting, on the other hand, might strongly violate some of your values. We'll continue to do more values work in this section, and you'll be able to see how you can use your values as the foundation of your motivation.

Unfortunately, as you start to look at and use your values, your practice will look like this:

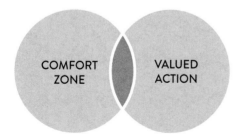

The eating skills that fit your values are way outside your comfort zone. Most of your food skill practice will feel uncomfortable. It's going to suck.

That being said, even while it feels uncomfortable, you'll be getting results. As long as you practice, you'll get results.

After a year of practice—often long after you've hit your goals—it'll start to feel more comfortable:

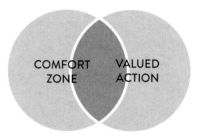

In the beginning, we need to create the psychological conditions in which you're able to do things that fit values outside of your comfort zone.

You'll notice, after a year of practice, many more of the things you value are within your comfort zone, but many still aren't.

The ENTIRE GAME is to get good at doing things that are currently uncomfortable.

Many of the things that are meaningful are uncomfortable at first. Growing and changing and trying a new approach is going to be really uncomfortable. Everything is uncomfortable when it's new.

I love the way gymnastics and movement coach Carl Paoli put it: "The goal is to chase the best way, not the most familiar way."

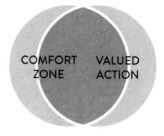

With practice, your valued actions around food become a lot more comfortable. That's the cool thing about practice. But I also want to be really clear about the kind of time frame we're talking about: Expect it to be years before this feels comfortable, before it becomes your new normal.

At that point, you'll find it's easy to maintain the results you've gotten. You'll be better at the skills; you'll be comfortable with them, and you'll even feel like doing the skills is simply an expression of who you are. Now you never need to worry about regaining weight again. You have those skills for life.

It's likely you'll spend a year of practice with many of the skills being fairly uncomfortable.

I want to say this again: *You can hit all of your goals* before you get really comfortable with the skills. As long as you're practicing, you'll get results.

You can get the results just by practicing.
You can get the results just by practicing.
You can get the results just by practicing.

It doesn't need to be perfect to work. It doesn't need to feel comfortable to work. You just need to be doing the practice.

Feeling comfortable likely won't come until *after* you've already gotten all of the results you want.

Leanness Results =
Uncomfortable practice

Comfort with Eating Skills =
Lots and lots and lots of uncomfortable practice

Don't worry; it will all be worth it. And, I'm going to give you all the tools you need to be successful practicing while it's uncomfortable.

THE DEFAULT SETTING OF MOTIVATION

The default setting for human beings is to look for motivation from one of two places:

1. **Reward or punishment;**

2. **Contingent self-esteem or guilt.**

Both are valid forms of motivation, but they're the forms of motivation that come with the lowest enjoyment and lowest wellbeing. They're the forms of motivation where the satisfaction is fleeting when you hit a goal. Blink and you'll miss the feeling of accomplishment. They're the kinds of motivation that really suck.

The feelings of accomplishment disappear so fast that people immediately lose motivation. Often when people hit a goal, they either quickly set a new and bigger goal, or they give up completely.

Setting a new and bigger goal sounds like the right thing to do, but it's really just getting on a hamster wheel. You end up running from one goal to the next and being shocked every time hitting the goal wasn't enough to change how you feel about yourself or your body.

Spoiler: The existential crisis that wasn't fixed with hitting the last goal won't be fixed by hitting the next goal.

- Punishment loses motivation the second the whip stops cracking;

- Reward loses motivation the second a reward is attained;

- Contingent self-esteem fades within weeks of hitting a goal;

- Guilt, which in the short-term motivates, turns into shame…which de-motivates.

You need to create a smarter plan. In Self Determination Theory, the motivations are lower on the self-determined side. We have 30-plus years of research showing that the more you pull from the less self-determined side, the weaker the motivation is, the faster the motivation fades, and the less satisfaction and wellbeing you derive from hitting goals…if you ever hit them.[244]

SELF DETERMINATION THEORY'S FOUR KINDS OF MOTIVATION			
← MORE EXTERNAL		MORE INTERNAL →	
Reward or Punishment	Contingent self-esteem or Guilt	Goals derived from your values	Values integrated into your sense of self

YOU HAVE TO WATCH OUT FOR *CONTINGENT SELF-ESTEEM* BEING YOUR ONLY FORM OF MOTIVATION.

Contingent Self-esteem
Being motivated by avoiding guilt and/or attempting to meet a societal standard or comparison

We all want to believe we'd finally feel worthy and good enough and loved and adored if we hit the right fitness level. We're preprogrammed by social media and TV—and often our friends and family—to believe that's the truth about life.

Contingent self-esteem is the default setting in the fitness field. We are always swimming against that current. If you don't intervene with your values, you will always backslide into feeling like fitness goals will give you self-esteem.

I'm going to give you some radical advice: Give up the pursuit of self-esteem and simply practice things that matter to you…and get better at them. Trade the endless and slippery pursuit of trying to feel great about yourself all the time, for the simple contentment that comes from doing things that matter to you, day in and day out. Take pride not in social comparison, but in your own progress and skill development.

Business philosopher Jim Rohn used to say: "The good will always be attacked. The weeds will always attack the garden."

It's like that with motivation; we have to find better motivation, and we have to defend it.

A BETTER PATH: SELF-DETERMINATION

On the flip side of punishment/reward and contingent self-esteem, we have more self-determined forms of motivation. These are much more robust, and they last longer.

- Goals that align with your values: Doing things that relate to a personally meaningful goal or value;

- Values integrated into your sense of self: Taking actions that are based on clarified values, integrated with your sense of self, and matter to you to express the kind of person you want to be.

On the following page, you'll see what that usually looks like in fitness.

SELF DETERMINATION THEORY'S FOUR KINDS OF MOTIVATION			
← MORE EXTERNAL		MORE INTERNAL →	
I work out so I can have a cookie afterward. or If I miss my workout, no carbohydrates tomorrow.	I work out to meet a societal standard of beauty. or I work out so I don't feel guilty.	I work out because I have a goal that aligns with my value of strength.	It's deeply important to me to be strong. Working out is an expression of being the kind of person I want to be.

At this point, you can probably see how you may have pulled from different forms of motivation at different times in your life. You might remember times when you tried to motivate yourself with rewards or punishments; that worked for a little while, and then it really started to suck. You might also remember times you worked out so you didn't feel guilty or because you wanted to meet a societal standard—and how completely miserable that was.

We know the left side of the chart are things that totally blow. It's okay to pull motivation from them once in a while or in the beginning, but they're too horrible to use as your only form of motivation.

You need motivation that doesn't suck: You need to add intrinsic motivation. Intrinsic motivation comes from clarifying your personal values.

A TALE OF TWO CLIENTS

SUSAN	MELISSA
Uses punishment and guilt as motivation Practices diet rules Repeats the diet cycle of failure, over and over again for decades. It gets more difficult every time, and she regains more weight, every time.	Uses her personal values for motivation Practices eating skills Eating skills get easier every month. She gets results every month. The whole process gets easier every year. Eventually, the eating skills and her leanness and strength are just an expression of who she is.

Your personal values and intrinsic motivation are related to three things:

- Autonomy
- Competence
- Relatedness

In Self Determination Theory, these are called "basic psychological needs." If you build these into your food skill and workout practices, you'll create the conditions to motivate yourself.[245,246]

Just remember:

- External motivation is the motivation to use if you want to repeat the diet cycle of failure.
- Internal motivation is the awesome kind of motivation you want to use for your Lean and Strong food skill practice and workout practice.

I'm going to give you a framework for making intrinsic motivation work for you. It's called the "*Lean and Strong Wise Five*."

THE WISE FIVE

Here we're going to dig into the psychology of intrinsic motivation when doing things outside your comfort zone.

This is the 30,000-foot view of weight loss. It isn't as immediately accessible as the earlier skills and Meta-skills. It won't change your relationship to your food and workout practice as immediately as The Ten Turning Points. This is the big picture. It's worth having this in the back of your head and reflecting on this from time to time, because this will change your relationship to your body, to fitness, and to food.

I realize at the ripe old age of 41, I'm probably too young to write anything "wise." Fortunately, none of this came from me. This all comes from either Self Determination Theory (SDT) or contextual behavioral science (CBS). Self Determination Theory gives us the science of intrinsic motivation. Contextual behavioral science gives us the skills for doing things that are hard and uncomfortable.

There are currently a half-dozen bestsellers on book shelves based on SDT or CBS. One of the best known is *Drive* by Daniel Pink, which is based on SDT. While I love his metaphors for SDT, I think he messed up a couple parts of it. Even so, it's amazing he got SDT into the hands of managers everywhere. *Emotional Agility* by Susan David, another huge business book, is based on CBS. It's rad that SDT and CBS are showing up in business books, but it's way past time we started seeing both in the fitness world.

The first three elements of The Wise Five are from SDT. Self Determination Theory has more than 30 years of extremely robust research behind it; I didn't invent it, but I'm smart enough to use what works.

1. **Autonomy**—We're going to call that "values."
2. **Competence**—We're going to call that "skills."
3. **Relatedness**—We're going to call that "connect."

The second two elements come from CBS, specifically Acceptance and Commitment Theory (ACT). They're actually one construct—psychological flexibility—but I've found my clients have an easier time applying them when we split it into two separate ideas.

1. **Psychological flexibility**—We're going to split that in two, and call it "acceptance" and "committed action."

We now have five evidence-based tools from psychology. They have a few decades of research behind them. Some of the research, like the research on psychological flexibility, have had major increases in the quantity of studies that have come out in the last three years that specifically relate to weight loss.

We're in the rare position where we have extraordinarily well-established tools, and their application to weight loss is cutting edge.

USING THE WISE FIVE

THE WISE FIVE— THE PURSUIT OF THESE IS ALWAYS CONSTRUCTIVE
VALUES
SKILLS
CONNECTION
ACCEPTING THOUGHTS AND FEELINGS
COMMITTED ACTION

Values—Base your food skill practice and strength training around your values.

Skills—Practice and get better at eating skills and strength training skills.

Connection—Listen to people, set healthy boundaries, be appropriately vulnerable, care about people.

Accept Thoughts and Feelings—Accept it's normal to have unwanted thoughts and uncomfortable feelings about food and your body. Don't numb thoughts and feelings with food. Feel your feelings.

Committed Action—Be willing to practice eating skills, guidelines, and workouts, even when it's hard, when you have unhelpful thoughts, or don't feel like it. Take action because it fits your values.

One thing you'll notice in this book is I teach a lot of things by using opposites. Sometimes, instead of explaining something to death, it's more effective to give you a comparison.

In this case, it's easier to understand The Wise Five when you can compare it to The Failure Five.

THE FAILURE FIVE VERSUS THE WISE FIVE

FAILURE FIVE	WISE FIVE
THE PURSUIT OF THESE IS OFTEN DESTRUCTIVE	**THE PURSUIT OF THESE IS ALWAYS CONSTRUCTIVE**
Reward or Punishment Try to control motivation	**Values** Practicing valued action
Self-esteem Try to control how I feel about myself	**Skills** Practicing skills
Status Try to control other people liking me	**Connection** Practicing prosocial behavior
Suppressing Unwanted Thoughts and Feelings Try to control thoughts and feelings	**Accepting Thoughts and Feelings** Practicing recognizing thoughts and feelings are normal
Force "Motivated" Thoughts and Feelings Try to control motivation	**Committed Action** Practicing taking action when it's hard

There are actually two different Failure Fives. This is the most common in the clients who hire me—it's The Failure Five related to *control*. There's another Failure Five related to *giving up* and we'll cover that later.

This can be looked at as a continuum from too much, to just right, to too little...like the groups at the top of the next page.

CONTINUUM OF WISE FIVE		
Failure Five	**Wise Five**	**Unfulfilled Five**
Trying to force and control self-determination	Actual self-determination	Opting out or giving up on self-determination
"Too much"	"Just right"	"Too little"

THE FAILURE FIVE

REWARD AND PUNISHMENT

This is the lowest form of motivation. Trying to control motivation with rewards and punishment is marginally effective in the short term. In the long term, it makes people hate life.

It's so future-oriented, you miss out on the present. This is one of the ways you motivate yourself in the diet cycle of failure: "I hate my life right now, but everything will be magical when I have abs." Usually, people never make it to their goals using rewards and punishments.

Reward and punishment are the most fleeting of motivations. Blink away from the carrot for a second, and you lose motivation. The second the whip stops cracking on your back, you lose motivation. It just doesn't last long enough for you to integrate your diet rules into your life. It's a short-term motivation for a short-term diet that literally causes a diet cycle of failure.

Even worse, rewards and punishments make you resent the actions you're taking. A meta-analysis of 128 research studies showed that even if you like and value what you're doing, if you're given rewards and punishments, you'll start to like it less.[247] Whatever you enjoyed about it is replaced with greedy reward seeking. Whatever you found meaningful about it is beaten out of you with

punishment. You'll enjoy what you're doing less, and you even like yourself less for doing it.

If you've ever been in a situation where a reward seemed meaningful, it's because of what you were doing, the people you were doing it with, or the work and skills you were developing were meaningful.

If a reward ever worked, it's because The Wise Five was underneath it holding it up. The reward, then, was just a bonus.

SELF-ESTEEM

It's a trap to use your fitness to try to like yourself more. People who have gotten ripped abs or whatever they thought would be amazing usually find they don't like themselves any more than they did before. Instead of liking themselves, they got a status symbol. Since their abs didn't make them like themselves more, they try to use them as a status symbol to coerce other people to like them, which is shallow and ineffective.

Sadly, the pursuit of self-esteem has been shown to take away everything meaningful in life. Pursuit of self-esteem lowers your valued action; it reduces skill practice, and it can hurt relationships.[248] The pursuit of self-esteem leads us to do things that make us feel good about ourselves, and avoid things with the potential to make us feel bad. The result is, we skip the most important kinds of practice when we aren't yet or aren't immediately good at things. The result is less practice, which keeps us from mastery.[249]

Five studies, including a longitudinal (long-term) study, found that pursuit of self-esteem related to poorer performance and quitting in the face of challenges.[250] Recently, studies have been comparing three things:

- **Self-esteem:** How much I like myself, how much I think I'm better than other people

- **Self-compassion:** How accepting and kind I can be to myself

- **Self-efficacy:** How much I feel like I will be effective at doing a task

Empirical research shows that the pursuit of self-compassion is related to increased self-esteem and self-efficacy.[251,252] Self-compassion offers all the benefits of self-esteem, without disadvantages like self-evaluation and ego-defensiveness.[253] Most relevant to us, between interventions for self-compassion and self-esteem, self-compassion is much more effective at positively impacting body image.[254,255]

You may notice there's a sticky conundrum: There's a difference between having self-esteem and pursuing self-esteem. *Having* self-esteem is generally considered positive, especially if it comes from a history of skill building and valued action, though it could be argued that's actually self-efficacy and not self-esteem. *Pursuing* self-esteem leads to lower wellbeing and ironically, lower self-esteem.

Paradoxically, the pursuit of self-esteem tends to reduce valued action, reduce connection, and reduce skill acquisition.[256] Trying to control how we feel about ourselves is less effective than simply doing what matters to us, connecting with people who matter to us, and building skills.

To sum it all up, if you want more self-esteem, you get all of the benefits and none of the problems if you instead pursue skill building and self-compassion.

STATUS

"Status" is where you use your fitness to make other people like you. Unfortunately, this usually backfires. People mostly envy people with status, which is massively different than liking them.

People don't feel awesome about themselves when they're around someone flaunting their status. Take social media, for example. It's been shown that following social media accounts of people with "perfect bodies" lowers the follower's wellbeing, worsens body image, and increases disordered eating.[257,258] Essentially, if you flaunt your new abs as a status symbol, you'll make other people feel worse.

Most of the fitness field revolves around status as motivation, and it's just wrong. It's a poor substitute for having quality relationships. Status is another fleeting form of motivation.

Research shows that pursuit of status, wealth, and physical attractiveness relate to lower vitality, wellbeing, and self-actualization. Conversely, pursuit of self-acceptance, community contribution, and physical health are related to higher wellbeing.[259]

And, if you're wondering if performance goals are the answer to body image status issues, it turns out they aren't. Trying to look cool by showing off your deadlift or bench press numbers isn't any healthier than trying to look cool by showing off your abs.[260]

Like self-esteem, this is another place where there's a difference between possession and pursuit. The possession of status can be super useful in that it can open significant opportunities we wouldn't otherwise have. In fact, possession of status, close friends, and skill competence all predict wellbeing.[261] It's just that the *pursuit* of status leads to lower wellbeing. If it sounds like a catch-22, it's not. The alternative is to pursue skill building, connection with others, and community contribution for their own sakes…and you may get a degree of status as a byproduct.

Ironically, studies show that people often gain status through demonstrating abilities to contribute to, cooperate with, and be generous with the groups they're a part of.[262]

Basically, if status and looking cool for others is your *only* source of motivation for fitness, it'll be tougher to succeed, and will be really terrible for actually feeling good about yourself. The word "only" is key. It's normal to want to look good; it's even normal to want status. It's just that things will massively suck for you if that's the only thing you have to pull from for motivation. Balance these by pulling from your values and the inherent satisfaction of skill building. Ground yourself with a bigger focus on your connection and contribution to others.

SUPPRESSING UNWANTED THOUGHTS AND FEELINGS

This has a variety of looks, but the way it shows up most commonly in fitness is forced positivity and "good vibes only." People feel they need to be up and happy all the time, but the human brain just isn't wired for that.[263] It's normal to be happy sometimes and sad other times.[264]

The issue here is, people who think they should force happy thoughts and suppress unhappy thoughts eventually get smashed. You can only white knuckle happy thoughts for so long. Suppressing negative thoughts and feelings has a harsh rebound effect. Many people who struggle with overeating overeat precisely when they have these emotional rebounds. The research on suppressing thoughts and feelings, unsurprisingly, mirrors the research on suppressing cravings. The people who have the biggest emotional suppression are those who always overeat the most when they snap.

We aren't robots—we can't be happy all the time. Looked at from a healthier perspective, the entire cornucopia of human emotions isn't only normal, but part of the beautiful ride of life. People often bond strongly when sharing intense sadness.

We often learn the most from hard and uncomfortable circumstances. People find enormous meaning in doing something for someone else, even when it isn't fun, and they don't enjoy the experience.

It's okay to cry at a funeral with the people we love. It's fine for paramedics not to enjoy cleaning a wound, but to do it because they care about patient health. It's fine that you don't jump out of bed with excitement to go to work on Monday morning, but you go anyway to provide for your family. It's okay to feel frustrated when something doesn't go your way. It's normal to be exhausted after a long night of taking care of a sick kid. It's okay not to want to work out. It's really fine if you look at the lunch you packed and don't feel like eating it. It's normal to feel all of these feelings. Cut yourself some slack.

The biggest and most damaging lie is that you should feel excited about all of these things. You don't. You might have heard you need to change your thoughts so that you want to do all of those things. You don't. Remember Monday morning: You don't always want to go to work; you go anyway. You don't go because you convinced yourself to want to in the moment; you go because it matters.

People who try to force positivity have worse life outcomes. Even in positive psychology, they call it "the tyranny of the positive attitude."[265] Second wave positive psychology is about embracing all of life's emotions and having positive *outcomes*, not positive *feelings*. Some of the most important personal growth can come out of sadness, loss, and failure. Many of the most meaningful things in our lives aren't easy or fun.[266,267]

Emotional eating develops from a myth that we're supposed to be happy every waking moment. It often starts with feeling bad, having some comfort food, and then feeling a little better. Once in a great while, that's totally fine, but when this is repeatedly practiced, people start becoming afraid of feeling bad. After a couple years, they may try to numb *all* their bad feelings with food.

People who expect to be happy all the time end up being afraid of being sad or frustrated or anxious or stressed out. They end up running away from very normal and common parts of the human experience.

The goal, of course, is to feel and honor your feelings—to be a complete human. If we don't practice being with unwanted emotions, we're doomed to emotionally eat for the rest of our lives.

FORCE MOTIVATED THOUGHTS AND FEELINGS

This is a part of the previous section. The big lie here is that you need to make yourself feel motivated or excited about doing something before you do it.

This means, for example, trying to get hyped about working out before working out. On days you're able to get hyped, you work out. On days when you just don't feel it, you can't work out. Since you believe you should be able to get excited about working out and that you even *need* to get excited about working out, you're caught off guard when it doesn't happen. You end up skipping a lot of workouts.

The feeling of motivation comes and goes in cycles. Weather has been used as an example a couple times in this book—sometimes it's summer and sometimes it's winter. If you only work out in the "summer" when you feel like it, you're going to miss half your workouts. Motivation is always up and down, and you can't rely on it as an indicator of what to do.

It works exactly the same with food. People try to get positive about eating the lunch they packed, and when they can't decide they want it today, they'll eat something else. You can't expect to have the feeling of wanting to practice your eating skills every day; it's not normal and it's not human.

You don't need to control your emotions and thoughts before taking actions that matter to you.

CONTROL IS THE PROBLEM, NOT THE SOLUTION

People fail with The Failure Five because they think control is the solution. Unfortunately, if they review their history, they'll find that control has always failed them:

1. You try to control your motivation with rewards and punishments, and start to hate what you're doing.

2. In trying to control your self-esteem, you feel worse.

3. You try to control who likes you by status, and they are repulsed instead.

4. You try to control your thoughts and emotions; it backfires—you lose control, and eat to numb your feelings and thoughts.

5. You try to control your thoughts and feelings to get motivated, and end up not doing what matters to you when you don't feel like it.

Most people don't know what to do if they don't pursue more control. That's where The Wise Five come in.

MORE FAILURE FIVE RESOURCES

If you want to nerd out on The Failure Five, I recommend a few resources:

- In the book *Popular: Finding Happiness and Success in a World That Cares Too Much about the Wrong Kinds of Relationships,* Mitch Prinstein outlines the destructive impact of pursuit of status (like having abs) versus like-ability (like relatedness). Essentially, status can open some doors, but it mostly distances us from people. It reduces our relatedness to others, lowers our likeability, and can lead to worse life outcomes due to personality conflicts.

- Jennifer Crocker and Lora Park, in their article *The Costly Pursuit of Self Esteem* from *Psychological Bulletin* of the American Psychological Association, outline how the three basic psychological needs from SDT— autonomy, competence, and relatedness—are all thwarted by the pursuit of self-esteem. That pursuit of self-esteem actually lowers autonomy and meaning in life, reduces the amount of competence-building practice people do, and drives wedges between people's relatedness to other people.

- Russ Harris, in his book *The Happiness Trap*, breaks down how the pursuit of happiness is often destructive and unfulfilling. We actually want to practice openness to feeling; taking actions consistent with our values is what gives us a meaningful life.

- Itai Ivtzan, Tim Lomas, Kate Hefferon, and Piers Worth in their textbook, *Second Wave Positive Psychology: Embracing the Dark Side of Life*, outline how life is about meaning, growth, and relationships. Our ability to experience a full range of human emotions, including "negative" emotions like sadness, is an important aspect of health. Transformational growth is often the result of great adversity.

THE WISE FIVE VALUES

Values are the key to intrinsic motivation. When you identify your values and take actions in alignment with them (like food skill practice and workouts), you're being your best version of yourself.

Values are essentially just what matters to you, what you stand for, and the kind of person you want to be. We want our values to dictate the actions we take, regardless of how we feel. Practicing taking actions in line with our values regardless of how we feel is the practice of getting out of our comfort zone, beating emotional eating, and living a meaningful life.

Simply taking action in line with our values significantly increases wellbeing. We just need to do the values reflections described later in this section and line up our food skill practice and workout practice with our values. It helps to reflect on how our values and practices line up weekly.

SKILLS

Building skills over time is phenomenal for our sense of self. Instead of self-esteem, we build self-efficacy. Self-efficacy is our belief in our abilities…based on our practice. It includes seeing our skills build over time, and overcoming obstacles in our skill practice.

We get deep contentment and meaning from practice. Neuroscientists believe we're wired for "effortful practice," that our wellbeing increases when we do things that are hard and that matter to us.

Skill building is often difficult and involves overcoming obstacles, but is meaningful and rewarding. Getting better at food and workout skills changes people's relationships to their bodies, their trust in their bodies, and how they feel about themselves.

CONNECTION

In research, this is called "relatedness" or "being pro-social." Ironically, the way most people think they'll be liked from fitness status only comes from being a better friend. We get more social capital from being better listeners than we do from abs. We feel better about ourselves from setting healthy boundaries than we do from abs. And we have a higher self-concept from taking care of people we care about than we do from how we look at the beach.

Being cool to people, ironically, looks exactly like The Wise Five:

1. **Values:** Give people the freedom to pursue what matters to them; talk to them about what matters to them.

2. **Skills:** Support them in growing and skill building in things that matter to them.

3. **Relatedness:** Hang with people who care about you and who care about some of the same things you do.

4. Let people feel their feelings. Let them know their feelings are normal and okay.

5. Support people in taking actions on things that matter to them.

Here I'm adapting relationship motivation theory (a sub-theory of Self Determination Theory) and acceptance and commitment therapy prosocial skills into The Wise Five. That's the foundation of The Wise Five; I just wanted you to know there's already precedent for applying SDT and ACT to relationship health.

Relationship skills are outside the scope of this book. Just keep in mind how important connection is to well-being.

Many people bring personal Tupperware meals to Thanksgiving dinner—theoretically in the name of leanness—only to alienate the people around them. Or they worry about going out to dinner with people because they don't know if they'll be able to order something healthy. That's not healthy; that's sad.

Your values need to include other people. Your values have to encompass connectedness and relatedness. No food skill practice should ever be at the expense of people you love. Many clients have gotten better relationships with their families by giving up diets and focusing on eating skills—they can actually be with people while eating. They don't have to be weird or over focused on food; they can focus on conversation and connection.

The real irony is that the clients I work with usually already have amazing relationships with family and close friends. The status they want to get from being super lean is about looking good for people they don't know or actually care about. Focus more on the people who already care about you and enjoy greater wellbeing.

ACCEPT THOUGHTS AND FEELINGS

It's normal for humans to have a whole cornucopia of thoughts and feelings. We have some thoughts that are useful (like planning), and some that aren't (like from the diet world). We have some emotions that are comfortable (happiness), and some emotions that are uncomfortable (sadness, frustration, anger). All emotions are normal parts of the human experience.

Ironically, it's the drive to "fix" our emotions and thoughts that drives emotional eating. Let me repeat that: It's not emotions that drive emotional eating; it's trying to *suppress* emotions that drives emotional eating.[268]

When people suppress or try to change their thoughts, it can work for a while, but they get a rebound of more of those thoughts and emotions. When people try to suppress cravings for foods, it can work for a while, then people rebound and eat more.

The people who most try to control their emotions are those who rebound the hardest with cravings and emotional eating. The research on all of that is covered in the defusion section on page 91.

As paradoxical as it may seem, the people who practice accepting their thoughts and feelings as normal are the people who emotionally eat the least and don't rebound. If you accept it's normal to be sad sometimes, you can be sad without eating to fix it.

Normal Human Pain

It's normal to be sad, angry, frustrated, or lonely. It's normal to have unhelpful thoughts sometimes.

Added Pain

There's an extra level of pain we normally put on top of normal pain when we add rumination about past pain, worry about future pain, or trying to control pain in the present. Trying to control thoughts and feelings actually adds pain, and makes things worse.

Acceptance frees you up to take different actions.[269] If you don't have to fix your thoughts and feelings, you can actually spend that energy participating in things that matter to you. You find you can be sad and still connect with friends. You can be frustrated and still practice your food skills or do your workouts. You can feel anxious and still go to a party. You can feel angry about something and still practice self-care.

"Willingness" might seem like a better word to you. Some of my clients hate the word "acceptance." If that's you, substitute it with "willingness." The concept is to be willing to feel all the normal human feelings when they come up. Be willing to ride them out, knowing that no emotion lasts forever.

Willingness is like the weather. Just like we're willing to drive to work when it's raining, we're willing to practice things that matter to us even when we're sad. In the same way it can be cloudy one day and sunny the next, we can be sad one day and happy the next. It all comes and goes. We want to be willing to just be, however something shows up that day—willing to feel all of the feelings that come and go. Choose to be willing to observe all of the thoughts that come and go. If we're willing to have them, they all come and go in their own time.

Self-compassion makes a huge difference. Self-compassion is being kind to ourselves even in the face of our own humanity. That can include responding to your own thoughts and feelings with kindness. Have compassion for yourself when negative thoughts and feelings come up. Think of how you'd be compassionate toward your best friend or one of your children, and apply that compassion to yourself. For many of us, self-compassion is the thing that facilitates willingness and acceptance.

I'm currently writing a book about tools to help with emotional eating, including an in-depth look at acceptance, willingness, and tools like defusion, and how these facilitate committed action. In the meantime, keep in mind *all of your feelings are normal*. For most people, learning to be with their feelings is a foundational skill practice. There's more on this later, but if you want a lot more on this before my next book comes out, read *A Liberated Mind* by Steven Hayes.

COMMITTED ACTION

Committed action pairs with accepting thoughts and feelings. We need to accept our thoughts and feelings because it's such an effective way to approach taking action. If we don't have to fix our thoughts and feelings, we can practice our eating skills and do our workouts even when it's hard.

This book is about committed action. All the skills practice, all the Meta-skills and workouts are committed action. Don't get so caught up in thinking about The Wise Five, you forget the whole point is to increase the frequency of your practice.

We're taking actions that support things that matter to us. We identify our values so we can line up our actions with them. And then we take action.

Lean and Strong is a *practice-based* system. The heart of the program is to increase frequency of behavior.

THE UNFULFILLED FIVE

When my clients fail, it's because of The Failure Five. I mostly work with people who are really motivated, but tend to drive that motivation from punishment, guilt, and status. They try and use black-and-white food rules… and they fail.

There's another end of the spectrum, though. I call the other end "The Unfulfilled Five." If The Failure Five are *too much* extrinsic motivation, The Unfulfilled Five are *too little* of any kind of motivation.

THE UNFULFILLED FIVE VERSUS THE WISE FIVE

THE UNFULFILLED FIVE VERSUS THE WISE FIVE	
THE PURSUIT OF THESE IS OFTEN DESTRUCTIVE	**THE PURSUIT OF THESE IS ALWAYS CONSTRUCTIVE**
Chaos No plan at all	**Values** Practicing valued action
Don't Try Skills Don't risk failure	**Skills** Practicing skills
Don't Try in Relationships Avoid vulnerability, boundaries, or connectedness	**Connect** Practicing prosocial behavior
Emotional Eating Numb unwanted thoughts and emotions through food	**Accept Thoughts and Feelings** Practice willingness to feel feelings and have thoughts
Wait for "Motivation" Only take action when "feeling like it"	**Committed Action** Practice taking action when it's hard

CHAOS

Often when people abandon diet rules, they abandon everything. They have no structure, no guidelines, and they don't track anything. With no plan and no direction, they always fail.

Sadly, the message we commonly get is there are only two modes in life: rules or free-for-all. We basically crush ourselves with the most rigid rules we can…until we explode and do whatever we want. Of course, neither way works very well.

You can't just throw your hands up and hope for the best. Chaos, ironically, is just as painful and ineffective as rigid rules and punishment.

DON'T TRY SKILLS

Some people are so afraid of failure, they won't try the skills. Skills are too new…too hard…too too.

This can come from either perfectionism or from a history of repeated failure. It doesn't actually matter where it comes from, though—it just doesn't work. While practicing doing nothing is safe and comfortable, it doesn't get us anywhere.

This is where the "get comfortable with being uncomfortable" from the beginning of the chapter kicks in. Food skill practice—or any new actions that align with our values—always start off uncomfortable. We run the risk of failure. In fact, practicing anything new and hard guarantees failure.

You can't avoid failure if you want to grow. You should expect to fail 20–30% of the time. It's not fun to fail, but it's necessary. The only way to learn skills is to try, fail, learn, and try again. Each time we get a little better.

Failure is a necessary part of learning.

DON'T TRY IN RELATIONSHIPS

Relationship skills are outside the scope of this book, but I have to mention them because they're a third of the psychological needs required for intrinsic motivation.

Basically, being cool to people—appropriate vulnerability, healthy boundaries, and staying connected—all take work. It's easier to avoid the work. But you'll have higher intrinsic motivation if you work at your relationships.

EMOTIONAL EATING

Numbing your feelings is a short-term solution. This isn't your fault.

The media and personal trainers on TV and magazines all tell us we should be happy all the time…we should never be sad. When we do feel sad, we assume it's wrong and we numb it with food.

It's normal to have a wide range of feelings.

It's normal to be happy sometimes and sad others.

It's normal to be excited sometimes, and low energy at others.

For humans, emotions are like the weather—changeable. It's okay to feel your feelings.

We get to honor our feelings by feeling them. Allowing ourselves to actually feel our feelings, frees us up to practice our eating skills even when we feel bad.

Living a meaningful life means taking action in line with our values, even when we have negative feelings.

WAIT FOR "MOTIVATION"

We make the mistake of thinking motivation is a feeling of wanting to do something. Worse, we get superstitious about that, thinking it should be required before taking actions that matter to us.

Often, we've been told if we know our "why" for doing something or have a big enough goal, it should make us want to do things. This is a really important error: Knowing why we're doing something has nothing to do with wanting to do it. In fact, the opposite is true: Knowing why (our values) should be the reason we do things when we *don't* want to and *don't* feel "motivated."

The feeling of motivation comes and goes like the weather. If we rely on good feelings to do what matters to us, we'll never do what matters consistently enough to get the results we want.

A NOTE TO PERSONAL TRAINERS

This book is written with the end-user in mind. That being said, I've met hundreds of trainers at workshops who told me they read my previous book, so I assume there will be a fair number of trainers reading this one as well.

This will be short and to the point, but I want the trainers reading this to understand how The Failure Five relates to coaching. The chart below should make sense after reading the previous sections on The Failure Five and the rest of the book.

THE COACH FAILURE FIVE VERSUS THE COACH WISE FIVE

COACHING THESE IS OFTEN DESTRUCTIVE	COACHING THESE IS ALWAYS CONSTRUCTIVE
Reward and Punishment Controlling clients—improper use of authority	**Autonomy Support** Supporting choice and investigating values
Self-esteem Fake or lazy praise	**Skill Learning Support** Give feedback on effective skill practice
Status Promoting client's pursuit of societal body ideals	**Relatedness** Letting clients know how you're similar to them—normalizing their struggles
The Tyranny of the Positive Attitude Telling clients to cheer up, be positive, try harder, or have a better attitude when they're struggling	**Accepting Thoughts and Feelings** Feel your own feelings Let your clients feel their feelings
Overly Outcome Goal Focused Having everything be about weight on the scale or how much weight gets lifted in workouts	**Supporting Committed Action** Setting practice frequency (action) goals, doing obstacle planning with them

It's a simple five-step process:

1. Don't foist The Failure Five on your clients. Practice The Wise Five yourself.

2. Practice The Wise Five yourself.

3. No, really, you absolutely must practice The Wise Five yourself.

4. Teach The Wise Five to your clients.

You have to use The Wise Five yourself. Do the hard work. You can share your own struggles with it to help normalize theirs. Here are some action steps to do with your clients to support The Wise Five in their food skill and workout practices:

- Listen to your clients talk about their food skill practice for the first 15 minutes of each session. Ask open-ended questions like, "What did you notice this week?" Listen more than talk.

- When they struggle with things, normalize their struggles. Let them know that most of your clients struggle with the same things. If you struggle with the same things, let them know. You can be a human, and let them be human.

- When you talk about committed action, think about changes you've wanted to make, but have struggled with—usually for trainers, that isn't fitness. Think about the marketing issue you didn't resolve, or that hard conversation in your life you still haven't had. Journal about the things in life that are hardest for you, and that you still have a hard time with. Relate that to the struggles your clients have.

- Let them feel their feelings. They're allowed to feel how they feel. They're allowed to have bad days. They're allowed to get frustrated. Let them feel their feelings. Normalize feeling feelings. Honor their feelings. Before the session is over, always redirect to future skill practice. We can feel our feelings, and do the work simultaneously.

- Give your clients choices about which eating skills to work on for the following week. I often give my clients a choice of three skills based on how the prior week went. Of course, working on the same skills again is always an option.

- Give them specific positive feedback. Precisely praise the skills they practiced and how much they practiced. Instead of "Good job," say "Really good work increasing the number of meals when you put your fork down between bites this week." Successful coaching takes listening and noting specifically what they did well.

- Have them circle values on the values list. Talk them through values reflections. Give them homework to journal about their values. Ask them how their values connected with their food skill practice and their workouts during the week. This should be a recurring conversation over years.

- Stop using the world "compliance" when talking about your clients. Compliance means "to yield to commands, to obey." Your work shouldn't be about them obeying you or obeying the program. Instead, use the word "concordance." Self-concordance means "to act in line with your values." Success isn't about them being compliant with the program; it's about them acting in concordance with their self-selected values.

- Always bring everything back to next week's skill practice. Which eating skills they are going to practice? How often they will practice? Where are they in their monthly workout plan? What days and times are they going to work out? What do they plan to progress or modify weight-wise in different exercises? Have them describe their

If/then plans to overcome specific obstacles they anticipate, with either food skills or workouts. Bring everything back to action.

SCOPE OF PRACTICE FOR PERSONAL TRAINERS REGARDING NUTRITION

DON'T DO THIS:

- Obviously saying certain foods treat medical conditions or will impact health in specific ways is an egregious scope of practice violation. Individualized nutrition recommendations or customized meal plans are also out, even though most trainers make this mistake.

- If you recommend cutting out certain foods or even whole macronutrients, you're treading on thin ice. On top of that, many countries and states have even stricter regulations on what you can and can't do as a personal trainer; check with your local laws to learn about this important issue. Always consider this: "Could I justify my credentials for making this recommendation to a judge and jury?"

- If someone has a medical nutrition issue that needs work or has in-depth questions about nutrition and health, refer out to a registered dietician.

DO THIS:

- You can discuss the relationship between total energy consumed and weight.

- Sharing your government's food guidelines are within your scope of practice. In the United States and Canada, that would be Canada's food guide and the United States' MyPlate guidelines. In other countries, you'll likely have to stick closely to your country's food guidelines.

- You can share nutrition information from other credible and well-known institutions. The World Health Organization and the American Heart Association are good examples. The "Healthy Eating Plate" from Harvard's T.H. Chan School of Public Health likely falls into this category as well.

- Ultimately, let clients make their own decisions about how they want to balance their meals.

- Instead of food content, focus on behavioral skills. Skills like eating slowly, noticing when full, and eating a meal every four to six hours are all reasonable recommendations.

- Double check the laws in your country or state.

SCOPE OF PRACTICE FOR PERSONAL TRAINERS REGARDING PSYCHOLOGY:

DON'T DO THIS:

- I shouldn't have to say this, but let me say it anyway: Mental health conditions are outside of a personal trainer's scope of practice. That should be obvious, but then again, we see trainers post on social media that "exercise is better than medication for depression." I hope that trainer ends up in jail. Obviously, we don't work with depression, anxiety, anorexia, bulimia, and so on.

- The gray areas are where clients are using food to cope with stress and emotions. Some people who are snacking because they're stressed out in the middle of a workday will likely respond really well to a skills-based approach.

- On the flip-side, someone who has more serious issues with eating and emotions or isn't making progress with these simple skills should be referred out. Referring out is really cool—counseling psychologists have a whole toolbox that personal trainers don't have.

DO THIS:

- In terms of psychology, personal trainers should mostly stick to letting clients explore their own reasons for motivation. Values work is great.

- Let clients feel their feelings. It can be really helpful for them to know that the thoughts and emotions they are having are normal. Clients can reflect on how their thoughts are just thoughts.

- You can share about the damaging nature of black-and-white diet rules and perfectionism.

- Ask questions, listen more than you talk, make it safe for them to explore, and let them sort out most of that for themselves. They do it all; you just listen.

For the most part, personal trainers should stick to behaviors. Whether you call them actions, skills, guidelines, or habits, that's the scope of a personal trainer in relationship to food and eating. The skills in this book work perfectly for that.

HOW DO I CONNECT WITH MY VALUES?

We're going to practice with a weekly values reflection in your journal.

Week One

1. Journal for five minutes about the kind of person you want to be around food and strength training. Think about what you'd do. Think about how you'd relate to your training and skills practice.

Finally, answer four questions:

   A. Who matters to me?

   B. What matters to me?

   C. Which character strengths do I admire?

   D. What do I want to stand for?

2. From those answers, select your values. If you're having trouble distinguishing your values, it might be helpful to review the intrinsic values versus external goals on page 193 or the values list on page 220.

Week Two

1. Pick one to three values from a values list.

2. Journal for 15–20 minutes about how those values relate to the kind of person you want to be, and why you chose those values over others. It's okay to reword the values to be personalized for you.

If you have trouble picking three or fewer values, use the 10–5–3 process. Circle your top ten. Then from those ten, underline your top five. Finally, from those five, put stars by the three most important to you right now.

In reality, it's okay to have lots of values. The issue, really, is that people have trouble focusing on more than three. If you talk to someone who is "trying to focus on these ten values," you find they're either overwhelmed by having so many, or they consistently forget all of them.

The point right now of having three is to be clear about what you're working on. You want to be able to remember them, and you want to be able to apply them to your food skill practice every day.

It's more effective to have fewer values that get remembered and applied to your practice. A dozen values you can't remember are useless.

EXAMPLE VALUES

CIRCLE YOUR TOP ONE TO THREE VALUES OR COME UP WITH YOUR OWN

Acceptance	Flexibility	Play
Adventure	Freedom	Reciprocity
Assertiveness	Friendship	Respect
Authenticity	Forgiveness	Resourcefulness
Balance	Fun	Responsibility
Beauty	Generosity	Romance
Caring	Gratitude	Safety
Challenge	Home	Self-awareness
Collaboration	Honesty	Self-care
Community	Humor	Self-discipline
Compassion	Humility	Self-expression
Connection	Industriousness	Self-respect
Contribution	Independence	Service
Cooperation	Intimacy	Skillfulness
Courage	Joy	Spirituality
Creativity	Justice	Stewardship
Curiosity	Kindness	Strength
Design	Knowledge	Supportiveness
Dignity	Leadership	Teamwork
Diversity	Learning	Tradition
Encouragement	Love	Trustworthiness
Ethics	Loyalty	Understanding
Equality	Mindfulness	Uniqueness
Excitement	Order	Usefulness
Exploration	Open-mindedness	Vision
Fairness	Optimism	Vulnerability
Faith	Patience	Wellbeing
Family	Persistence	Wholeheartedness
Fitness	Personal Development	Wisdom

Week Three

1. Look at the one to three values you picked last week.

2. Journal topic (write for at least five minutes): *How do the eating skills you're practicing right now express your values?*

Week Four

1. Reflect on the one to three values you picked the first week. You can reevaluate and choose different values if you prefer. You can search the internet for other values lists and pull from those as well. Just keep it to one to three values. Don't get caught up in picking the "right" values. The best way to figure out your values is practice, followed by reflection, which you're going to do for months. It's better to figure it out over time, through practice and reflection, than it is to try to get the "perfect" values up front.

2. Journal topic (write for at least five minutes): *What will your life look like five years from now if you continue to practice skills that match your values?*

Week Five

1. Look at your one to three values.

2. Journal topic (write for at least five minutes): *What was a tough choice you had to make with your eating skills or workouts this week? How do your values relate to that choice? Looking at your values, would you make the same choice again, or would you do something different in the future?*

Week Six

1. Pick two values for each area of your life:

    A.   Personal growth, health and fitness

    B.   Relationships and family

    C.   Work and career or education

    D.   Fun, play, relaxation

2. Journal topic (write for at least five minutes): *Do any of your values compete? Does the kind of person you want to be in other areas of your life impact who you want to be in health and fitness?*

Week Seven

1. Take a look at your values in any of the four areas of your life.

2. Journal topic (write for at least five minutes): *What skill practice would be in the direction of those values?*

Week Eight

1. Consider your food and fitness-related values.

2. Journal topic (write for at least five minutes): *What is your current skill practice missing in relationship to those values? What is your skill practice totally nailing in relationship to those values?*

Week Nine

1. Take at least five minutes to review your previous journal entries.

Week Ten

1. Look at your values in all four areas of your life.

2. Journal topic (write for at least five minutes): *What do you want the epitaph on your gravestone to be?*
   The old joke goes that no one really wants the epitaph on their gravestone to read "finally lost the last 15 pounds." Usually they want it to read something like, "loving parent and great friend," or "caring and honest," or "volunteered in the community."

While this may seem a little morbid, it's a good way to cut through the status-based fitness ideas we've been sold all our lives, and really get at the kind of person we want to be.

Week Eleven

1. Reflect again on your food and fitness values.

2. Journal topic (write for at least five minutes): *How do practicing your food values positively impact other areas of your life? How do they positively impact people around you?*

Week Twelve

1. Look at your food and fitness values.

2. Journal topic (write for at least five minutes): *What will your life look like if you continue practicing these values for the next ten years?*

Week Thirteen

1. Pick two values for each area of your life:

   A. Personal growth, health and fitness

   B. Relationships and family

   C. Work and career or education

   D. Fun, play, relaxation

2. Journal topic (write for at least five minutes): *Are these the same values you picked last time you did this practice? What's the same? What's different? Why do these values matter to you going forward?*

ADVANCED VALUES REFLECTIONS: TAKING PERSPECTIVE

Perspective taking is one of the most powerful reflections we can do. We're often too close to our goals and obstacles to be objective, which is one of the reasons talking to a friend or a coach can be so helpful. We can actually do the same thing for ourselves by imagining a different perspective and journaling from that perspective.

Week One: Asking for Advice

1. Look at your food and fitness values.

2. Imagine you're 20 years older and wiser.

3. Journal topic (write for at least five minutes): *What advice would the older and wiser you give you about your values, food skill practice, and workouts right now?*

Week Two: Giving Advice

1. Consider your food and fitness values.

2. Imagine you're talking with a really good friend who has those same values.

3. Journal topic (write for at least five minutes): *What advice would you give your good friend about food values, food skill practice, and workouts right now?*

Week Three: Asking for Advice

1. Reflect on your food and fitness values.

2. Imagine you're talking to the wisest and most compassionate person you know.

3. Journal topic (write for at least five minutes): *What advice would they give you about your values and your eating skills and workouts right now?*

Week Four: Giving Advice

1. Look at your food and fitness values.

2. Imagine a child or teenager going through the same things you are and who has the same values. It can be your son or daughter, or a niece or nephew, or a child of a friend. If this young person came to you and asked about food skill practice, workouts, and values, what advice would you give?

3. This can be really powerful because we're smarter and more compassionate about the

needs of kids. People would never impose many of the meaner impulses they have about their bodies, their weight, and food on a kid they care about—often they'd counsel the opposite of their own impulses. This is an important conflict to sort out: Firstly, you may have to actually give some wise and compassionate advice someday. Secondly, it's useful to think about what it would look like for you to do with your wise and compassionate counsel, to follow your own advice.

4. Journal topic (write for at least five minutes): *What advice would you give that child about the values and food skill practice and workouts right now?*

Week Five: Connection to Others

1. Look at your food and fitness values.

2. Think about a family member, a good friend, your coworkers, or a community you're a part of.

3. Journal topic (write for at least five minutes): *How will it help you make a difference for others if you approached your food, fitness, and body from a values perspective? How would it make a difference to approach your relationships with them from the perspective of your values?*

LIGHTNING ROUND: ONE-MINUTE DAILY REFLECTIONS

Many of my clients have found they do better by doing those reflections in really short bursts—literally one minute each day.

They'll pick any of the reflections daily and write for one minute—whatever they think, whatever comes up.

Most of the research I've read has utilized weekly values reflections. But the majority of the clients I work with do super short reflections almost every day.

The first benefit: If they do a one-minute reflection four or five days per week, it seems to keep their values top-of-mind.

The second benefit: For many people, it's easier to blurt out a one-minute reflection, just whatever comes to mind. This develops into deep insight over time. The additive effect of short reflections can sometimes be easier to manage than trying to come up with something brilliant once a week or trying to carve out five or more minutes in one sitting.

The one-minute versions work so well for my clients that in the future I'm considering recommending those over the weekly reflections. Sometimes what works in real life is slightly different from what's been tested in research. Feel free to try both for yourself and see which fits your life better.

If you go the one-minute route, you can still use the weekly prompts.

VALUES REFLECTION FOR LIFE

I hope you continue to journal about your values for the rest of your life. You may gain insight into them over years. Or you may notice your expression of your values changes over decades. For example, the value of "family" is expressed in different ways at 12 years old than at 32 years old…to 52…to 72. It's the same value, but the actions you take to express it will be different.

Other places you can look for value reflection prompts:

People you really admire: What are their values? What actions do they take that line up with their values? What obstacles did they have to overcome to consistently express their values?

People in books and movies who inspire you: What are their values? What are the actions they take in line with their values? What obstacles did they have to overcome to consistently express their values?

EXAMPLE CLIENT VALUES LISTS

With so many things, I've found that giving you examples of values clients have chosen before can help. Here are some values my clients have recently chosen for themselves:

- Adventure, calm, caring
- Creativity, fun, peace
- Consistency, connection, self-compassion
- Gentleness, honesty, and caring
- Discipline, wellbeing, persistence
- Creativity, curiosity, wisdom
- Curiosity, persistence, and trustworthiness
- Humor, persistence, and forgiveness
- Balance, growth, knowledge
- Family, loyalty, determination, strength
- Perseverance, balance, family
- Legacy, improvisation, intelligence
- Balance, joy, and choice

The values people choose often sound drastically different from how people normally approach diets and crushing workouts. You'll notice they can apply to multiple areas of your life, not just fitness. If you approach your food skill practice from that place, you'll probably hit all your fitness goals. Lastly, you'll see the way you approach food and fitness will be an expression of the person you want to be, what you stand for, and what matters to you.

PARENTING AS A METAPHOR FOR VALUES

People don't set a goal to get their kids to 18 years old, and then the job will be done.

You don't have a couple tough days parenting and think, "I'll just start again next week." Or "You kids have to fend for yourself; I'm going to try again in January."

You don't parent when it's exciting and stop when it's hard.

Parenting doesn't have an end date. You're a parent for life, even though how you express being a parent changes drastically every decade.

Interestingly, parents score lower on reports of fun, comfort, and pleasantness in life, and score higher on meaning in life. It's not that it's easier or more fun—it's that it really matters to them.

Let's look at how you can take that approach to your values in fitness:

- Your lean and strong values are a direction. They don't have an end date.

- Your lean and strong values are your values on days when it you feel motivated and they're still your values on days you don't feel motivated.

- Your lean and strong values are your values because they matter to you, not because they're more fun.

EMERGENCY ROOM DOCTOR AS A METAPHOR FOR VALUES

As we talked about earlier, emergency room doctors don't set a goal for how many people they're going to save each day (that would be super weird). They get up and save as many lives as they can, because it's who they are.

If someone dies in the emergency room, they don't throw up their hands and say, "I'll just start again next week." They don't let everyone else die that night because "I'm a perfectionist." If something bad happens, they go to the next patient and again do their best.

They don't do it when it's exciting and stop when it's hard. People's lives are on the line—they do it when it's exciting *and* when it's hard.

Being an emergency room doctor doesn't have an end date. The docs get up and do it again tomorrow.

It's a super difficult, super stressful, highly emotional job. They don't do it because it's fun or comfortable; they do it because it matters to them.

Let's look at how you can take that approach to your values in fitness:

- Your lean and strong values are a direction. They don't have an end date.

- Your lean and strong values are your values even after you mess up.

- Your lean and strong values are your values because they matter to you, not because they're comfortable or easy.

THE ULTIMATE BLACK BELT LEVEL OF VALUES WORK

We now have all these eating skills for you to work on. We have all these workouts. The majority of my clients find, whichever values they personally identified, the eating skills and workouts match their values. That's pretty awesome.

The eating skills give them a way to live their values, in action, in their lives.

The workouts give them a way to live their values, in action, in the gym.

In essence, I've given you a ton of *structure* to live your values. Structure is super useful for having a place to start, for learning and developing skills.

It isn't the ultimate end, though. The ultimate end is always flexibility. The goal is to be able to freestyle.

My highest-level clients get to a point where they don't always need to be practicing specific skills. Instead, they're practicing making decisions from their values.

If they value longevity, they can use that value as a way to make decisions about any meal, any balance of food, or any treat in the moment. If they value longevity, they can immediately discard workout programs that are clearly too much or too stupid. If they value longevity, they can always find what's smart and reasonable in a program, and discard things that are extreme, dangerous, and short-sighted.

At first, this higher level has a cost. That cost is *thinking*. It takes more energy to make decisions. This is also a fairly high level of decision making.

I get it; people don't want to make every decision based on: "How does this meal express who I want to be as a person?" But if you make *some* decisions from there, it's amazing how good you can get at it.

People tend to find out really cool things, like:

- Sometimes I want to have a glass of wine on the back porch after a long day. Most of the time, I want to read, or sit quietly, or go for a walk, or hug a pet. Sometimes I want to eat the slice of cake. In fact, I wouldn't be the kind of person I really want to be if I didn't have a slice of cake on my birthday. It fits my values to have cake on my birthday. It's the kind of example I want to set for my kids to have cake on my birthday. It doesn't fit my values to eat so much cake that I feel gross and have trouble sleeping because "it's a free day." That actually doesn't fit my values.

All of a sudden, the continuum from "clean" to "dirty" food starts to seem ridiculous. Most people know it doesn't fit their personal values to have treats all the time, nor does it fit their values not to have them at all.

You get to sort it through…*from your values.*

THE WORK AND THE MISTAKES

This is work.

It's also the most important work you will ever do for your health and fitness. When you're clear about *who you want to be* with food, you have a filter for making decisions about food and fitness. You have a true north.

You'll totally make mistakes, and you'll learn. It's wonderful to try something and upon reflection, realize you went too far one way or the other. It's okay to find out you made a call based on your values and accidentally ate too little…or too much. It's okay to have a treat for a special day, and later realize it sucked. It's okay to realize you missed your grandma's special pie, and that next time you'll have it.

This kind of trial and error is the best way to test your values in action.

The journaling and the reflection on your values is really, really valuable.

It's just as valuable to try making decisions from those values in real life.

What you'll learn from *trying it out* will be everything. Living from your values requires practice. Learn by doing.

The cycle of reflection and practice is huge.

Don't make the mistake of practice without reflection.

Don't make the mistake of reflection without practice.

You need both. Practice, then reflect.

Then practice some more. Then reflect again.

ACCEPTING THOUGHTS AND FEELINGS

"The desire for more positive experience is itself a negative experience.

And, paradoxically, the acceptance of one's negative experience is itself a positive experience."

~ **Mark Manson**

The Subtle Art of Not Giving A F*ck

"Don't erect a wall to protect you from experiencing life. The same wall that keeps out your disappointment also keeps out the sunlight of enriching experiences. So let life touch you."

~ **Jim Rohn**

LASTING WEIGHT LOSS WITH THIS ONE WEIRD TRICK!

The internet is littered with stupid articles saying you can lose weight fast with one weird trick. It's always something stupid like some magically wonderful cleanse you need to drink, or some magically evil food you need to avoid. If there's anything to avoid in weight loss, it's that kind of magical thinking.

That being said, I have a remarkably simple and obvious thing for you to do to create easier and more lasting weight loss forever—to have a better life.

It sounds really silly, but motivation science shows that when we have more meaning, better relationships, and do things that are more engaging, we are more intrinsically motivated to take care of ourselves.

Now, I know you probably already have a meaningful life and great relationships, and do things that are engaging. So, this isn't exactly about having more of that. It's about taking the things that make all of those things work and applying them to your health and fitness. You want to connect meaning and engagement and relationships to your fitness.

It's odd we never think to take the things that work for us in every other great areas of our lives and apply them to fitness. Instead, we have fitness pros telling us to approach this from ways that are punishing and terrible. It's not your fault for not doing things that work in other areas of your life.

MATURITY AND IMMATURITY

Metacognition means "thinking about thinking." It's a higher level of maturity.

It's immature to assume every thought is true, should be positive, and is a command. It's very mature to be able to notice your thoughts as thoughts often being automatic echoes from other people or from your past.

Low-level, Immature Thinking:

- My thoughts are true.
- My thoughts are me.
- My thoughts are urgent commands.
- My thoughts are all helpful.
- I need to control my thoughts.
- I need to control my emotions.

High-level, Mature Thinking:

- Sometimes it's unhelpful to evaluate if a thought is true or false.
- Some of my thoughts come from me; some are from other people; some are from media and society, and many are from diet culture.
- My thoughts are just thoughts.
- Some thoughts are helpful, and some thoughts are unhelpful.
- It's normal to have wanted thoughts and unwanted thoughts.
- It's normal to have helpful thoughts and unhelpful thoughts.
- It's normal to have positive emotions and negative emotions.
- If I control my thoughts, they'll usually rebound into emotional eating.
- If I control my emotions, they'll usually rebound into emotional eating.
- I can always take action toward what matters to me, regardless of my thoughts.
- I can always take action toward what matters to me, regardless of my emotions.

ACCEPTANCE IS NOT CONTROL

We covered a lot of this in the section on defusion, but here's a quick review.

For people who have low or moderate issues with cravings and emotional eating, changing and controlling thoughts works, but for people with bigger issues with cravings and emotional eating, thought control and changing thoughts makes things worse. If you struggle with cravings or emotional eating, you'll have significantly bigger rebound eating.[270,271,272,273]

Thought and emotion suppression just doesn't work for anyone. Suppressing cravings leads to a huge eating rebound.[274]

In long-term behavioral weight-loss trials, acceptance has always been as effective,[275] or more effective, than standard treatments including controlling and changing thoughts. For people with more external eating (you want food if you see it), emotional eating, or cravings eating, acceptance is clearly more effective.[276,277,278] Those results hold up even at two-year follow-ups.[279]

The big takeaway is this—if you have a friend who does really well with thought control, cool; it totally works for some people. If you always rebound after thought control—you aren't alone—acceptance will work significantly better for you.

If control hasn't worked for you in the past, more control isn't the answer. Try going the opposite way and using acceptance.

IT'S LAZY TO LABEL ALL FEELINGS AS "FAT" OR "STRESS"

It's mature to be accurate about the feelings you're having. You may look at yourself in the mirror and have really hard feelings like disgust, disappointment, frustration, or loneliness. But those are actual emotions, distinct and more accurate than "fat."

You may have physical sensations like feeling bloated, but that's also not "feeling fat." Everyone experiences a gross feeling when they're bloated. That's called "feeling bloated." It's a physical sensation, not an emotion. When you feel bloated, you should expect not to feel awesome and not feel great in your clothes. It's like having a headache—no one feels great when they have a headache, but they don't mistake it for "feeling fat."

When you have emotions, like sadness, disgust, loneliness, anger, fear, or frustration, you can check in:

- Are these thoughts coming from idealized body standards or diet culture?

- Are these thoughts coming from me feeling out of alignment with my personal values?

- Is it a combination of both?

If it's from some sort of diet culture or idealized standard, remember, in our diet obsessed culture, it's normal to have those thoughts. We're surrounded by this input from both friends and media; it would be weird not to have these thoughts sometimes, similar to how we're constantly surrounded by ideas about how we should be more successful.

It's normal to have those thoughts.

It's mature to notice them as thoughts and recognize where they came from.

If it's that you're out of alignment with your values, then:

1. Know it's normal and okay to have those thoughts and feelings;

2. Remember you don't have to change those thoughts and feelings;

3. The responsible thing to change is your *actions*.

ACCEPTING EMOTIONS IS NOT ACCEPTING SITUATIONS

A 2017 paper outlined three studies on acceptance and psychological health. The first study had a really cool sample with 1,003 participants, both men and women, multiple ethnicities, and a wide variety of socioeconomic backgrounds. They found acceptance of thoughts and feelings robustly predicted wellbeing and life satisfaction. They controlled for other explanations, measuring four different factors of mindfulness, the ability to reevaluate thoughts, and even baseline stress levels, and found acceptance predicted wellbeing independently.[280]

The researchers also noted that acceptance of *situations* wasn't required, only acceptance of *thoughts and emotions*. That means a person could work to change a situation (like working on eating skills and doing workouts) while still accepting the thoughts and emotions.

They found that accepting thoughts and emotions reduced experiences of sadness and stress. What's even cooler, they found that acceptance didn't change other emotions like joy or contentedness. Essentially, they found acceptance was all upside. They replicated the correlational results of the first study in a second laboratory study, and then a third long-term (longitudinal) study, and the results were consistent across all three.

JOY, SADNESS, ANGER, DISGUST, AND FEAR

The best example of accepting emotions comes from the Pixar movie, *Inside Out*. In the movie, a young girl named Riley struggles with her feelings about her parents moving to a new city. Most of the movie is set inside her head, with the main characters being her feelings: Joy, Sadness, Disgust, Anger, and Fear.

The movie starts off with the very common assumption that joy is the "best" emotion. This is the idea that more joy is better, and the other feelings—especially sadness—are the "wrong" emotions to have. The crux of the hero's journey is Joy finding out she isn't the right emotion—that a healthy person has all of the emotions at one time or another. Sometimes we even have multiple emotions at the same time, all mixed together.

The fun part of the movie is the interplay between the characters Joy and Sadness. Joy, of course, we all love; she's fun and great and adventurous and exciting. On the other hand, Sadness has this amazing ability to connect people and bond them together. And, being with Sadness actually makes the other characters feel better.

I ask my "emotional eating" clients to watch that movie. Emotional eating, at the base level, is predicated on the idea that people should be happy all the time. Emotional eating is about *numbing* sadness, anger, disgust, and fear.

Acceptance is the ability to be with all of your emotions, not just those you want. Sadness and anger are normal and healthy; humans aren't built for *constant* happiness. People who seem constantly happy are either being fake or they're on drugs. There's no constant happiness in normal human physiology.

Normal and healthy is a balance of all the emotions. Normal people are happy when things are awesome, and they're sad when things are terrible.

- It's not about being Debbie Downer, where everything sucks all of the time.

- It's also not about being that super fake and obnoxious fitness trainer who's pretending to be happy every minute.

The most common feedback I get after doing workshops or first sessions with clients is about how upbeat and positive I am. I actually think my ability to be authentically happy comes from my willingness to be sad. When I think about my mom dying, I cry. When I think about trainers fat shaming clients, I get angry. Sometimes while writing this book, I was really frustrated.

People often ask me: Josh, why do you talk so much about accepting sadness when you seem so happy? In truth, it was when I became able to cry more that I started laughing more. When I became able to feel and process anger in healthy ways, I became able to feel peaceful. One way to think about it is that these are two sides of the same coin.

Things aren't that dichotomous, though. Sometimes you can feel multiple things at the same time. You can feel things…and take actions totally unrelated to your feelings. Emotions don't work in perfect opposites; it's more like they're just all part of the human experience.

The emotions in *Inside Out* were based on Paul Ekman's six basic emotions, which were later shortened to five for the movie, as "surprise" and "fear" ended up being too similar as characters. There are also other models of emotion mapping—for example, the feelings wheel shown on page 96.

In 2017, Alan Cowen and Dacher Keltner (who also consulted on *Inside Out*) ran a study where they identified 27 discreet emotions: admiration, adoration, aesthetic appreciation, amusement, anger, anxiety, awe, awkwardness, boredom, calmness, confusion, craving, disgust, empathetic pain, entrancement, excitement, fear, horror, interest, joy, nostalgia, relief, romance, sadness, satisfaction, sexual desire, and surprise.

However, the idea is less about having a perfect list of distinct emotions and more about giving you a list to pick from. Often, clients who have a habit of trying to numb emotions—whether through food or TV or social media—initially have a hard time identifying them.

In every case, identifying an emotion makes it seem less urgent. It makes it seem less like a thing that needs to be immediately fixed. Identifying an emotion, like thought labeling, creates defusion, which we covered in detail on page 91.

That defusion allows us to take different actions. We get to simultaneously acknowledge and honor our emotions without being bullied by them.

Emotion menu based on the work of Cowen and Keltner:

Admiration	Adoration	Aesthetic Appreciation
Amusement	Anger	Anxiety
Awe	Awkwardness	Boredom
Calmness	Confusion	Craving
Disgust	Emphathetic Pain	Entrancement
Excitement	Fear	Horror
Interest	Joy	Nostalgia
Relief	Romance	Sadness
Satisfaction	Sexual Desire	Surprise

Labeling your feelings provides a bit of distance, a little perspective. The only way out of difficult emotions is through. Identifying your emotions gives you the ability to sit with them. You may plan some time for self-care to take care of yourself. Or you may just accept that it's normal to have emotions.

Emotional eating is about suppressing everything that isn't joy. As you can see in the menus and feelings wheels and the movie *Inside Out*, there are many normal human emotions besides joy.

Your choice is to be completely driven out of control with emotional eating, or learn to sit patiently with your emotions.

The feelings wheel, thought labeling, metacognitive meditation, or journaling about your emotions are tools to help you get enough distance from your thoughts that you can sit with them. They give you a higher-level thinking about your thoughts.

Thinking about thinking gives you power.

BE CAPTAIN MARVEL

Captain Marvel is another great movie about emotions. For six years, her mentor Yon-Rogg (played by Jude Law), told her she had to control her emotions. He was constantly telling her he's trying to make her the "best version of herself," and that requires keeping her emotions in check.

Captain Marvel (played by Brie Larson) starts the movie having tried—and repeatedly failing—to do this.

Of course, over the course of the movie, she lets go of that. It's a cool arc in that her growth isn't about learning something new or gaining some skill; it's about returning to being herself. She connects with her friend Maria Rambau and her daughter, whom she loves. She connects to her values and doing what she thinks is right. And she connects back to her emotions.

Captain Marvel is able to feel her feelings and she's able to do the things that matter to her. Ironically, several characters attempt to bait her into doing stupid things over her emotions, and she never takes the bait, especially in one of the climactic fight scenes. She never made a bad decision based on her emotions. At every point she makes the decision that best fits her values.

She was vulnerable and she was strong. She was kind and she was courageous. She cared and she was brave. She felt her emotions and she made smart decisions. That's being a superhero.

Be like Captain Marvel: She felt her feelings, and she took actions in line with her values. You can do both.

GRIT AND EMOTIONAL EATING

Grit is the ability to feel emotions, and take actions that matter to you anyway.

We're often told grit is suppressing emotions, changing emotions, having the "right" emotions, or having no emotions. It's not any of those. You might have heard courage isn't the absence of fear; courage is acting in the presence of fear. Grit is like that.

And that's the key to working through emotional eating. Once people know they're okay having all the emotions and thoughts, it frees them up to take completely new actions even in the presence of those thoughts and emotions. They do more work. They get more practice. That's why they hit their fitness goals.

The skill of accepting *all* emotions is tightly related to the skill of doing better work, more work, and more consistent work. That's grit.

ACCEPTANCE REDUX

RIGID/CONTROL (DON'T DO THIS)	FLEXIBILITY/DEFUSION (DO THIS)
Try to suppress thoughts	Noticing thoughts as thoughts, and letting them come and go in their own time. Practice your eating skills, even in the presence of hard thoughts—the same way you go to work on Monday morning, even if you think, "I don't want to."
Try to suppress emotions	Think of thoughts like the weather, knowing sometimes it's rainy, and sometimes it's sunny. We can't control emotions like we can't control the weather; they both change on their own, and it's okay.
Try to change "bad" thoughts to "good" thoughts	Use a metaphor like monsters on the bus. Know passengers (thoughts) get on and off the bus all the time. Your job is just to drive the bus. Sometimes monsters ("bad" thoughts) get on the bus, and our job is just to let them ride. Continue driving to our goals and values, regardless of which passengers (thoughts) get on and off.

RIGID/CONTROL (DON'T DO THIS)	FLEXIBILITY/DEFUSION (DO THIS)
Try to be happy all of the time	Think about the movie *Inside Out,* and all of the different emotions (joy, sadness, disgust, fear, and anger) she had within her. It was healthier for her to express joy sometimes and express sadness other times—they both had a place in her life.
Try to suppress cravings for certain foods	Remember it's normal to crave highly palatable foods, and cravings come and go. Re-engage with the eating skills you're practicing, or with your work, or with the people you're with. Engage in what's going on right now, even in the presence of cravings.
Eat to numb out hard emotions	Use a feelings wheel to name which feelings you're feeling. Journal about your feelings. Then continue to practice your eating skills, even in the presence of hard emotions.
Eat to manage stress	Remember it's normal to want to use food when feeling stressed. It's okay to let those feelings come and go. You can accept that stress is normal, and wanting to eat is normal, and then not eat. Or you can do some other activity that fits your values, like going for a walk to give yourself a break, then come back to doing what you have to do.

COMMITTED ACTION

As covered earlier, committed action is the pair to accepting thoughts and feelings. Committed action allows us to change our behaviors—increasing food skill practice, getting in our workouts, and taking whatever other actions fit our values.

Here is where we do what matters to us even when it's hard and even in the presence of unwanted thoughts and uncomfortable feelings. Sometimes people get caught up in the accepting part without adding the action part—but we need to do the actions that matter to us.

This whole book is about committed action toward all the skills and guidelines, all the Meta-skills, and all the workouts. The game we're playing is to get in the frequency of those practices that fit our values. Every page is about what actions to take and strategies for being successful with those actions.

Remember: *Everything comes down to frequency of practice.*

- We don't do values reflections just because it's a fun journal exercise. We do values work so we can take committed action in line with our values.

- We don't build skills without any context. We build skills so we're effective in taking committed actions in line with our values.

- We don't just pay lip service to connection. We commit to taking actions in our relationships that are in line with our values.

- We don't accept our thoughts and feelings just because it allows us to be a healthy and complete human. We accept our thoughts and feelings so we can take actions that are in line with our values, even when they're really hard.

The Wise Five aren't an entirely cerebral exercise. The Wise Five always have to come back to action.

YOU *HAVE* THE CRITIC AND YOU *ARE* THE FIGHTER

"It is not the critic who counts; not the man who points out how the strong man stumbles, or where the doer of deeds could have done them better.

"The credit belongs to the man who is actually in the arena, whose face is marred by dust and sweat and blood; who strives valiantly; who errs, who comes short again and again, because there is no effort without error and shortcoming; but who does actually strive to do the deeds; who knows great enthusiasms, the great devotions; who spends himself in a worthy cause; who at the best knows in the end the triumph of high achievement, and who at the worst, if he fails, at least fails while daring greatly, so that his place shall never be with those cold and timid souls who neither know victory nor defeat."

~ Theodore Roosevelt

That quote from Teddy Roosevelt perfectly sums up the interplay between accepting thoughts and emotions and taking committed action if we look at it in an unconventional way. We just need to see we're both the critic and the man or women in the arena.

If you've ever done anything difficult, you've met your inner critic, where you felt all the thoughts about doubt, all the concerns, and noticed all your failures. In anything you've ever been successful at, you've also been the person in the arena—striving and persisting through all the ups and downs and things going well or not going well.

Emotional eating is how we try to silence the critic. The biggest problem is our unwillingness to hear the critic, our desire to control the critic, and the fact that we can't accept that all humans have an inner critic. We've been sold the lie that successful people don't have an inner critic.

We need to learn to notice the critic as what he is—just a critic. The critic criticizes—that's his job. Having an inner critic is simply part of being human. In relation to eating skills and working out, our inner critic comes entirely from the diet world. With all the dieting and body shaming messages we've heard in our lives, everyone has that critic.

Sometimes we hear the critic's voice booming through the speakers and across the arena. Sometimes we make the mistake of thinking the critic is our own voice, or we make the mistake of worrying the critic is telling the truth. We wonder if the critic is our coach giving us commands. Of course, the critic is none of those; the critic is simply the critic, saying things that are unhelpful.

Truly, the critic does not count. The credit does go to the man or woman in the arena. No matter how loudly the critic criticizes, we're who gets to choose what we do in the arena. We get to choose our actions, whether we're going to listen to the critic or listen to our values. We can strive for great deeds—we can dare gtreatly; we can spend ourselves in worthy cause.

Our first job is to recognize the voice of the critic as the voice of the critic. Our second job is to get to our practice in the arena in spite of what the critic says. Our values, our skill practice, our relationships—all of the actions that matter to us are in the arena. That's where we make our stand.

VULNERABILITY, COURAGE, AND BRENÉ BROWN

Daring Greatly is one of my favorite books ever. Brené Brown based her book on that Teddy Roosevelt quote. The book is about vulnerability and courage, describing how they're two sides of the same coin—that we can't have courage without being vulnerable.

These twin concepts, vulnerability and courage, are another great way to look at accepting thoughts and feelings and committed action. Acceptance is extremely vulnerable. It's literally the courage to be with ourselves, exactly as we are. Committed action is the courage to take action when it's hard, and braving the vulnerability of success and failure that comes with practice.

In *Rising Strong*, the same author talks about the "messy middle" of any great story—the part where the main character is lost and struggling. Everyone wants to skip to the end where the hero has everything figured out, but that's not how life works. We need the courage and vulnerability to push through that messy middle.

Acceptance is about allowing your journey to be messy, like it always is in the middle. Committed action means we continue to move forward in spite of the messiness.

AVOID IMPOSSIBLE STANDARDS AND "I CAN DO IT ALL"

Red Light (stop)

Yellow Light (caution)

Green Light (go)

Reflecting and rating is a super helpful tool for my clients to evaluate their life stress.

- **Red Light Life Stress**—This is when your house burns down, you lose your job, or a family member is in critical condition in the hospital. In this case, working on eating skills and work-outs might be completely inappropriate. Just like a red light at a stoplight, when you see you're at a red light in your life, stop working on the stuff in this book. Handle the stresses first.

- **Yellow Light Life Stress**—This is when you have long hours or a big project at work. Maybe your kids are sick or they have extra things you need to drive them to and from. It could be you're arguing with a family member or close friend. In these times, it's like seeing a yellow light: Proceed with caution. You can still pursue your food skill practice and workouts, but you might need to moderate it in light of everything going on in your life.

- **Green Light Life Stress**—This is when everything in your life is awesome. Your relationships are great. Work is going great. Everyone is healthy. You have a normal amount of free time. When you get a green light in life stress, just like a green light when driving—go! This is when you can rock out on your food skill practice and workouts.

This idea gives you a way to acknowledge how much is going on in your life. You might notice you spend a fair bit of time in yellow. It's a problem when we act like we're always in green, and we set up totally unrealistic expectations for the kind of time and energy required and the possible progress of strength and leanness.

When you're in red, it's appropriate to put all of this completely aside. I've had clients who felt like they were "off their plan" or apologized for not practicing when they had major life events. It's good to acknowledge when it's time not to practice.

Some people find it useful to mark on the tracker when they're in a yellow or green light situation. The most important part, though, is just to note what's going on in your life, and adjust your practice accordingly.

This is a concept Dan John used in Intervention for consulting with athletes about life stress that was adapted from the Navy's medical readiness for deployment assessment.

THE WISE FIVE AND BODY IMAGE

You don't have to figure out if what you think about your body is true or untrue.

Either way, focusing on it excessively is the part that's unworkable.

In our culture, it would be weird to love your body every minute—even with a "perfect" body. We're hit with too many messages telling us to fix ourselves and about what's wrong with us.

So, instead of trying to convince yourself you love your body every minute of every day—

1. Notice thoughts about negative body image.

2. Remember those are normal in our body-obsessed culture.

3. Realize it's unworkable to spin them over and over again.

4. Go do something that matters to you.

5. Seriously, go do something that matters to you, whether it's connecting with someone you care about, expressing yourself creatively, doing work that matters to you, taking care of yourself, contributing to others, or work on a skill you're learning.

You need to have other things in your life that are important to you, that you participate in, and you need to weigh those equally.

It's simply unworkable to pin all of your self-worth on one external thing, and focus on it all the time. Have other things you care about.

You can work on your fitness and not have it be your only sense of self-worth. Similarly, people can work on a career and work toward getting a raise or a promotion without basing their entire sense of self-worth on their income or job title.

THE WAR OF BODY IMAGE

Imagine a battlefield with diet-world body hate on one side and body love on the other. Imagine those two sides in a drawn-out, terrible trench warfare. Sometimes body hate gains some ground; other times body love gains some ground. Mostly, the fight just rages on, and neither side really wins.

The normal perspective is to get in there and fight. Try to figure out which side is "right" or "true," then fight for one side or the other, and try to change the battle. You might find no matter which side you fight for, the war just starts up again later.

The Wise Five perspective is just to notice the war. Step outside of it, like you're watching it on TV. You're no longer surprised when it shows up because it shows up all the time. You don't have to pick a side; you don't have to fight. If you just let it do its thing, it's just like having the TV on in the background.

Acceptance is when we know it's normal for the war of body image to go on. Instead of getting in and fighting in the war, simply let it be, like a war movie on TV just going in the background. It's actually fairly peaceful if you just let it be.

Committed action is knowing you can do all the things that matter to you in your life, even if the body image war is sometimes on TV in the background. You can still connect with your friends; you can practice skills for things that matter to you, and you can be the kind of person you want to be.

The body image war will sometimes be on TV. Just let that go on in the background while you focus on *making your life bigger*.

GROUNDHOG DAY

Groundhog Day is one of my favorite movies ever, because it's about The Wise Five.

Bill Murray's character, Phil, starts off the movie doing The Wise Five. He's basically all about himself, and he tries to force Andie McDowell's character, Rita, to fall in love with him through status and contrived situations.

As the movie progresses and as he's forced to relive the same day over and over, he discovers he can't engineer a way to make her love him. In Wise Five lingo, that means he figures out he can't control connection.

Instead, even though he's forced to live the same day over and over, he chooses not to be the same person each time. He starts to learn skills like ice sculpting and playing piano; he learns about everyone in town; he really listens to people. He starts to fix all the problems that happen in that town. He becomes a really good person.

1. **Values:** In the beginning, he clearly values only status. By the end, he values community and people.

2. **Skills:** He takes lessons and practices playing piano and ice sculpting.

3. **Connection:** In the beginning, he doesn't care about or pay attention to anyone else. By the end, he learns about everyone in town and finds out what matters to them. He even organizes his day around helping people.

4. **Acceptance:** He goes through a period of intense despair, but eventually he accepts his feelings. After that, he can spend his time practicing skills that matter to him and taking care of people.

5. **Committed Action:** He tries out the day seemingly hundreds of different ways. He catches the kid falling out of the tree even though the kid never thanks him. He takes actions that fit his values even though he knows they don't make any difference, and he'll have to start over every day. He takes those only because they make up the kind of person he wants to be.

Groundhog Day is a funny movie that pulls together all the elements of The Wise Five in clever ways. As much as I love watching '80s comedies just for the sake of watching '80s comedies, this one is secretly deep. If you want a cool illustration of The Failure Five, it's Bill Murray's character at the beginning of the movie. Then for a depiction of The Wise Five, it's him at the end of the movie.

WHO GETS RESULTS RAPIDLY?

The people who practice the skills and work out the most consistently get the best results the fastest.

Ironically, the only people who are able to practice the most frequently and most consistently are people who do higher-level work:

- The Meta-skills: If/Then planning, values reflection, and flexibility

- The Ten Turning Points: Practicing excellence instead of perfectionism, self-care instead of punishment, and goldilocksing instead of doing too much

- The Wise Five: Clarify your values, accept your thoughts and feelings, commit to taking action even when it's hard.

The people who want to hold onto their perfectionism suffer the most and have the most weekly starts and stops. The people who don't goldilocks based on the red/yellow/green situations in their lives have more big failures and quit the most often. The people who keep going back to dieting or who try to turn the guidelines and skills into diet rules similarly have many time-consuming starts and stops.

Most people do too much, take off like a rocket, and then repeatedly crash and burn. People who *do* goldilocks their skills and workout practice so they're engaging do really well. Tailoring the skills to your current level helps you make faster progress.

People who practice excellence do really well, and the people who embrace The Wise Five do the best. Really, the people who just follow the program get the fastest results. They are the people who embrace that it's going to be new and uncomfortable, and that they're going to make mistakes and who get in the most practice.

And the people who get in the most practice win.

Rapid results occur when you practice the skills and Meta-skills and embrace the crucial Turning Points and The Wise Five. It's the same as moving slowly and steadily and just resisting it less.

But, of course, I don't really care how long it takes you to build these into your life. If it takes a while to practice through old habits and normal resistance, that's okay. As long as you're making measurable progress in your skill and Meta-skill practice, you're doing awesome. It'll all come together as your skills increase. Similarly, if you're reflecting on your Turning Points and your Wise Five, it will all come together in time.

NERDY ESSAY ABOUT BODY ACCEPTANCE AND BODY CHANGE

Thesis: You must look a certain way to have value. You're not good enough. The only legitimate goal is to change how you look.

Antithesis: You should have no goals or values around how you look. To accept yourself completely, you must resist any desire to change.

Synthesis: Personal autonomy: Whatever you want for yourself—whatever fits your personal values—is what matters. You may simultaneously accept yourself and where you are, and also take actions that cause change.

The original construct of the fitness field was essentially that you don't look good enough, and fitness is about fixing that. Then, there was an equal and opposite reaction in some movements of body positivity that you should completely accept yourself, and any pursuit of change is betraying that acceptance.

I'd argue for the middle:

- Whatever you want, you can want. Don't let people provide things for you to want.

- Acceptance and change, paradoxically, work really well together. We now have a ton of evidence—specifically from research into contextual behavioral sciences like ACT and DBT—that acceptance and change are an effective combination.

THE BIGGEST LOSER WAS THE WORST THING TO HAPPEN TO THE FITNESS WORLD

The Biggest Loser reinforced a cultural conversation that people who are overweight should hate themselves and be constantly berated and punished into losing weight.

It's not that this doesn't work. Clearly, from the results on the show, it worked in a way. The problem with trying to "hate yourself" fit is the punishment and berating needs to be nearly constant. You have to be locked on location somewhere; otherwise the sheer horribleness of it will overtake you.

1. First, none of us are locked on a virtual island with people constantly yelling at us. We will never have enough structure to make that work.

2. Second, that's completely terrible. Even if it worked, the cost to your quality of life is too high.

3. Third, we have a better way.

Ironically, people get more motivational mileage out of caring about something than they do hating themselves.

NERDY, SCIENCY BACKGROUND

The "hating yourself" side of motivation falls into the two categories we talked about at the beginning of this section: reward and punishment and contingent self-esteem or guilt.

On the flip side, we have internalized values.

More practically, just think about it:

- Do you take care of your kids because you hate yourself or because you care about your kids?

- Did you go to college because you hate yourself or because you care about education?

- Do you go to the doctor because you hate yourself or because you care about health?

The whole idea that you're supposed to hate your body so much you make it fit is ridiculous. People do things they care about.

Do you take better care of your best friend or your worst enemy?

This isn't a philosophical discussion about how we should take care of everyone. Just, realistically, we take care of our good friends because we care about them. We don't do much for our worst enemies because we don't care about them.

Our bodies are the same: We take better care of them if we care about them.

I'M NOT ASKING YOU TO LOVE YOUR BODY

I'm not asking you to like your body more. I'm asking you to take care of it.

Punishing or hating yourself fit doesn't work. Identifying what you care about and learning how to take actions consistently with what you care about is the real work of motivation.

The "punishment and hating your body" style of motivation doesn't work for very long. It's certainly never worked long enough to get results. If that started you on your journey to fitness, that's fine, but it's time to grow up. It's time to identify what you care about and take measurable actions consistent with those things. Fitness is simply a matter of taking those actions—of taking care of yourself.

That's easier said than done, which is why the rest of the book is about the skills, planning, turning points, and psychology of taking those actions.

DON'T LET ANYONE TELL YOU YOUR GOAL WEIGHT

People often ask what their goal weight should be. Sometimes they ask what their "happy weight" would be. I resist answering those questions because it's not up to me to tell you what you should want. You should run from any trainer or coach who tries to tell your goals.

Here's a perspective that might be useful in sorting this out for yourself: Think about your "values weight." Instead of a number on the scale, think about a frequency of acting in line with your values. You end up where you end up. Your "values weight" is simply whatever weight you settle at when your actions—your skill practice—are in line with *your personal values*. That's it.

Consider all the things you value in your life.

Consider the kind of person you want to be.

Be that person.

Many people aren't currently living in line with their values in relation to food, and by simply pulling their actions in line with their values, they lose weight. Getting leaner and stronger is often a natural byproduct of being the kind of person you want to be. That's a very, very cool way to approach this: being the kind of person you want to be. Only you get to say who that is.

It's important to remember you can't do it all. And you can't be perfect. Clarifying your values means balancing your priorities.

Honestly, I could be bigger, leaner, and stronger if I didn't write books or go back to school to study psychology. But those things matter to me, and right now they matter to me more than being three percent leaner. I mostly eat and work out to maintain my sanity while I'm doing this much work. I'm acting in line with my values—all of my values, including contribution, connection, and education,

This is different for everyone. I'm sure you have commitments with family, career, and community along with your values like strength and health. You need to find your own balance. True up your actions to your values and your personal balance. Being the person you want to be on a daily basis is a bigger goal.

DON'T LET ANYONE TELL YOU YOUR GOAL STRENGTH

Similarly, don't let anyone tell you how strong you need to get. Don't let people set arbitrary goals for you. Most people reading this probably aren't on a professional sports team or are training for the Special Forces. Those people have legitimate standards they have to meet. Most of us don't.

We just need to determine our values. If the kind of person you want to be is someone who values strength, you're going to strength train. You probably value intelligent planning and reasonable expectations, and you're going to follow the programs in this book. You probably care about progress, so you're going to track your weights, and make progress over time.

That's actually enough. Look at your values. Take actions in line with your values. You will absolutely get stronger. As strong as you are today, taking actions in line with your values will get you as strong as you ought to be.

What's the alternative? Taking actions that aren't in line with your values? Sure, you could do something stupid, like more volume or weight than you can handle in an effort to force faster progress, but usually people doing that just get hurt. The best you can do is smart programming, and then see where it takes you.

Focus on actions in line with your values. Show up for the kind of person you want to be by doing the workouts. Focus on being the kind of person you want to be, and see how that expresses itself in the weight room. You get to live your values in your strength training, every session. You get to be the kind of person you want to be, in action, in your workout today.

CREATE YOURSELF

I think it's funny any time I read about someone "finding" themselves, because it's easier to create yourself from your values.

Similarly, whenever someone is going into an uncomfortable situation, people often suggest, "Just be yourself." I always found myself wondering what that meant. Did it mean I was supposed to be uncomfortable and awkward?

In reality, "finding" or "being" yourself is simply clarifying your values and acting in line with them. My biggest values include connecting with people and making a difference. The funny thing is, I can be my same uncomfortable and awkward self and still connect with lots of people, and make a difference. I can accept I often feel awkward, and I can also take actions like speaking on stage in front of 300 people, or coaching people every day because it's important to me to make a difference.

Similarly, you can have all the thoughts and cravings you have now and still take actions in line with your values. You can be the kind of person you want to be, even while being an imperfect human. There's nothing to fix about you; you just may have some values to clarify and some actions to change. You can do those things, being the totally human you that you are.

We all have things we just sort of fell into. We have thoughts about ourselves and what we're capable of that we mostly got from other people. We have concepts of what we should want out of life, mostly coming from TV. We have all these things we do that are mostly just habit. That's the "you" that you sort of fell into.

You can create something else. Create yourself by clarifying your personal values. That's all there is to it—clarify your values, then start taking actions in line with them.

Just don't fall into the trap of your values or your best version of yourself being some perfect, idealized, robot version of yourself. People always assume their best version of themselves would be the one who's able to meet all of society's standards for beauty, productivity, socializing, buying things, and parenting…all at the same time.

That "everything all the time" is no one's best self. That perfect person can't connect with people because no one else is perfect. Values are inherently flexible and allow for your humanity and imperfections.

Allow yourself to be a human. Forgive yourself for your mistakes and the normal shortcomings of being human. Take actions in line with your values as often as possible, even in all of your humanity.

In those actions, you're being the "you" that you created. Values don't have a beginning or an end. Any time you're taking actions in line with your values, you're living your values. You can be the person you want to be—today. You can be that *right now*. It's not a far-off, someday, maybe thing. If you take actions in line with your values right now, you're living those values. You are being the "you" that you created, right now, today.

Notice how your values in food and fitness expand out into the rest of your life. Ideally, your fitness, the skills in this book, and The Wise Five all make it possible for you to express yourself as the kind of person you want to be in your life. Hopefully, it frees you up to be more engaged in your family, friends, career, hobbies, and community. It's predictable that these will become fully integrated—it's circular—such that your value-based engagement in other areas of your life makes fitness easier too.

LEAN AND STRONG FOR LIFE DEPENDS ON THE WISE FIVE

The Wise Five are simple to list, yet demand a lifetime of practice.

THE FAILURE FIVE	THE WISE FIVE
Reward or Punishment	Values
Self-esteem	Skills
Status	Connection
Suppressing Unwanted Thoughts and Feelings	Accepting Thoughts and Feelings
Force "Motivated" Thoughts and Feelings	Committed Action

They fall into a continuum:

CONTINUUM OF THE WISE FIVE		
Trying to force and control self-directedness	Actual self-directedness	Opting out or giving up on self-directedness
The Failure Five	The Wise Five	The Unfulfilled Five

We have enough evidence from three decades of research into Self Determination Theory and contextual behavioral science to know pursuing The Wise Five is an effective path to wellbeing. Practicing The Wise Five is the path to increased intrinsic motivation to get lean and strong.

Similarly, we know pursuing The Failure Five reduces wellbeing. Practicing The Failure Five reduces intrinsic motivation to eat well and work out.

The Wise Five is the highest view from which to look at your leanness and strength. The Wise Five are the psychology of getting lean and strong. Often, even the best books on habits and food still skip motivation science, and that might be the missing piece for you.

The Wise Five are about making your food and fitness a meaningful part of your life that add to all the other parts of life that matter to you.

CONCLUSION

There are five levels to *Lean and Strong:*

Don't Diet   The first step is to stop doing things that don't work
Eating Skills and Workout Skills   What skills to practice to get lean and strong
Meta-skills   How to practice the skills so your practice is successful each week
The Ten Turning Points   How to think about your skills practice so you don't sabotage your results every eight weeks
The Wise Five   Understanding intrinsic motivation and how it works

As mentioned in the beginning of the book, most diet books don't take a big enough view to actually make a difference for people. They start at dieting or habits and they don't even get that right.

However, you now have all five levels required for the behavior changes you need to get lean and strong. It's likely some of these levels are completely new to you—that should be exciting! Now you have a complete system with all of the tools you need.

You can look at it like this:

What not to do

Diet

What to do

The eating skills and workout skills

How

The Meta-skills

What to think

The Ten Turning Points

Motivation and behavior science

The Wise Five

Anytime you get lost with food, just come back to practicing the skills. When it omes down to it, there are only four.

	DURING MEALS	BETWEEN MEALS
LISTEN TO YOUR BODY	Notice when getting full, and stop when full	Distinguish true hunger versus cravings, boredom, tiredness, emotions, or thoughts
USE A GUIDELINE	Plate healthy and balanced portions	Eat a balanced meal every four to six hours, without snacking in between

Anytime you hit an obstacle, use The Meta-skills and The Ten Turning Points. Make sure your leanness and strength practice is good for life with The Wise Five.

You now have the most complete system currently available. You have the most up-to-date research translated into a system. This might be the first time in your life you have everything you need. It will be an exciting adventure to see what new results you can get, how you build your relationship to your body, your fitness and food changes, and how connecting your values to your practice adds a new level of meaning to your leanness and strength.

Whatever matters to you, you have a system to take actions consistent with that.

Being lean and strong is about being successful with your eating skills and workout program. Being lean and strong should be a meaningful part of your life that adds to and supports all the people and things you value, that you stand for, and that matter to you.

THE REAL LEAN AND STRONG

There are multiple definitions of lean. The first, and most obvious, is that of having a healthy and athletic ratio of muscle to fat. That's likely the reason you purchased this book, and you've been provided the tools to get that.

Importantly, though, lean has another definition: to be efficient, economical, and agile in pursuit of your goals. While people often start this book with the former, they finish it with the latter. Where people might initially struggle with rigidness and perfectionism, a lean mind is marked by flexibility and self-compassion.

Similarly, there are multiple definitions of strong. When people think of working out, they think of strength in terms of physical power—the muscles' ability to produce force.

By now, you might be seeing strength show up in other places. The word "strong" can also be used to describe a person's character, when he or she is courageous, clear, and resilient.

In that way, being strong might be the ability to accept and be with your thoughts and emotions. Being strong might boil down to being clear about your personal values, and taking actions in line with your values even when it's hard.

Lean: Being efficient, economical, and agile, in pursuit of your goals
(*The Ten Turning Points*)

Strong: Doing what matters to you, even when it's hard
(*The Wise Five*)

A NOTE FROM THE AUTHOR

This book was supposed to be a quick update to *Fat Loss Happens on Monday,* but it grew into this monster. I realized pretty quickly that just new skills and workouts weren't going to be enough, that it would take looking at a few different levels, like The Meta-skills and The Wise Five. I think it ended up being complete, but I hope along the way it didn't lose readability. I'm always concerned that it's a rare reader who makes it this far.

Similar to the first book, I started writing it back home, on the Central Coast of California. I was lucky enough to take a few weeks off of client work, and hike during the day and write at night. Some magical "ah ha" moments happen while I'm hiking, but only if I'm writing 2,000—2,500 words per day in a flow.

There's a little peninsula overlooking the estuary and the back bay near home. Sitting on that bench was where I figured out I could organize all of this by skills and guidelines, and by between meals and during meals. The next day, I threw out most of what I'd previously written… and started over. I don't know how most people write, but it seems like I have to write about 60,000 words before I can figure out how the book is supposed to work.

Months later, back in Denver, I was stuck on the book's organization. At that point, it was three sections: Lean, Strong, and Wise. But it just didn't work. The meat was in there, but it was a convoluted mess. I remember walking through the snow in the neighborhood, all bundled up in my puffy jacket, wool hat, boots, and gloves—tromping through the snow, looking at the Christmas lights, and wondering if my book would ever come together. Then it just sort of hit me, and I'm pulling off my gloves, dropping them in the snow, and frantically typing into my phone, "The book has five sections: 1) ~~Diet~~, 2) Skills, 3) Meta-skills, 4) Turning Points, 5) Psychology."

It went through a couple more iterations, but that quick note, with my fingers turning blue and snow landing on the phone screen, pulled together the whole book. Starting again, reorganizing everything, I had to constantly reminding myself, *this is what the work looks like in real life.* Those flashes of inspiration, while elating, usually mean doubling the work. It's a glorious kind of suffering, and I totally love it.

I think maybe there is something to that—the magic happens in the reflection and the rest, but the magic only happens after a ton of work. That probably applies to leanness and strength as well: Reflection matters a great deal, but it's also only useful after having done the work.

I'm pretty lucky, in that my coaching informs my writing, and my coaching gets sharper by organizing it in writing. It's circular, and I can't imagine it any other way. I'm really stoked that I get to do two things that make a difference for people, and that I've practiced both enough to be pretty good at them.

One thing that isn't circular: I'm an awesome listener. I kind of lament that I can't somehow translate that into this book for you because there's a component of my clients getting results that comes from me just listening to them in a way where they can sort out what matters to them.

On one of the best days of my life, back in 2004, I realized I could make a difference for people just by listening to them. Before that, making a difference had always seemed like it would take amazing charisma or brilliant knowledge, neither of which I had. But I could listen. Specifically, I could listen for what mattered to people, and in the listening, they seemed to get clearer for themselves...and that made a difference. Sometimes they didn't work out their concerns, but somehow it started to seem a little more okay, even though nothing got fixed. I want everyone to know that any time they want to make a difference, just listening to someone might be enough.

I wrote this book for people who wanted to get leaner and stronger, but I hope it makes a difference in another way too. I hope to have some impact on the fitness profession toward being kinder, more professional, and more effective. The diet field, especially, can be a total dumpster fire. Or is it a cesspool? As Dan John often reminds us, "We can do better." It was my intention that the delivery is kind; the references make it professional, and the organization is effective.

I look at it like this—diets work for a small circle of people. My first book, *Fat Loss Happens on Monday*, worked for a large circle of people. It's my experience that the tools in this book work for a significantly larger circle. There are already enough people trying to create the optimal diet for the people in the smallest circle. I think my job is to keep making the circle bigger.

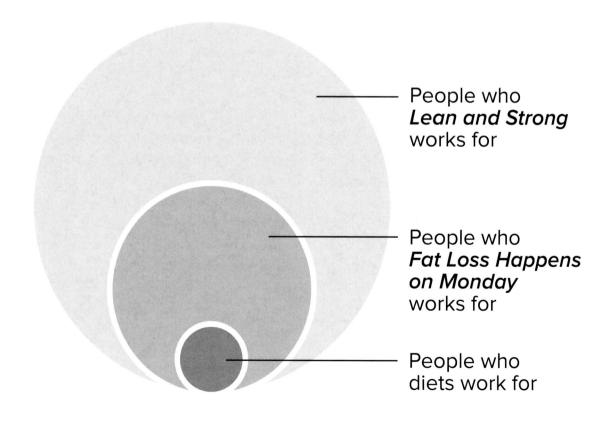

People who
Lean and Strong
works for

People who
*Fat Loss Happens
on Monday*
works for

People who
diets work for

POST CREDITS SCENE

This is going to be my favorite and most effective tool for managing emotional eating, stress eating, and cravings. If you have issues with any of those, make this tool the centerpiece of your food skill practice.

Okay, so I'm a huge nerd. I love *Marvel* movies. The best part, of course, is the post-credits scene. That's where you get a funny clip or a preview of what's to come as a reward through waiting through all the credits. It's a solid Easter egg for the real nerds, like after the first *Avengers* movie, where we first got a glimpse of Thanos, who would almost a decade later appear in *Infinity War* and *Endgame*.

This is the post credits scene for *Lean and Strong*. It's my clients' favorite defusion tool. The defusion tool is called "Let the Monsters Ride the Bus." I like it so much, I've joked about naming the upcoming book on emotional eating after it. So, here you're getting a really effective tool and a preview of the next book.

This is an adaptation of the extremely popular ACT metaphor, "Passengers on the Bus," from Hayes, Strosahl, and Wilson's *Acceptance and Commitment Therapy: An experiential approach to behavior change*. Some version of this metaphor has shown up in nearly every ACT book ever written because it's so elegant and efficient. Here's how I like to explain it:

"Let the Monsters Ride the Bus"

Imagine you're a bus driver. You're driving your bus in the direction of your values and goals. As you're driving, you stop at stops and passengers get on and off at different times. These passengers represent your thoughts, while the driving represents your actions.

Sometimes, cool passengers get on the bus. These are really cool thoughts, like, "Wow, I'm really feeling myself today!" or "Things sure are going well." They can also be emotions like joy, delight, peace, tranquility, determination, or inspiration. These passengers get on and off the bus, in their own time and at their own stops.

Other times, you stop at a stop and a monster gets on the bus. The monsters can be thoughts like, "I feel fat," or "This isn't working," or "I blew my diet." They can also be emotions like sadness, anger, frustration, or loneliness. They can even be cravings for desserts, or treats, or getting seconds. The monsters also get on and off in their own time and at their own stops.

When we get cool passengers, it seems easy to drive our route in the direction of our values. The cool passengers make us feel good about our actions and it's really easy. If we just had these cool passengers forever, it would be pretty easy to hit our goals.

When we get monsters, it seems hard to drive the bus. The monsters are always yelling at us, and telling us to take unplanned turns away from our goals and values.

Sometimes, we stop the bus and turn around to fight with the monsters, and try to push them off of the bus. Of course, to fight with the monsters, it means we stopped driving toward our goals and we're facing the other way.

Other times, we don't want to hear the monsters yelling anymore, so we eat food until we sort of numb them. This is a pretty big turn away from our route—we're driving the opposite direction of our goals and values. But food is really effective at numbing and turning down the volume, and of course, if we eat to handle the monsters, it turns into a lot of extra eating.

The mistake people make is thinking they need to fight the monsters or eat to numb them. People have been taught they need to fight the monsters. For many people, fighting the monsters doesn't work. Not only are they stopped and not driving toward their goals, but it also seems like the more they fight the monsters, the bigger the monsters get. The next thing they know, they find themselves eating to numb them.

The fix is hard and counterintuitive, but it is also extremely effective:

Let the monsters ride the bus.

What no one tells you is that you can continue to drive toward your goals and values even with monsters on the bus. The cool passengers get on the bus, ride for a while and get off…and the monsters will also get on the bus, ride around for a while, and then get off! They'll all get on and off in their own time. Our only job is to continue driving the bus toward our values.

I don't know who originally added "monsters" to the "passengers on the bus" metaphor, but I totally love it.

My big addition to the metaphor is the word LET. "*Let* the Monsters Ride the Bus" makes a huge difference because everyone misunderstands this metaphor the first time they hear it. People have heard they're supposed to fight the monsters so many times that even after hearing a metaphor about *not* fighting them, they still assume they're supposed to fight.

When people embrace *letting* the monsters ride the bus, they find they have a really powerful tool for taking actions in line with their values, consistently, even when it's hard. This is a master key for working with cravings and emotional eating.

The way to use this metaphor is simple: When you have cravings or uncomfortable thoughts that make you want to eat to fix them, imagine those thoughts as monsters. Practice taking actions in line with your values even while you let the monsters ride the bus.

Using the metaphor—imagining the thoughts as monsters—is a defusion technique. Letting them ride the bus is acceptance. Imagining the thoughts as monsters gives you the distance you need to make new choices, and take new actions.

Defusion is a skill, and skills require practice. It's a higher-level skill, and might require lots of practice. Many people report that practicing defusion actually makes their cravings *worse* for the first couple of weeks they try using it. That's okay, because we aren't trying to make the cravings go away; we're trying to practice your skills *in spite of cravings*. We're trying to let the cravings "ride the bus."

Some people struggle with visualization and imagining metaphors. If that's you, that's okay. You can do just as well by labeling your thoughts "thought monsters" or "your inner critic." You might even say to yourself or write in a journal, "I notice I'm having the thought that _____." These are all ways to create defusion—that distance—from your thoughts. Even if you have trouble seeing it, it's effective just to label them "monsters."

After a few months of practice, many clients report that this skill completely changed their lives in relation to food. Nothing will ever be the same for them, as long as they live. It gets easier and becomes more natural to use this skill at three months, six months, and a year, and people see dramatic differences in their weight because of it.

Put "Let the Monsters Ride the Bus" on your food skill tracker. Then track every time you use the metaphor by imagining your unwanted thoughts, cravings, or emotions as monsters. Track it; it's a practice.

The point of letting the monsters ride the bus is that *you can keep driving the bus toward your values.*

Defusion means separating your thoughts from your actions. Imagine your thoughts as monsters, but then keep driving. Driving could be practicing your food skills; it could be going to the gym to do a workout, or it could be any of the items on the self-care list.

Letting the monsters ride the bus is about freeing yourself up to drive: Go do something that matters to you.

Josh Hillis

APPENDIX ONE
EATING SKILLS
AND GUIDELINES PROGRAMS

BEGINNER: WEEKS ONE THROUGH FOUR

WEEK ONE		DAY:	M	T	W	TH	F	SA	SU
		DATE:							
DURING MEALS	Put the fork down between bites								
	Plating: Increase protein								
BETWEEN MEALS	Notice hunger for 30 minutes before a meal								
	Eat a meal every four to six hours (no snacks)								

WEEK TWO		DAY:	M	T	W	TH	F	SA	SU
		DATE:							
DURING MEALS	Put the fork down between bites								
	Plating: Increase vegetables								
BETWEEN MEALS	Notice hunger for 30 minutes before a meal								
	Eat a meal every four to six hours (no snacks)								

WEEK THREE	DAY:	M	T	W	TH	F	SA	SU
	DATE:							
DURING MEALS	Put the fork down between bites							
	Plating: One serving of carbohydrates							
BETWEEN MEALS	Notice hunger for 30 minutes before a meal							
	Eat a meal every four to six hours (no snacks)							

WEEK FOUR	DAY:	M	T	W	TH	F	SA	SU
	DATE:							
DURING MEALS	Put the fork down between bites							
	Plating: One tablespoon of fat							
BETWEEN MEALS	Notice hunger for 30 minutes before a meal							
	Eat a meal every four to six hours (no snacks)							

INTERMEDIATE: WEEKS ONE THROUGH FOUR

WEEK ONE	DAY:	M	T	W	TH	F	SA	SU
	DATE:							
DURING MEALS	Put the fork down between bites							
	Plating: Increase protein							
BETWEEN MEALS	Eat a meal every four to six hours (no snacks)							
	Wait ten minutes before eating a snack							

WEEK TWO	DAY:	M	T	W	TH	F	SA	SU
	DATE:							
DURING MEALS	Put the fork down between bites							
	Plating: Increase vegetables							
BETWEEN MEALS	Eat a meal every four to six hours (no snacks)							
	Wait ten minutes before eating a snack							
PLANNING	If: Then:							

WEEK THREE	DAY:	M	T	W	TH	F	SA	SU
	DATE:							
DURING MEALS	Put the fork down between bites							
	Plating: One serving of carbohydrates							
BETWEEN MEALS	Eat a meal every four to six hours (no snacks)							
	Wait ten minutes before eating a snack							
PLANNING	If: Then:							
TURNING POINT	Practice excellence and self-compassion							

WEEK FOUR	DAY:	M	T	W	TH	F	SA	SU
	DATE:							
DURING MEALS	Put the fork down between bites							
	Plating: One tablespoon of fat							
BETWEEN MEALS	Eat a meal every four to six hours (no snacks)							
	Wait ten minutes before eating a snack							
PLANNING	If: Then:							
TURNING POINT	Practice excellence and self-compassion							
WISE FIVE	Values (list three)							

INTERMEDIATE: WEEKS FIVE THROUGH EIGHT

WEEK FIVE	DAY: DATE:	M	T	W	TH	F	SA	SU
DURING MEALS	Plate balanced meals							
	Check in with your stomach mid-meal							
BETWEEN MEALS	Eat a meal every four to six hours without snacking in between							
	Distinguish true hunger from cravings, boredom, tiredness, emotions, or thoughts							

WEEK SIX	DAY: DATE:	M	T	W	TH	F	SA	SU
DURING MEALS	Put the fork down between bites							
	Notice when full, and stop							
BETWEEN MEALS	Eat a meal every four to six hours without snacking in between)							
	Distinguish true hunger from cravings, boredom, tiredness, emotions, or thoughts							
PLANNING	If: Then:							

WEEK SEVEN		DAY:	M	T	W	TH	F	SA	SU
		DATE:							
DURING MEALS	Plate balanced meals								
	Notice when full, and stop								
BETWEEN MEALS	Eat a meal every four to six hours without snacking in between								
	Distinguish true hunger from cravings, boredom, tiredness, emotions, or thoughts								
PLANNING	If: Then:								
TURNING POINT	Engagement/flow/goldilocksing								

WEEK EIGHT		DAY:	M	T	W	TH	F	SA	SU
		DATE:							
DURING MEALS	Put the fork down between bites								
	Notice when full, and stop								
BETWEEN MEALS	Eat a meal every four to six hours without snacking in between								
	Distinguish true hunger from cravings, boredom, tiredness, emotions, or thoughts								
PLANNING	If: Then:								
TURNING POINT	Engagement/flow/goldilocksing								
WISE FIVE	Values (List three)								

INTERMEDIATE: WEEKS NINE THROUGH TWELVE

WEEK NINE	DAY:	M	T	W	TH	F	SA	SU
	DATE:							
DURING MEALS	Plate balanced meals							
	Notice when full, and stop							
BETWEEN MEALS	Distinguish true hunger from cravings, boredom, tiredness, emotions, or thoughts							
	Practice deliberate self-care instead snacking							

WEEK TEN	DAY:	M	T	W	TH	F	SA	SU
	DATE:							
DURING MEALS	Plate balanced meals							
	Notice when full, and stop							
BETWEEN MEALS	Distinguish true hunger from cravings, boredom, tiredness, emotions, or thoughts							
	Practice deliberate self-care instead snacking							
PLANNING	If:							
	Then:							

WEEK ELEVEN	DAY:	M	T	W	TH	F	SA	SU
	DATE:							
DURING MEALS	Plate balanced meals							
	Notice when full, and stop							
BETWEEN MEALS	Distinguish true hunger from cravings, boredom, tiredness, emotions, or thoughts							
	Practice deliberate self-care instead snacking							
PLANNING	If: THEN:							
TURNING POINT	Weight loss comes from self-care							

WEEK TWELVE	DAY:	M	T	W	TH	F	SA	SU
	DATE:							
DURING MEALS	Plate balanced meals							
	Notice when full, and stop							
BETWEEN MEALS	Distinguish true hunger from cravings, boredom, tiredness, emotions, or thoughts							
	De-fusion from unwanted thoughts, feelings, and cravings							
PLANNING	If: Then:							
TURNING POINT	Weight loss comes from self-care							
WISE FIVE	Values (List three)							

ADVANCED: WEEKS ONE THROUGH FOUR

WEEK ONE	DAY:	M	T	W	TH	F	SA	SU
	DATE:							
DURING MEALS	Plate balanced meals							
	Wait ten minutes before getting seconds							
BETWEEN MEALS	Distinguish true hunger from cravings, boredom, tiredness, emotions, or thoughts							
	De-fusion from unwanted thoughts, feelings, and cravings							

WEEK TWO	DAY:	M	T	W	TH	F	SA	SU
	DATE:							
DURING MEALS	Put down the fork between bites							
	Notice that flavor enjoyment is different from fullness							
BETWEEN MEALS	Notice and wait through normal hunger 30 minutes before eating							
	De-fusion from unwanted thoughts, feelings, and cravings							
PLANNING	If: Then:							

WEEK THREE	DAY:	M	T	W	TH	F	SA	SU
	DATE:							
DURING MEALS	Eat without screens							
	Practice five senses mindfulness while eating							
BETWEEN MEALS	Flexibility: Saying "yes" sometimes and "no" other times							
	De-fusion from unwanted thoughts, feelings, and cravings							
PLANNING	If: Then:							
TURNING POINT	(pick one)							

WEEK FOUR	DAY:	M	T	W	TH	F	SA	SU
	DATE:							
DURING MEALS	Notice when full, and stop							
	Check in on fullness one hour after eating							
BETWEEN MEALS	Self-care: coping, self-soothing, fun activities, and hobbies							
	De-fusion from unwanted thoughts, feelings, and cravings							
PLANNING	If: Then:							
TURNING POINT	(pick one)							
WISE FIVE	Values (List three)							

ADVANCED: WEEKS FIVE THROUGH EIGHT

WEEK FIVE	DAY: DATE:	M	T	W	TH	F	SA	SU
DURING MEALS	Wait ten minutes before getting seconds							
	Do something engaging immediately after eating							
BETWEEN MEALS	Get engaged with what's going on right now							
	De-fusion from unwanted thoughts, feelings, and cravings							

WEEK SIX	DAY: DATE:	M	T	W	TH	F	SA	SU
DURING MEALS	Practice five senses experience of the meal							
	Notice that flavor enjoyment is different from fullness							
BETWEEN MEALS	Self-care: coping, self-soothing, fun activities, and hobbies							
	De-fusion from unwanted thoughts, feelings, and cravings							
PLANNING	If: Then:							

WEEK SEVEN		DAY:	M	T	W	TH	F	SA	SU
		DATE:							
DURING MEALS	Wait ten minutes before having seconds								
	Do something engaging immediately after eating								
BETWEEN MEALS	Get engaged with what's going on right now								
	De-fusion from unwanted thoughts, feelings, and cravings								
PLANNING	If: Then:								
TURNING POINT	(pick one)								

WEEK EIGHT		DAY:	M	T	W	TH	F	SA	SU
		DATE:							
DURING MEALS	Stop before eating too much								
	Do something engaging immediately after eating								
BETWEEN MEALS	Self-care: coping, self-soothing, fun activities, and hobbies								
	De-fusion from unwanted thoughts, feelings, and cravings								
PLANNING	If: Then:								
TURNING POINT	(pick one)								
WISE FIVE	Values (List three)								

ADVANCED: WEEKS NINE THROUGH TWELVE

WEEK NINE	DAY: DATE:	M	T	W	TH	F	SA	SU
DURING MEALS	Notice when full, and stop							
	Plate balanced portions							
BETWEEN MEALS	Distinguish between hunger and stress							
	De-fusion from unwanted thoughts, feelings, and cravings							

WEEK TEN	DAY: DATE:	M	T	W	TH	F	SA	SU
DURING MEALS	Notice when full, and stop							
	Plate balanced portions							
BETWEEN MEALS	Distinguish between hunger and stress							
	De-fusion from unwanted thoughts, feelings, and cravings							
PLANNING	If: Then:							

WEEK ELEVEN	DAY: DATE:	M	T	W	TH	F	SA	SU
DURING MEALS	Notice when full, and stop							
	Plate balanced portions							
BETWEEN MEALS	Distinguish between hunger and stress							
	De-fusion from unwanted thoughts, feelings, and cravings							
PLANNING	If: Then:							
TURNING POINT	(pick one)							

WEEK TWELVE	DAY: DATE:	M	T	W	TH	F	SA	SU
DURING MEALS	Notice when full, and stop							
	Plate balanced portions							
BETWEEN MEALS	Distinguish between hunger and stress							
	De-fusion from unwanted thoughts, feelings, and cravings							
PLANNING	If: Then:							
TURNING POINT	(pick one)							
WISE FIVE	Values (List three)							

LIFETIME

WEEK ONE	DAY: DATE:	M	T	W	TH	F	SA	SU
DURING MEALS	Plate balanced portions							
	Notice when full, and stop							
BETWEEN MEALS	Eat a meal every four to six hours, without snacking in between							
	Distinguish between hunger and stress							
WISE FIVE	Values (List three)							

WEEK TWO	DAY: DATE:	M	T	W	TH	F	SA	SU
DURING MEALS	Plate balanced portions							
	Notice when full, and stop							
BETWEEN MEALS	Eat a meal every four to six hours, without snacking in between							
	Distinguish between hunger and stress							
WISE FIVE	Values (List three)							

WEEK THREE	DAY: DATE:	M	T	W	TH	F	SA	SU
DURING MEALS	Plate balanced portions							
	Notice when full, and stop							
BETWEEN MEALS	Eat a meal every four to six hours, without snacking in between							
	Distinguish between hunger and stress							
WISE FIVE	Values (List three)							

WEEK FOUR	DAY: DATE:	M	T	W	TH	F	SA	SU
DURING MEALS	Plate balanced portions							
	Notice when full, and stop							
BETWEEN MEALS	Eat a meal every four to six hours, without snacking in between							
	Distinguish between hunger and stress							
WISE FIVE	Values (List three)							

HOW TO FIX SNACKING BETWEEN MEALS

WEEK ONE	DAY: DATE:	M	T	W	TH	F	SA	SU
DURING MEALS	Put the fork down between bites							
	Plate balanced portions							
BETWEEN MEALS	If I want a snack, I'll wait ten minutes							
	Distinguish hunger from boredom, stress, tiredness, or emotions							
PLANNING	If: I get tired in the afternoon Then: I'm going to have some black coffee							
TURNING POINT	Perfectionism versus excellence in practice							
VALUES (LIST THREE)	Reasonableness, strength, vulnerability							

WEEK TWO	DAY: DATE:	M	T	W	TH	F	SA	SU
DURING MEALS	Eat enough at meals							
	Eat without screens							
BETWEEN MEALS	Eat a meal every four to six hours							
	Wait until hungry, then eat a meal							
PLANNING	If: I get bored at work THEN: I'm going to walk for five mintues							

WEEK TWO	DAY:	M T W TH F SA SU
	DATE:	
TURNING POINT	Weight loss as punishment versus self-care	
VALUES (LIST THREE)	Reasonableness, strength, vulnerability	

This is an example of a tracker set up specifically to fix snacking between meals.

Not snacking between meals starts with making sure you're getting enough food and balanced macronutrients at meals. You'll never fix snacking if you chronically eat too little at meals. When trying to fix snacking, it's actually better to eat a little too much at meals. Snacks always add up to more calories than just having solid meals.

Then, we want to make sure you hit psychological fullness—eating without screens and putting your fork down between bites have both been shown to reduce snacking. Researchers believe it has to do with the memory of eating.

Waiting ten minutes before having a snack is one of the most powerful ways to break the habit of snacking. Our biggest issue is, we don't put any space between a craving and a snack, between stimulus and response. We get a craving; we immediately eat.

If we give ourselves a little waiting time, often that alone is enough to break the pattern. It can literally be that simple.

It also doubles as time to check in with ourselves to see what's really going on. That's when we can distinguish between being actually hungry and eating a meal versus just being tired, bored, stressed, or emotional.

HOW TO FIX GETTING SECONDS

WEEK ONE	DAY: DATE:	M	T	W	TH	F	SA	SU
DURING MEALS	Put the fork down between bites							
	Plate balanced portions							
BETWEEN MEALS	Wait ten minutes before getting seconds							
	Do some deliberate self-care after eating							
PLANNING	If: I want seconds Then: I'm going to remember I always want seconds right after a meal, but then I feel full and satisfied ten minutes later							
TURNING POINT	Values versus goals							
VALUES (LIST THREE)	Self-care, self-awareness, courage							

WEEK TWO	DAY: DATE:	M	T	W	TH	F	SA	SU
DURING MEALS	Eat enough at meals							
	Eat without screens							
BETWEEN MEALS	Wait ten minutes before getting seconds							
	Do some deliberate self-care after eating							

WEEK TWO		DAY:	M	T	W	TH	F	SA	SU
		DATE:							
PLANNING	If: I want seconds Then: I'm going to leave the table or kitchen and go do something fun or relaxing								
TURNING POINT	Weight loss as punishment versus self-care								
VALUES (LIST THREE)	Self-care, self-awareness, courage								

This is an example of a tracker set up specifically to fix grazing.

When trying to fix grazing or going back for seconds, it's always better to make one good-sized plate—make sure it's enough. Then you'll know you've had enough, and there's no reason to graze or go back for seconds.

Waiting ten minutes before getting seconds is simplest way to fix that. Note that getting seconds requires eating *enough at meals*. You have to plate enough that you don't need seconds. Also, note that if you're still hungry after ten minutes, you should eat more.

The ten-minute trick gives you time to notice you're full. Get up and do something else instead of staring at more food. Everyone always wants to have seconds. It's normal to want seconds. Just go do something else. You'll be successful with this when you break the pattern of automatically getting seconds.

I can't stress this enough: *If you're still hungry after 10 minutes, eat more.* This isn't a magic trick to get you not to be hungry. If you need more food, eat it. Then next time, remember you really need to plate more food to begin with. It's a learning experience.

Plating balanced portions goes with plating enough—set your food up in such a way you're actually getting the nutrition you need.

FILL-IN CUSTOM SKILL AND GUIDELINES TRACKER

WEEK ONE	DAY:	M	T	W	TH	F	SA	SU
	DATE:							
DURING MEALS								
BETWEEN MEALS								

WEEK TWO	DAY:	M	T	W	TH	F	SA	SU
	DATE:							
DURING MEALS								
BETWEEN MEALS								
PLANNING	If:							
	Then:							

WEEK THREE	DAY:	M	T	W	TH	F	SA	SU
	DATE:							
DURING MEALS								
BETWEEN MEALS								
PLANNING	If:							
	Then:							
TURNING POINT								

WEEK FOUR	DAY:	M	T	W	TH	F	SA	SU
	DATE:							
DURING MEALS								
BETWEEN MEALS								
PLANNING	If:							
	Then:							
TURNING POINT								
VALUES (LIST THREE)								

WEEK FIVE	DAY:	M	T	W	TH	F	SA	SU
	DATE:							
DURING MEALS								
BETWEEN MEALS								

WEEK SIX	DAY:	M	T	W	TH	F	SA	SU
	DATE:							
DURING MEALS								
BETWEEN MEALS								
PLANNING	If: Then:							

WEEK SEVEN	DAY:	M	T	W	TH	F	SA	SU
	DATE:							
DURING MEALS								
BETWEEN MEALS								
PLANNING	If:							
	Then:							
TURNING POINT								

WEEK EIGHT	DAY:	M	T	W	TH	F	SA	SU
	DATE:							
DURING MEALS								
BETWEEN MEALS								
PLANNING	If:							
	Then:							
TURNING POINT								
VALUES (LIST THREE)								

WEEK NINE	DAY:	M	T	W	TH	F	SA	SU
	DATE:							
DURING MEALS								
BETWEEN MEALS								

WEEK TEN	DAY:	M	T	W	TH	F	SA	SU
	DATE:							
DURING MEALS								
BETWEEN MEALS								
PLANNING	If:							
	Then:							

WEEK ELEVEN	DAY:	M	T	W	TH	F	SA	SU
	DATE:							
DURING MEALS								
BETWEEN MEALS								
PLANNING	If: Then:							
TURNING POINT								

WEEK TWELVE	DAY:	M	T	W	TH	F	SA	SU
	DATE:							
DURING MEALS								
BETWEEN MEALS								
PLANNING	If: Then:							
TURNING POINT								
VALUES (LIST THREE)								

APPENDIX TWO
WARMUPS

You are going to have two kinds of warmups: general warmups and specific warmups. The general warmups for beginner, intermediate, and advanced are listed below. For any move that has two sides, *the number listed is for each side.*

BEGINNER WARMUP

360° Breathing	1x60 seconds
Quad T-Spine Rotations	1x8
Hip Flexor Stretch	1x8
Two-leg Dumbbell Hip Bridge	1x8
Goblet Squats	1x8

INTERMEDIATE WARMUP

360° Breathing	1x60 seconds
Quad T-Spine Rotations	8
Hip Flexor Stretch	8
Single-leg Dumbbell Hip Bridge	8
Bear Crawl	1x30–60 seconds

Specific warmups are done right before any particularly heavy exercise

ADVANCED WARMUP

360° Breathing	1x60 seconds
Bretzel	2x8
Bear Crawl	1x30 seconds forward 1x30 seconds backward
Kettlebell Swings	2x8

Specific warmups are done right before a particularly heavy exercise

Breathing is the foundation. It's easy to get stuck in the habit of breathing into your shoulders and chest, instead of your diaphragm. That primarily chest and shoulders breathing is often a result of stress, and often can tighten up our shoulders and hips considerably. Taking a minute to work on deep breathing will increase your movement quality, prepare you to breathe properly doing your workout. It also works as a transition time to get out of the possible stress of work mode, kids mode, or errands mode, and get into workout mode. It's a really great minute to actually relax. Take more than a minute if you need more, and feel free to take a few minutes of 360° breathing after the workout if you'd like.

After breathing, you'll get into thoracic spine mobility, hip mobility, and warming up your lower and upper body. It's pretty short, and with the core work right after, should be enough. For particularly heavy exercises, like deadlifts and squats, you might want to do a specific warmup immediately before that exercise.

SPECIFIC WARMUP INFORMATION

If you're intermediate or advanced, and lifting fairly heavy, it makes sense to do some specific warmup sets. For your warmup sets, you'll do two sets of five reps. The first set will be 50% of the weight in your work sets, and the second set will be 75% of the weight in your work sets.

Note: I keep saying "percentage of the working weight" because I want to be clear that, if you're doing ten repetition sets that day, "100%" is 100% of your ten-rep work sets for that day's workout. I don't want there to be any confusion with people who are used to calculating weights off of their one-rep max, which isn't what we're talking about here.

Specific Warmup	1x5 reps @ 50% of the weight for work sets 1x5 reps @ 75% of the weight for work sets
Work Sets (the sets listed on the workout card)	3x10 @ 100% of working weight

Example: 3 sets of 10 with a 200 pound Trap Bar Deadlift

Specific Warmup	1x5 @ 100 pounds 1x5 @ 150 pounds
Work Sets (the sets listed on the workout card)	3x10 @ 200 pounds

This is a way to get your body ready for that specific movement, without tiring yourself out. Use half the reps of the work set for that phase, and a percentage of your working weight, work up a little. If you're feeling particularly tight on a given day, or it's cold outside, you might add another warmup set or two at 85-90% of the working weight.

Don't worry about getting the percentages just right, warmups sets don't need a lot of precision. Grab whatever the easiest combination of weights gets you sort of close to those percentages.

The idea is just to get a couple of easier sets where you can:

- Get your body ready for that specific movement

- Work up to being ready for that specific work weight

- Check in with your body, and see how it feels doing that particular movement on that day

360° BREATHING

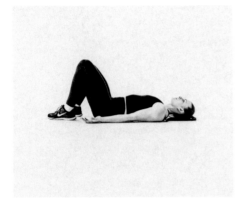

Start

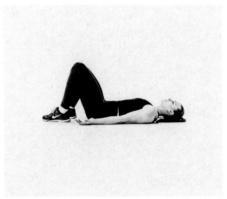

Finish

- Slightly press your low back toward the floor

- Breathe in through your nose

- Feel the air fill up at your low back

- Then the sides of your body

- And then your belly

- Take a long, slow exhale

TWO-LEG DUMBBELL HIP BRIDGE

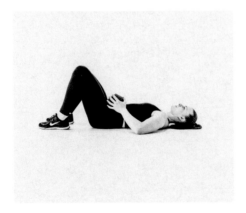

Start

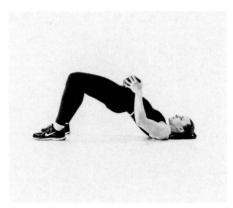

Finish

- Lower your hips

- Flex your butt

- Drive the dumbbell up to the ceiling

APPENDIX THREE
BEGINNER WORKOUTS

There are 12 workouts to do over the course of each month, so you'll do about three workouts per week.

The first page includes all of the "odd" workouts—1, 3, 5, 7, 9, 11.

The second page has the "even" workouts—2, 4, 6, 8, 10, 12.

You'll flip the page *every other* workout to do the workouts in numerical order.

To be clear:

1. Do three workouts per week.

2. Do the workouts in numerical order: 1, 2, 3, 4, 5…just like counting.

It could look like:

1. Workout one on Monday

2. Workout two on Wednesday

3. Workout three on Friday

…and so on.

The actual days you do the workouts are unimportant, but try to avoid doing two back to back if you can. That being said, doing two workouts on back-to-back days is still better than skipping a workout.

Notice how the volume of work (the number of sets of each exercise) increases over the course of the month. You'll start off with two sets of everything, and by the end of the month, you'll be doing three or four sets of everything.

All of the exercises are grouped either in supersets (two exercises back to back) or trisets (three exercises back to back to back). Do all of the exercises in that group, and then rest. In the trisets, the first two are strength exercises; the third, in italics, is a mobility exercise.

For exercises that are single-arm or single-leg, the repetitions listed are to be done on *both sides*.

Do three workouts per week, in numerical order. Week one, do workouts 1, 2, and 3. Week two, do workouts 4, 5, and 6. Use this sheet as a tracker to write down the weight used for each exercise in the box for that workout, underneath the sets and reps.

BEGINNER—MONTH ONE, ODD WORKOUTS

	WORKOUT 1	WORKOUT 3	WORKOUT 5	WORKOUT 7	WORKOUT 9	WORKOUT 11
BAND DEAD BUGS	2x5	2x5	2x5	2x8	2x8	2x8
DOUBLE-DUMBBELL BENCH PRESSES	2x20	2x20	2x20	3x15	3x15	3x15
ROMANIAN DEADLIFTS	2x20	2x20	2x20	3x15	3x15	3x15
HIP FLEXOR STRETCHES	2x8	2x8	2x8	3x8	3x8	3x8
SINGLE-DUMBBELL ROWS	2x20	2x20	2x20	3x15	3x15	3x15
GOBLET SQUATS	2x20	2x20	2x20	3x15	3x15	3x15
T-SPINE ROTATIONS	2x8	2x8	2x8	3x8	3x8	3x8
ONE-ARM KETTLEBELL SWINGS	1x10	2x10	3x10	4x10	5x10	5x10

When three exercises are grouped together, do those back-to-back as a tri-set. For exercises on one leg or one arm, sets listed are for each side.

BEGINNER—MONTH ONE, EVEN WORKOUTS

	WORKOUT 2	WORKOUT 4	WORKOUT 6	WORKOUT 8	WORKOUT 10	WORKOUT 12
PALLOF PRESSES	2x10	2x10	2x10	3x10	3x10	3x10
						:
SINGLE-CABLE ROWS	2x20	2x20	2x20	3x15	3x15	3x15
GOBLET SQUATS	2x20	2x20	2x20	3x15	3x15	3x15
T-SPINE ROTATIONS	2x8	2x8	2x8	3x8	3x8	3x8
45° INCLINE DOUBLE-DUMBBELL BENCH PRESSES	2x20	2x20	2x20	3x15	3x15	3x15
ROMANIAN DEADLIFTS	2x20	2x20	2x20	3x15	3x15	3x15
HIP FLEXOR STRETCHES	2x8	2x8	2x8	3x8	3x8	3x8
WALK	5–10 minutes	5–10 minutes	5–10 minutes	5–10 minutes	5–10 minutes	5–10 minutes

Do three workouts per week, in numerical order. Week one, do workouts 1, 2, and 3. Week two, do workouts 4, 5, and 6. Use this sheet as a tracker to write down the weight used for each exercise in the box for that workout, underneath the sets and reps.

BEGINNER—MONTH TWO, ODD WORKOUTS

	WORKOUT 1	WORKOUT 3	WORKOUT 5	WORKOUT 7	WORKOUT 9	WORKOUT 11
BAND DEAD BUGS	2x8	2x8	2x8	2x10	2x10	2x10
DOUBLE-DUMBBELL BENCH PRESSES	3x12	3x12	3x12	3x10	3x10	3x10
ROMANIAN DEADLIFTS	3x12	3x12	3x12	3x10	3x10	3x10
HIP FLEXOR STRETCHES	3x8	3x8	3x8	3x8	3x8	3x8
SINGLE-DUMBBELL ROWS	3x12	3x12	3x12	3x10	3x10	3x10
GOBLET SQUATS	3x12	3x12	3x12	3x10	3x10	3x10
T-SPINE ROTATIONS	3x8	3x8	3x8	3x8	3x8	3x8
WALK	5–10 minutes	5–10 minutes	5–10 minutes	5–10 minutes	5–10 minutes	5–10 minutes

When three exercises are grouped together, do those back-to-back as a tri-set. For exercises on one leg or one arm, sets listed are for each side.

BEGINNER—MONTH TWO, EVEN WORKOUTS

	WORKOUT 2	WORKOUT 4	WORKOUT 6	WORKOUT 8	WORKOUT 10	WORKOUT 12
PALLOF PRESSES	2x10	2x10	2x10	3x10	3x10	3x10
SINGLE-ARM LAT PULLDOWNS	3x12	3x12	3x12	3x10	3x10	3x10
SPLIT SQUATS	3x12	3x12	3x12	3x10	3x10	3x10
T-SPINE ROTATIONS	3x8	3x8	3x8	3x8	3x8	3x8
45° INCLINE DOUBLE-DUMBBELL BENCH PRESSES	3x12	3x12	3x12	3x10	3x10	3x10
ONE-ARM KETTLEBELL SWINGS	3x12	3x12	3x12	3x10	3x10	3x10
HIP FLEXOR STRETCHES	3x8	3x8	3x8	3x8	3x8	3x8
WALK	5–10 minutes	5–10 minutes	5–10 minutes	5–10 minutes	5–10 minutes	5–10 minutes

Do three workouts per week, in numerical order. Week one, do workouts 1, 2, and 3. Week two, do workouts 4, 5, and 6. Use this sheet as a tracker to write down the weight used for each exercise in the box for that workout, underneath the sets and reps.

BEGINNER—MONTH THREE, ODD WORKOUTS

	WORKOUT 1	WORKOUT 3	WORKOUT 5	WORKOUT 7	WORKOUT 9	WORKOUT 11
BAND DEAD BUGS	3x10	3x10	3x10	3x10	3x10	3x10
DOUBLE-DUMBBELL BENCH PRESSES	4x8	4x8	4x8	4x5	4x5	4x5
SPLIT-STANCE DEADLIFTS	4x8	4x8	4x8	4x5	4x5	4x5
HIP FLEXOR STRETCHES	4x8	4x8	4x8	4x8	4x8	4x8
SINGLE-DUMBBELL ROWS	4x8	4x8	4x8	4x5	4x5	4x5
DOUBLE KETTLEBELL SQUATS	4x8	4x8	4x8	4x5	4x5	4x5
T-SPINE ROTATIONS	4x8	4x8	4x8	4x8	4x8	4x8
WALK	5–10 minutes	5–10 minutes	5–10 minutes	5–10 minutes	5–10 minutes	5–10 minutes

When three exercises are grouped together, do those back-to-back as a tri-set. For exercises on one leg or one arm, sets listed are for each side.

BEGINNER—MONTH THREE, EVEN WORKOUTS

	WORKOUT 2	WORKOUT 4	WORKOUT 6	WORKOUT 8	WORKOUT 10	WORKOUT 12
PALLOF PRESSES	2x10	2x10	2x10	3x10	3x10	3x10
SINGLE-ARM LAT PULLDOWNS	4x8	4x8	4x8	4x5	4x5	4x5
SPLIT SQUATS	4x8	4x8	4x8	4x5	4x5	4x5
T-SPINE ROTATIONS	4x8	4x8	4x8	4x8	4x8	4x8
45° INCLINE DOUBLE-DUMBBELL BENCH PRESSES	4x8	4x8	4x8	4x5	4x5	4x5
ROMANIAN DEADLIFTS	4x8	4x8	4x8	4x5	4x5	4x5
HIP FLEXOR STRETCHES	4x8	4x8	4x8	4x8	4x8	4x8
WALK	5–10 minutes	5–10 minutes	5–10 minutes	5–10 minutes	5–10 minutes	5–10 minutes

APPENDIX FOUR
INTERMEDIATE WORKOUTS

There are 12 workouts to do over the course of each month, so you'll do about three workouts per week.

The first page includes all of the odd workouts—1, 3, 5, 7, 9, 11.

The second page has the even workouts—2, 4, 6, 8, 10, 12.

You'll flip the page every other workout to do the workouts in numerical order.

It could look like:

- Workout one on Monday
- Workout two on Wednesday
- Workout three on Friday

…and so on.

The actual days you do the workouts are unimportant, but try to avoid doing two back to back if you can. That being said, doing two workouts on back-to-back days is still better than skipping one.

Notice how the volume of work—the number of sets of each exercise—increases over the course of the month. You'll start off with two sets of everything, and by the end of the month, you'll be doing three or four sets of everything.

All of the exercises are grouped either in supersets (two exercises back to back) or trisets (three exercises back to back to back). Do all of the exercises in that group, and then rest. In the trisets, the first two are strength exercises; the third, in italics, is a mobility exercise.

For exercises that are single-arm or single-leg, the repetitions listed are to be done on *each side*.

Pushups are listed as "max reps." This means to do the maximum number of repetitions you can with *perfect form*. If your form breaks, stop. Or, if it's easier, you can think about it like stopping when you feel like you could do only one more rep.

If you can't do a pushup from your toes, you can do pushups with your hands elevated, like on a bench, railing, or table. If you can do more than 20 pushups for three sets, move to a harder pushup variation. If you need harder pushup variations, check out spiderman pushups, archer pushups, band pushups, or weighted vest pushups in my first book, *Fat Loss Happens on Monday*.

Assisted chin-ups can be done with a band as shown on page 334, or with an assisted pull-up machine if your gym has one. If you aren't ready for assisted chin-ups, substitute chins with high cable rows.

The deadlifts in the intermediate program are all listed as trap bar deadlifts. If you don't have a trap bar, or if it's your preference, feel free to use a barbell.

Do three workouts per week, in numerical order. Week one, do workouts 1, 2, and 3. Week two, do workouts 4, 5, and 6. Use this sheet as a tracker to write down the weight used for each exercise in the box for that workout, underneath the sets and reps.

INTERMEDIATE LOW VOLUME—MONTH ONE, ODD WORKOUTS

	WORKOUT 1	WORKOUT 3	WORKOUT 5	WORKOUT 7	WORKOUT 9	WORKOUT 11
BAND DEAD BUGS	2x10	2x10	2x10	3x10	3x10	3x10
TRAP BAR DEADLIFTS	2x10	2x10	2x10	3x10	3x10	3x10
PUSHUPS	2x max	2x max	2x max	3x max	3x max	3x max
HIP FLEXOR STRETCHES	2x8	2x8	2x8	3x8	3x8	3x8
SINGLE-CABLE ROWS	2x10	2x10	2x10	3x10	3x10	3x10
SPLIT SQUATS	2x10	2x10	2x10	3x10	3x10	3x10
T-SPINE ROTATIONS	2x8	2x8	3x8	3x8	3x8	3x8
ONE-ARM KETTLEBELL SWINGS	1x10	2x10	3x10	4x10	5x10	5x10

When three exercises are grouped together, do those back-to-back as a tri-set. For exercises on one leg or one arm, sets listed are for each side.

INTERMEDIATE LOW VOLUME—MONTH ONE, EVEN WORKOUTS

	WORKOUT 2	WORKOUT 4	WORKOUT 6	WORKOUT 8	WORKOUT 10	WORKOUT 12
PALLOF PRESSES	2x10	2x10	2x10	3x10	3x10	3x10
ASSISTED CHIN-UPS	2x10	2x10	2x10	3x10	3x10	3x10
DOUBLE-KETTLEBELL FRONT SQUATS	2x10	2x10	2x10	3x10	3x10	3x10
T-SPINE ROTATIONS	2x8	2x8	2x8	3x8	3x8	3x8
75° INCLINE DOUBLE-DUMBBELL BENCH PRESSES	2x10	2x10	2x10	3x10	3x10	3x10
ONE-KETTLEBELL COSSACK DEADLIFTS	2x10	2x10	2x10	3x10	3x10	3x10
HIP FLEXOR STRETCHES	2x8	2x8	2x8	3x8	3x8	3x8
ONE-ARM KETTLEBELL SWINGS	1x10	2x10	3x10	4x10	5x10	5x10

Do three workouts per week, in numerical order. Week one, do workouts 1, 2, and 3. Week two, do workouts 4, 5, and 6. Use this sheet as a tracker to write down the weight used for each exercise in the box for that workout, underneath the sets and reps.

INTERMEDIATE LOW VOLUME—MONTH TWO, ODD WORKOUTS

	WORKOUT 1	WORKOUT 3	WORKOUT 5	WORKOUT 7	WORKOUT 9	WORKOUT 11
KETTLEBELL DEAD BUGS	2x12	2x12	2x12	3x12	3x12	3x12
DUMBBELL BENCH PRESSES	2x20	2x20	2x20	3x20	3x20	3x20
SINGLE-LEG DUMBBELL HIP BRIDGES	2x 10–20	2x 10–20	2x 10–20	3x 10–20	3x 10–20	3x 10–20
HIP FLEXOR STRETCHES	2x8	2x8	2x8	3x8	3x8	3x8
GOBLET SQUATS	2x20	2x20	2x20	3x20	3x20	3x20
DUMBBELL BENT-OVER ROWS	2x20	2x20	2x20	3x20	3x20	3x20
T-SPINE ROTATIONS	2x8	2x8	2x8	3x8	3x8	3x8
ONE-ARM KETTLEBELL SWINGS	:30 work :30 rest x2 minutes	:30 work :30 rest x3 minutes	:30 work :30 rest x4 minutes	:30 work :30 rest x5 minutes	:30 work :30 rest x5 minutes	:30 work :30 rest x5 minutes

When three exercises are grouped together, do those back-to-back as a tri-set. For exercises on one leg or one arm, sets listed are for each side.

INTERMEDIATE LOW VOLUME—MONTH TWO, EVEN WORKOUTS

	WORKOUT 2	WORKOUT 4	WORKOUT 6	WORKOUT 8	WORKOUT 10	WORKOUT 12
HORIZONTAL CABLE ROTATIONS	2x12	2x12	2x12	3x12	3x12	3x12
SINGLE-ARM LAT PULLDOWNS	2x20	2x20	2x20	3x20	3x20	3x20
WALKING LUNGES	2x20	2x20	2x20	3x20	3x20	3x20
T-SPINE ROTATIONS	2x8	2x8	2x8	3x8	3x8	3x8
45° INCLINE DOUBLE-DUMBBELL BENCH PRESSES	2x20	2x20	2x20	3x20	3x20	3x20
ROMANIAN DEADLIFTS	2x20	2x20	2x20	3x20	3x20	3x20
HIP FLEXOR STRETCHES	2x8	2x8	2x8	3x8	3x8	3x8
ONE-ARM KETTLEBELL SWINGS	:30 work :30 rest x2 minutes	:30 work :30 rest x2 minutes	:30 work :30 rest x4 minutes	:30 work :30 rest x4 minutes	:30 work :30 rest x6 minutes	:30 work :30 rest x6 minutes

Do three workouts per week, in numerical order. Week one, do workouts 1, 2, and 3. Week two, do workouts 4, 5, and 6. Use this sheet as a tracker to write down the weight used for each exercise in the box for that workout, underneath the sets and reps.

INTERMEDIATE LOW VOLUME—MONTH THREE, ODD WORKOUTS

	WORKOUT 1	WORKOUT 3	WORKOUT 5	WORKOUT 7	WORKOUT 9	WORKOUT 11
BALL BODY SAWS	2x8	2x8	2x8	3x8	3x8	3x8
TRAP BAR DEADLIFTS	2x8	2x8	2x8	3x8	3x8	3x8
SINGLE-ARM KETTLEBELL FLOOR PRESSES	2x8	2x8	2x8	3x8	3x8	3x8
T-SPINE ROTATIONS	2x8	2x8	2x8	3x8	3x8	3x8
DOUBLE-CABLE ROWS	2x8	2x8	2x8	3x8	3x8	3x8
DOUBLE-DUMBBELL REAR-FOOT-ELEVATED SPLIT SQUATS	2x8	2x8	2x8	3x8	3x8	3x8
HIP FLEXOR STRETCHES	2x8	2x8	2x8	3x8	3x8	3x8
ONE-ARM KETTLEBELL SWINGS	20	20, 15	20, 15, 10	20, 15, 10, 5	20, 15, 10, 5	20, 15, 10, 5

When three exercises are grouped together, do those back-to-back as a tri-set. For exercises on one leg or one arm, sets listed are for each side.

INTERMEDIATE LOW VOLUME—MONTH THREE, EVEN WORKOUTS

	WORKOUT 2	WORKOUT 4	WORKOUT 6	WORKOUT 8	WORKOUT 10	WORKOUT 12
PALLOF PRESSES	2x8	2x8	2x8	3x8	3x8	3x8
ASSISTED CHIN-UPS	2x8	2x8	2x8	3x8	3x8	3x8
BARBELL BACK SQUATS	2x8	2x8	2x8	3x8	3x8	3x8
T-SPINE ROTATIONS	2x8	2x8	2x8	3x8	3x8	3x8
75° INCLINE DOUBLE-DUMBBELL BENCH PRESSES	2x8	2x8	2x8	3x8	3x8	3x8
SPLIT-STANCE DEADLIFTS	2x8	2x8	2x8	3x8	3x8	3x8
HIP FLEXOR STRETCHES	2x8	2x8	2x8	3x8	3x8	3x8
ONE-ARM KETTLEBELL SWINGS	20	20, 15	20, 15, 10	20, 15, 10, 5	20, 15, 10, 5	20, 15, 10, 5

Do three workouts per week, in numerical order. Week one, do workouts 1, 2, and 3. Week two, do workouts 4, 5, and 6. Use this sheet as a tracker to write down the weight used for each exercise in the box for that workout, underneath the sets and reps.

INTERMEDIATE MEDIUM VOLUME—MONTH ONE, ODD WORKOUTS

	WORKOUT 1	WORKOUT 3	WORKOUT 5	WORKOUT 7	WORKOUT 9	WORKOUT 11
BAND DEAD BUGS	2x10	3x10	3x10	3x10	3x10	3x10
TRAP BAR DEADLIFTS	2x10	3x10	3x10	3x10	3x10	4x10
PUSHUPS	2x max	3x max	3x max	3x max	3x max	4x max
HIP FLEXOR STRETCHES	2x8	3x8	3x8	3x8	3x8	4x8
SINGLE-CABLE ROWS	2x10	3x10	3x10	3x10	3x10	4x10
SPLIT SQUATS	2x10	3x10	3x10	3x10	3x10	4x10
T-SPINE ROTATIONS	2x8	3x8	3x8	3x8	3x8	4x8
ONE-ARM KETTLEBELL SWINGS	1x10	2x10	3x10	4x10	5x10	5x10

When three exercises are grouped together, do those back-to-back as a tri-set. For exercises on one leg or one arm, sets listed are for each side.

INTERMEDIATE MEDIUM VOLUME—MONTH ONE, EVEN WORKOUTS

	WORKOUT 2	WORKOUT 4	WORKOUT 6	WORKOUT 8	WORKOUT 10	WORKOUT 12
PALLOF PRESSES	2x10	3x10	3x10	3x10	3x10	3x10
ASSISTED CHIN-UPS	2x10	3x10	3x10	3x10	3x10	4x10
DOUBLE-KETTLEBELL FRONT SQUATS	2x10	3x10	3x10	3x10	3x10	4x10
T-SPINE ROTATIONS	2x8	3x8	3x8	3x8	3x8	4x8
75° INCLINE DOUBLE-DUMBBELL BENCH PRESSES	2x10	3x10	3x10	3x10	3x10	4x10
ONE-KETTLEBELL COSSACK DEADLIFTS	2x10	3x10	3x10	3x10	3x10	4x10
HIP FLEXOR STRETCHES	2x8	3x8	3x8	3x8	3x8	4x8
ONE-ARM KETTLEBELL SWINGS	1x10	2x10	3x10	4x10	5x10	5x10

Do three workouts per week, in numerical order. Week one, do workouts 1, 2, and 3. Week two, do workouts 4, 5, and 6. Use this sheet as a tracker to write down the weight used for each exercise in the box for that workout, underneath the sets and reps.

INTERMEDIATE MEDIUM VOLUME—MONTH TWO, ODD WORKOUTS

	WORKOUT 1	WORKOUT 3	WORKOUT 5	WORKOUT 7	WORKOUT 9	WORKOUT 11
KETTLEBELL DEAD BUG	2x12	3x12	3x12	3x12	3x12	3x12
DOUBLE-DUMBBELL BENCH PRESSES	2x15	3x15	3x15	3x15	3x15	4x15
SINGLE-LEG DUMBBELL HIP BRIDGES	2x15	3x15	3x15	3x15	3x15	4x15
HIP FLEXOR STRETCHES	2x8	3x8	3x8	3x8	3x8	4x8
GOBLET SQUATS	2x15	3x15	3x15	3x15	3x15	4x15
DUMBBELL BENT-OVER ROWS	2x15	3x15	3x15	3x15	3x15	4x15
T-SPINE ROTATIONS	2x8	3x8	3x8	3x8	3x8	4x8
ONE-ARM KETTLEBELL SWINGS	:30 work :30 rest x2 minutes	:30 work :30 rest x2 minutes	:30 work :30 rest x4 minutes	:30 work :30 rest x5 minutes	:30 work :30 rest x6 minutes	:30 work :30 rest x6 minutes

When three exercises are grouped together, do those back-to-back as a tri-set. For exercises on one leg or one arm, sets listed are for each side.

INTERMEDIATE MEDIUM VOLUME—MONTH TWO, EVEN WORKOUTS

	WORKOUT 2	WORKOUT 4	WORKOUT 6	WORKOUT 8	WORKOUT 10	WORKOUT 12
HORIZONTAL CABLE ROTATIONS	2x12	3x12	3x12	3x12	3x12	3x12
SINGLE-ARM LAT PULLDOWNS	2x15	3x15	3x15	3x15	3x15	4x15
WALKING LUNGES	2x15	3x15	3x15	3x15	3x15	4x15
T-SPINE ROTATIONS	2x8	3x8	3x8	3x8	3x8	4x8
45° INCLINE DOUBLE-DUMBBELL BENCH PRESSES	2x15	3x15	3x15	3x15	3x15	4x15
SINGLE-LEG DUMBBELL HIP BRIDGES	2x 10–15	3x 10–15	3x 10–15	3x 10–15	3x 10–15	4x 10–15
HIP FLEXOR STRETCHES	2x8	3x8	3x8	3x8	3x8	4x8
ONE-ARM KETTLEBELL SWINGS	:30 work :30 rest x2 minutes	:30 work :30 rest x2 minutes	:30 work :30 rest x4 minutes	:30 work :30 rest x4 minutes	:30 work :30 rest x6 minutes	:30 work :30 rest x6 minutes

Do three workouts per week, in numerical order. Week one, do workouts 1, 2, and 3. Week two, do workouts 4, 5, and 6. Use this sheet as a tracker to write down the weight used for each exercise in the box for that workout, underneath the sets and reps.

INTERMEDIATE MEDIUM VOLUME—MONTH THREE, ODD WORKOUTS

	WORKOUT 1	WORKOUT 3	WORKOUT 5	WORKOUT 7	WORKOUT 9	WORKOUT 11
BALL BODY SAWS	2x8	3x8	3x8	3x8	3x8	3x8
TRAP BAR DEADLIFTS	2x5	3x5	3x5	3x5	3x5	4x5
SINGLE-KETTLEBELL FLOOR PRESSES	2x5	3x5	3x5	3x5	3x5	4x5
HIP FLEXOR STRETCHES	2x8	3x8	3x8	3x8	3x8	4x8
SINGLE-CABLE ROWS	2x5	3x5	3x5	3x5	3x5	4x5
REAR-FOOT-ELEVATED SPLIT SQUATS	2x5	3x5	3x5	3x5	3x5	4x5
T-SPINE ROTATIONS	2x8	3x8	3x8	3x8	3x8	4x8
ONE-ARM KETTLEBELL SWINGS	20	20, 15	20, 15, 10	20, 15, 10, 5	20, 15, 10, 5	20, 15, 10, 5

When three exercises are grouped together, do those back-to-back as a tri-set. For exercises on one leg or one arm, sets listed are for each side.

INTERMEDIATE MEDIUM VOLUME—MONTH THREE, EVEN WORKOUTS

	WORKOUT 2	WORKOUT 4	WORKOUT 6	WORKOUT 8	WORKOUT 10	WORKOUT 12
PALLOF PRESSES	2x8	3x8	3x8	3x8	3x8	3x8
CHIN-UPS OR ASSISTED CHIN-UPS	2x5	3x5	3x5	3x5	3x5	4x5
BARBELL BACK SQUATS	2x5	3x5	3x5	3x5	3x5	4x5
T-SPINE ROTATIONS	2x8	3x8	3x8	3x8	3x8	4x8
75° INCLINE DOUBLE-DUMBBELL BENCH PRESSES	2x5	3x5	3x5	3x5	3x5	4x5
SPLIT-STANCE DEADLIFTS	2x5	3x5	3x5	3x5	3x5	4x5
HIP FLEXOR STRETCHES	2x8	3x8	3x8	3x8	3x8	4x8
ONE-ARM KETTLEBELL SWINGS	20	20, 15	20, 15, 10	20, 15, 10, 5	20, 15, 10, 5	20, 15, 10, 5

Do three workouts per week, in numerical order. Week one, do workouts 1, 2, and 3. Week two, do workouts 4, 5, and 6. Use this sheet as a tracker to write down the weight used for each exercise in the box for that workout, underneath the sets and reps.

INTERMEDIATE HIGH VOLUME—MONTH ONE, ODD WORKOUTS

	WORKOUT 1	WORKOUT 3	WORKOUT 5	WORKOUT 7	WORKOUT 9	WORKOUT 11
BAND DEAD BUGS	2x10	3x10	3x10	3x10	3x10	3x10
DEADLIFT VARIATIONS	Romanian 2x12	Trap Bar 2x5	Trap Bar 3x5	Romanian 3x12	Trap Bar 4x5	Trap Bar 4x5
HIP FLEXOR STRETCHES	2x8	3x8	3x8	3x8	3x8	4x8
PUSHUPS	2x max	2x max	3x max	3x max	3x max	4x max
SINGLE-LEG DUMBBELL HIP BRIDGES	2x12	2x12	3x12	3x12	3x12	4x12
T-SPINE ROTATIONS	2x8	3x8	3x8	3x8	3x8	4x8
SINGLE-CABLE ROWS	2x12	2x12	3x12	3x12	3x12	4x12
SPLIT SQUATS	2x12	2x12	3x12	3x12	3x12	4x12
BRETZEL STRETCHES	2x8	3x8	3x8	3x8	3x8	4x8
ONE-ARM KETTLEBELL SWINGS	1x10	2x10	3x10	4x10	5x10	5x10

When three exercises are grouped together, do those back-to-back as a tri-set. For exercises on one leg or one arm, sets listed are for each side.

INTERMEDIATE HIGH VOLUME—MONTH ONE, EVEN WORKOUTS

	WORKOUT 2	WORKOUT 4	WORKOUT 6	WORKOUT 8	WORKOUT 10	WORKOUT 12
PALLOF PRESSES	2x10	3x10	3x10	3x10	3x10	3x10
CHIN-UPS VARIATIONS	Single-Arm Lat Pulldown 2x12	Chin-Ups or Assisted Chin-ups 2x5–15	Chin-Ups or Assisted Chin-ups 3x3–5	Single-Arm Lat Pulldown 3x12	Chin-Ups or Assisted Chin-ups 4x5–15	Chin-Ups or Assisted Chin-ups 4x3–5
T-SPINE ROTATIONS	2x8	3x8	3x8	3x8	3x8	4x8
75° INCLINE DOUBLE-DUMBBELL BENCH PRESSES	2x12	2x12	3x12	3x12	3x12	4x12
ONE-KETTLEBELL COSSACK DEADLIFTS	2x12	2x12	3x12	3x12	3x12	4x12
HIP FLEXOR STRETCHES	2x8	3x8	3x8	3x8	3x8	4x8
DUMBBELL ROWS	2x12	2x12	3x12	3x12	3x12	4x12
DOUBLE KETTLEBELL FRONT SQUATS	2x12	2x12	3x12	3x12	3x12	4x12
BRETZEL STRETCHES	2x8	3x8	3x8	3x8	3x8	4x8
ONE-ARM KETTLEBELL SWINGS	1x10	2x10	3x10	4x10	5x10	5x10

Do three workouts per week, in numerical order. Week one, do workouts 1, 2, and 3. Week two, do workouts 4, 5, and 6. Use this sheet as a tracker to write down the weight used for each exercise in the box for that workout, underneath the sets and reps.

INTERMEDIATE HIGH VOLUME—MONTH TWO, ODD WORKOUTS

	WORKOUT 1	WORKOUT 3	WORKOUT 5	WORKOUT 7	WORKOUT 9	WORKOUT 11
KETTLEBELL DEAD BUGS	2x12	3x12	3x12	3x12	3x12	3x12
DEADLIFT VARIATIONS	Romanian 2x12	Trap Bar 2x5	Trap Bar 3x5	Romanian 3x12	Trap Bar 4x5	Trap Bar 4x5
HIP FLEXOR STRETCHES	2x8	2x8	3x8	3x8	4x8	4x8
DUMBBELL BENCH PRESS	2x20	2x20	3x20	3x20	3x20	3x20
SINGLE-LEG DUMBBELL HIP BRIDGES	2x20	2x20	3x20	3x20	3x20	3x20
T-SPINE ROTATIONS	2x8	2x8	3x8	3x8	3x8	3x8
DUMBBELL ROWS	2x20	2x20	3x20	3x20	3x20	3x20
GOBLET SQUATS	2x20	2x20	3x20	3x20	3x20	3x20
BRETZEL STRETCHES	2x8	2x8	3x8	3x8	3x8	3x8
ONE-ARM KETTLEBELL SWINGS	:30 work :30 rest x2 minutes	:30 work :30 rest x2 minutes	:30 work :30 rest x4 minutes	:30 work :30 rest x4 minutes	:30 work :30 rest x6 minutes	:30 work :30 rest x6 minutes

When three exercises are grouped together, do those back-to-back as a tri-set. For exercises on one leg or one arm, sets listed are for each side.

INTERMEDIATE HIGH VOLUME—MONTH TWO, EVEN WORKOUTS

	WORKOUT 2	WORKOUT 4	WORKOUT 6	WORKOUT 8	WORKOUT 10	WORKOUT 12
CABLE HORIZONTAL ROTATIONS	2x12	3x12	3x12	3x12	3x12	3x12
CHIN-UPS VARIATIONS	Single-Arm Lat Pulldown 2x12	Chin-Ups or Assisted Chin-ups 2x5–15	Chin-Ups or Assisted Chin-ups 3x3–5	Single-Arm Lat Pulldown 3x12	Chin-Ups or Assisted Chin-ups 4x5–15	Chin-Ups or Assisted Chin-ups 4x3–5
T-SPINE ROTATIONS	2x8	2x8	3x8	3x8	4x8	4x8
45° INCLINE DOUBLE-DUMBBELL BENCH PRESSES	2x20	2x20	3x20	3x20	3x20	3x20
ROMANIAN DEADLIFTS	2x20	2x20	3x20	3x20	3x20	3x20
HIP FLEXOR STRETCHES	2x8	2x8	3x8	3x8	3x8	3x8
SINGLE-CABLE ROWS	2x20	2x20	3x20	3x20	3x20	3x20
WALKING LUNGES	2x20	2x20	3x20	3x20	3x20	3x20
BRETZEL STRETCHES	2x8	2x8	3x8	3x8	3x8	3x8
ONE-ARM KETTLEBELL SWINGS	:30 work :30 rest x2 minutes	:30 work :30 rest x2 minutes	:30 work :30 rest x4 minutes	:30 work :30 rest x4 minutes	:30 work :30 rest x6 minutes	:30 work :30 rest x6 minutes

Do three workouts per week, in numerical order. Week one, do workouts 1, 2, and 3. Week two, do workouts 4, 5, and 6. Use this sheet as a tracker to write down the weight used for each exercise in the box for that workout, underneath the sets and reps.

INTERMEDIATE HIGH VOLUME—MONTH THREE, ODD WORKOUTS

	WORKOUT 1	WORKOUT 3	WORKOUT 5	WORKOUT 7	WORKOUT 9	WORKOUT 11
BALL BODY SAWS	2x8	3x8	3x8	3x8	3x8	3x8
DEADLIFT VARIATIONS	Romanian 2x12	Barbell 2x5	Trap Bar 3x5	Romanian 3x12	Barbell 4x5	Trap Bar 4x5
HIP FLEXOR STRETCHES	2x8	2x8	3x8	3x8	4x8	4x8
DUMBBELL BENCH PRESS	2x8	3x8	3x8	3x8	3x8	4x8
SINGLE-LEG DEADLIFTS	2x8	3x8	3x8	3x8	3x8	4x8
T-SPINE ROTATIONS	2x8	3x8	3x8	3x8	3x8	4x8
DOUBLE-CABLE ROWS	2x8	3x8	3x8	3x8	3x8	4x8
REAR-FOOT-ELEVATED SPLIT SQUATS	2x8	3x8	3x8	3x8	3x8	4x8
BRETZEL STRETCHES	2x8	3x8	3x8	3x8	3x8	4x8
ONE-ARM KETTLEBELL SWINGS	20	20, 15	20, 15, 10	20, 15, 10, 5	20, 15, 10, 5	20, 15, 10, 5

When three exercises are grouped together, do those back-to-back as a tri-set. For exercises on one leg or one arm, sets listed are for each side.

INTERMEDIATE HIGH VOLUME—MONTH THREE, EVEN WORKOUTS

	WORKOUT 2	WORKOUT 4	WORKOUT 6	WORKOUT 8	WORKOUT 10	WORKOUT 12
PALLOF PRESSES	2x8	3x8	3x8	3x8	3x8	3x8
CHIN-UPS VARIATIONS	Single-Arm Lat Pulldown 2x12	Chin-Ups or Assisted Chin-ups 2x5–15	Chin-Ups or Assisted Chin-ups 3x3–5	Single-Arm Lat Pulldown 3x12	Chin-Ups or Assisted Chin-ups 4x5–15	Chin-Ups or Assisted Chin-ups 4x3–5
T-SPINE ROTATIONS	2x8	2x8	3x8	3x8	4x8	4x8
SINGLE-KETTLEBELL MILITARY PRESSES	2x8	3x8	3x8	3x8	3x8	4x8
SPLIT-STANCE DEADLIFTS	2x8	3x8	3x8	3x8	3x8	4x8
HIP FLEXOR STRETCHES	2x8	3x8	3x8	3x8	3x8	4x8
BARBELL SQUATS	2x8	3x8	3x8	3x8	3x8	4x8
DUMBBELL ROWS	2x8	3x8	3x8	3x8	3x8	4x8
BRETZEL STRETCHES	2x8	3x8	3x8	3x8	3x8	4x8
ONE-ARM KETTLEBELL SWINGS	20	20, 15	20, 15, 10	20, 15, 10, 5	20, 15, 10, 5	20, 15, 10, 5

APPENDIX FIVE
ADVANCED WORKOUTS

The big difference between the intermediate and advanced workouts is that you'll be working on multiple repetition ranges each week. Each week, you'll have one day focused on leanness, one day focused on strength, and one day focused on endurance.

In the first month, that looks like:

- Workout one on Monday, sets of *10 repetitions*

- Workout two on Wednesday, sets of *6 repetitions*

- Workout three on Friday, sets of *15 repetitions*

In the medium and high-volume programs, you'll also have a strength focus at the beginning—either deadlifts or chin-ups. That first focus set will have its own rep scheme, and the variation will change.

All the exercises are grouped either in supersets (two exercises back to back) or trisets (three exercises back to back to back). Do all of the exercises in that group, and then rest. In the trisets, the first two are strength exercises; the third, in italics, is a mobility exercise.

For exercises that are single-arm or single-leg, the repetitions listed are to be done on each side.

Pushups are listed as "max." This means to do the maximum number of repetitions you can with *perfect form*. If you can do more than 20 pushups for three sets, move to a harder pushup variation. And, if you can already do more than 20 reps per set, I'm sure you already know a few harder pushup variations you could do. If you want some more ideas, check out spiderman pushups, archer pushups, band pushups, or weighted vest pushups in my first book, *Fat Loss Happens on Monday*. If you're really advanced, you might find that combining them works really well, like pushups with a band *and* a weighted vest, or archer pushups *with* a weighted vest.

Folks are going to be in lots of different places for the chin-ups. Some will be doing assisted chin-ups for the 5–15 rep days, and regular chin-ups for the 3–5 rep days. Others will do regular chin-ups for the 5–15 rep days and add weight with a weighted vest or dip belt on the 3–5 rep days. Given that this is the advanced program, if you need to do weighted chin-ups, I trust you've been around the gym long enough to sort that out for yourself.

Do three workouts per week, in numerical order. Week one, do workouts 1, 2, and 3. Week two, do workouts 4, 5, and 6. Use this sheet as a tracker to write down the weight used for each exercise in the box for that workout, underneath the sets and reps.

ADVANCED LOW VOLUME—MONTH ONE, ODD WORKOUTS

	WORKOUT 1	WORKOUT 3	WORKOUT 5	WORKOUT 7	WORKOUT 9	WORKOUT 11
BALL BODY SAWS	2x8	2x8	2x8	3x8	3x8	3x8
TRAP BAR DEADLIFTS	2x10	2x6	2x15	3x10	3x6	3x15
PUSHUPS	2x max	2x max	2x max	3x max	3x max	3x max
HIP FLEXOR STRETCHES	2x8	2x8	2x8	3x8	3x8	3x8
SINGLE-CABLE ROWS	2x10	2x6	2x15	3x10	3x6	3x15
SPLIT SQUATS	2x10	2x6	2x15	3x10	3x6	3x15
BRETZEL STRETCHES	2x8	2x8	2x8	3x8	3x8	3x8
ONE-ARM KETTLEBELL SWINGS	1x10	2x10	3x10	4x10	5x10	5x10

When three exercises are grouped together, do those back-to-back as a tri-set. For exercises on one leg or one arm, sets listed are for each side.

ADVANCED LOW VOLUME—MONTH ONE, EVEN WORKOUTS

	WORKOUT 2	WORKOUT 4	WORKOUT 6	WORKOUT 8	WORKOUT 10	WORKOUT 12
HORIZONTAL CABLE ROTATIONS	2x8	2x8	2x8	3x8	3x8	3x8
ASSISTED CHIN-UPS	2x15	2x10	3x6	3x15	3x10	3x6
DOUBLE-KETTLEBELL SQUATS	2x15	2x10	3x6	3x15	3x10	3x6
T-SPINE ROTATIONS	2x8	2x8	3x8	3x8	3x8	3x8
SINGLE-KETTLEBELL MILITARY PRESSES	2x15	2x10	3x6	3x15	3x10	3x6
ONE-KETTLEBELL COSSACK DEADLIFTS	2x15	2x10	3x6	3x15	3x10	3x6
BRETZEL STRETCHES	2x8	2x8	3x8	3x8	3x8	3x8
ONE-ARM KETTLEBELL SWINGS	1x10	2x10	3x10	4x10	5x10	5x10

Do three workouts per week, in numerical order. Week one, do workouts 1, 2, and 3. Week two, do workouts 4, 5, and 6. Use this sheet as a tracker to write down the weight used for each exercise in the box for that workout, underneath the sets and reps.

ADVANCED LOW VOLUME—MONTH TWO, ODD WORKOUTS

	WORKOUT 1	WORKOUT 3	WORKOUT 5	WORKOUT 7	WORKOUT 9	WORKOUT 11
KETTLEBELL DEAD BUGS	2x10	2x10	3x10	3x10	3x10	3x10
DUMBBELL BENCH PRESSES	2x12	2x8	3x20	3x12	3x8	3x20
SINGLE-LEG DUMBBELL HIP BRIDGES	2x12	2x8	3x20	3x12	3x8	3x20
HIP FLEXOR STRETCHES	2x8	2x8	3x8	3x8	3x8	3x8
DOUBLE-KETTLEBELL SQUATS	2x12	2x8	3x20	3x12	3x8	3x20
DUMBBELL BENT-OVER ROWS	2x12	2x8	3x20	3x12	3x8	3x20
BRETZEL STRETCHES	2x8	2x8	3x8	3x8	3x8	3x8
ONE-ARM KETTLEBELL SWINGS	:30 work :30 rest x2 minutes	:30 work :30 rest x2 minutes	:30 work :30 rest x4 minutes	:30 work :30 rest x5 minutes	:30 work :30 rest x6 minutes	:30 work :30 rest x6 minutes

When three exercises are grouped together, do those back-to-back as a tri-set. For exercises on one leg or one arm, sets listed are for each side.

ADVANCED LOW VOLUME—MONTH TWO, EVEN WORKOUTS

	WORKOUT 2	WORKOUT 4	WORKOUT 6	WORKOUT 8	WORKOUT 10	WORKOUT 12
HIGH TO LOW CABLE ROTATIONS	2x10	2x10	3x10	3x10	3x10	3x10
SINGLE-ARM LAT PULLDOWNS	2x20	2x12	3x8	3x20	3x12	3x8
WALKING LUNGES	2x20	2x12	3x8	3x20	3x12	3x8
T-SPINE ROTATIONS	2x8	2x8	3x8	3x8	3x8	3x8
45° INCLINE DOUBLE-DUMBBELL BENCH PRESSES	2x20	2x12	3x8	3x20	3x12	3x8
ROMANIAN DEADLIFTS	2x20	2x12	3x8	3x20	3x12	3x8
BRETZEL STRETCHES	2x8	2x8	3x8	3x8	3x8	3x8
ONE-ARM KETTLEBELL SWINGS	:30 work :30 rest x2 minutes	:30 work :30 rest x2 minutes	:30 work :30 rest x4 minutes	:30 work :30 rest x4 minutes	:30 work :30 rest x6 minutes	:30 work :30 rest x6 minutes

Do three workouts per week, in numerical order. Week one, do workouts 1, 2, and 3. Week two, do workouts 4, 5, and 6. Use this sheet as a tracker to write down the weight used for each exercise in the box for that workout, underneath the sets and reps.

ADVANCED LOW VOLUME—MONTH THREE, ODD WORKOUTS

	WORKOUT 1	WORKOUT 3	WORKOUT 5	WORKOUT 7	WORKOUT 9	WORKOUT 11
BALL BODY SAWS	2x12	2x12	3x12	3x12	3x12	3x12
BARBELL DEADLIFTS	2x8	2x5	3x12	3x8	3x5	3x12
SINGLE-ARM KETTLEBELL FLOOR PRESSES	2x8	2x5	3x12	2x8	3x5	3x12
HIP FLEXOR STRETCHES	2x8	2x8	3x8	3x8	3x8	3x8
DOUBLE-KETTLEBELL ROWS	2x8	2x5	3x12	3x8	3x5	3x12
REAR-FOOT-ELEVATED SPLIT SQUATS	2x8	2x5	3x12	3x8	3x5	3x12
BRETZEL STRETCHES	2x8	2x8	3x8	3x8	3x8	3x8
ONE-ARM KETTLEBELL SWINGS	20	20, 15	20, 15, 10	20, 15, 10, 5	20, 15, 10, 5	20, 15, 10, 5

When three exercises are grouped together, do those back-to-back as a tri-set. For exercises on one leg or one arm, sets listed are for each side.

ADVANCED LOW VOLUME—MONTH THREE, EVEN WORKOUTS

	WORKOUT 2	WORKOUT 4	WORKOUT 6	WORKOUT 8	WORKOUT 10	WORKOUT 12
LOW TO HIGH CABLE ROTATIONS	2x12	2x12	3x12	3x12	3x12	3x12
BARBELL SQUATS	2x12	2x8	3x5	3x12	3x8	3x5
CHIN-UPS OR ASSISTED CHIN-UPS	2x12	2x8	3x5	3x12	3x8	3x5
T-SPINE ROTATIONS	2x8	2x8	3x8	3x8	3x8	3x8
SINGLE-KETTLEBELL MILITARY PRESSES	2x12	2x8	3x5	3x12	3x8	3x5
SPLIT-STANCE DEADLIFTS	2x12	2x8	3x5	3x12	3x8	3x5
BRETZEL STRETCHES	2x8	2x8	3x8	3x8	3x8	3x8
ONE-ARM KETTLEBELL SWINGS	20	20, 15	20, 15, 10	20, 15, 10, 5	20, 15, 10, 5	20, 15, 10, 5

Do three workouts per week, in numerical order. Week one, do workouts 1, 2, and 3. Week two, do workouts 4, 5, and 6. Use this sheet as a tracker to write down the weight used for each exercise in the box for that workout, underneath the sets and reps.

ADVANCED MEDIUM VOLUME—MONTH ONE, ODD WORKOUTS

	WORKOUT 1	WORKOUT 3	WORKOUT 5	WORKOUT 7	WORKOUT 9	WORKOUT 11
BALL BODY SAWS	2x8	2x8	2x8	3x8	3x8	3x8
DEADLIFT VARIATIONS	Romanian 2x12	Barbell 2x5	Trap Bar 3x5	Romanian 3x12	Barbell 3x5	Trap Bar 4x5
HIP FLEXOR STRETCHES	2x8	2x8	3x8	3x8	3x8	4x8
PUSHUPS	2x max	2x max	3x max	3x max	3x max	4x max
SINGLE-LEG DUMBBELL HIP BRIDGES	2x10	2x5	3x15	3x10	3x5	3x15
T-SPINE ROTATIONS	2x8	2x8	3x8	3x8	3x8	3x8
SINGLE-CABLE ROWS	2x10	2x5	3x15	3x10	3x5	3x15
SPLIT SQUATS	2x10	2x5	3x15	3x10	3x5	3x15
BRETZEL STRETCHES	2x8	2x8	3x8	3x8	3x8	3x8

When three exercises are grouped together, do those back-to-back as a tri-set. For exercises on one leg or one arm, sets listed are for each side.

ADVANCED MEDIUM VOLUME—MONTH ONE, EVEN WORKOUTS

	WORKOUT 2	WORKOUT 4	WORKOUT 6	WORKOUT 8	WORKOUT 10	WORKOUT 12
HORIZONTAL CABLE ROTATIONS	2x8	2x8	2x8	3x8	3x8	3x8
CHIN-UP VARIATIONS	Single-Arm Lat Pulldown 2x12	Chin-ups 2x5–15	Chin-ups 3x3–5	Single-Arm Lat Pulldown 3x12	Chin-ups 3x5–15	Chin-ups 4x3–5
T-SPINE ROTATIONS	2x8	2x8	2x8	3x8	3x8	4x8
DOUBLE-KETTLEBELL SQUATS	2x15	2x10	3x5	3x15	3x10	3x5
DUMBBELL ROWS	2x15	2x10	3x5	3x15	3x10	3x5
HIP FLEXOR STRETCHES	2x8	2x8	3x8	3x8	3x8	3x8
SINGLE-KETTLEBELL MILITARY PRESSES	2x15	2x10	3x5	3x15	3x10	3x5
ONE-KETTLEBELL COSSACK DEADLIFTS	2x15	2x10	3x5	3x15	3x10	3x5
BRETZEL STRETCHES	2x8	2x8	3x8	3x8	3x8	3x8

Do three workouts per week, in numerical order. Week one, do workouts 1, 2, and 3. Week two, do workouts 4, 5, and 6. Use this sheet as a tracker to write down the weight used for each exercise in the box for that workout, underneath the sets and reps.

ADVANCED MEDIUM VOLUME—MONTH TWO, ODD WORKOUTS

	WORKOUT 1	WORKOUT 3	WORKOUT 5	WORKOUT 7	WORKOUT 9	WORKOUT 11
KETTLEBELL DEAD BUGS	2x10	2x10	3x10	3x10	3x10	3x10
DEADLIFT VARIATIONS	Romanian 2x12	Barbell 2x5	Trap Bar 3x5	Romanian 3x12	Barbell 3x5	Trap Bar 4x5
HIP FLEXOR STRETCHES	2x8	2x8	3x8	3x8	3x8	4x8
DOUBLE-DUMBBELL BENCH PRESSES	2x12	2x8	3x20	3x12	3x8	3x20
SINGLE-LEG DUMBBELL HIP BRIDGES	2x12	2x8	3x20	3x12	3x8	3x20
T-SPINE ROTATIONS	2x8	2x8	3x8	3x8	3x8	3x8
DOUBLE-KETTLEBELL SQUATS	2x12	2x8	3x20	3x12	3x8	3x20
DUMBBELL ROWS	2x12	2x8	3x20	3x12	3x8	3x20
BRETZEL STRETCHES	2x8	2x8	3x8	3x8	3x8	3x8
ONE-ARM KETTLEBELL SWINGS	:30 work :30 rest x2 minutes	:30 work :30 rest x2 minutes	:30 work :30 rest x4 minutes	:30 work :30 rest x4 minutes	:30 work :30 rest x6 minutes	:30 work :30 rest x6 minutes

When three exercises are grouped together, do those back-to-back as a tri-set. For exercises on one leg or one arm, sets listed are for each side.

ADVANCED MEDIUM VOLUME—MONTH TWO, EVEN WORKOUTS

	WORKOUT 2	WORKOUT 4	WORKOUT 6	WORKOUT 8	WORKOUT 10	WORKOUT 12
HIGH TO LOW CABLE ROTATIONS	2x10	2x10	2x10	3x10	3x10	3x10
CHIN-UP VARIATIONS	Single-Arm Lat Pulldown 2x12	Chin-ups 2x5–15	Chin-ups 3x5–15	Single-Arm Lat Pulldown 3x12	Chin-ups 3x5–15	Chin-ups 4x3–5
T-SPINE ROTATIONS	2x8	2x8	3x8	3x8	3x8	3x8
SINGLE-CABLE ROWS	2x20	2x12	3x8	3x20	3x12	3x8
WALKING LUNGES	2x20	2x12	3x8	3x20	3x12	3x8
HIP FLEXOR STRETCHES	2x8	2x8	3x8	3x8	3x8	3x8
45° INCLINE DOUBLE-DUMBBELL BENCH PRESSES	2x20	2x12	3x8	3x20	3x12	3x8
ROMANIAN DEADLIFTS	2x20	2x12	3x8	3x20	3x12	3x8
BRETZEL STRETCHES	2x8	2x8	3x8	3x8	3x8	3x8
ONE-ARM KETTLEBELL SWINGS	:30 work :30 rest x2 minutes	:30 work :30 rest x2 minutes	:30 work :30 rest x4 minutes	:30 work :30 rest x4 minutes	:30 work :30 rest x6 minutes	:30 work :30 rest x6 minutes

Do three workouts per week, in numerical order. Week one, do workouts 1, 2, and 3. Week two, do workouts 4, 5, and 6. Use this sheet as a tracker to write down the weight used for each exercise in the box for that workout, underneath the sets and reps.

ADVANCED MEDIUM VOLUME—MONTH THREE, ODD WORKOUTS

	WORKOUT 1	WORKOUT 3	WORKOUT 5	WORKOUT 7	WORKOUT 9	WORKOUT 11
BALL BODY SAWS	2x12	2x12	2x12	3x12	3x12	3x12
DEADLIFT VARIATIONS	Romanian 2x12	Barbell 2x5	Trap Bar 3x5	Romanian 3x12	Barbell 3x5	Trap Bar 3x5
HIP FLEXOR STRETCHES	2x8	2x8	3x8	3x8	4x8	4x8
DOUBLE-DUMBBELL BENCH PRESSES	2x8	2x4	3x12	3x8	3x4	3x12
SINGLE-LEG DEADLIFTS	2x8	3x4	3x12	3x8	3x4	3x12
T-SPINE ROTATIONS	2x8	2x8	3x8	3x8	3x8	3x8
DOUBLE-CABLE ROWS	2x8	3x4	3x12	3x8	3x4	3x12
SPLIT SQUATS	2x8	3x4	3x12	3x8	3x4	3x12
BRETZEL STRETCHES	2x8	2x8	3x8	3x8	3x8	3x8
ONE-ARM KETTLEBELL SWINGS	20	20, 15	20, 15, 10	20, 15, 10, 5	20, 15, 10, 5	20, 15, 10, 5

When three exercises are grouped together, do those back-to-back as a tri-set. For exercises on one leg or one arm, sets listed are for each side.

ADVANCED MEDIUM VOLUME—MONTH THREE, EVEN WORKOUTS						
	WORKOUT 2	WORKOUT 4	WORKOUT 6	WORKOUT 8	WORKOUT 10	WORKOUT 12
LOW TO HIGH CABLE ROTATIONS	2x12	2x12	2x12	3x12	3x12	3x12
CHIN-UP VARIATIONS	Single-Arm Lat Pulldown 2x12	Chin-ups 2x5–15	Chin-ups 3x3–5	Single-Arm Lat Pulldown 3x12	Chin-ups 3x5–15	Chin-ups 4x3–5
T-SPINE ROTATIONS	2x8	2x8	3x8	3x8	3x8	4x8
BARBELL SQUATS	2x12	2x8	3x4	3x12	3x8	3x4
DUMBBELL ROWS	2x12	2x8	3x4	3x12	3x8	3x4
HIP FLEXOR STRETCHES	2x8	2x8	3x8	3x8	4x8	4x8
SINGLE-KETTLEBELL MILITARY PRESSES	2x12	2x8	3x4	3x12	3x8	3x4
SPLIT-STANCE DEADLIFTS	2x12	2x8	3x4	3x12	3x8	3x4
BRETZEL STRETCHES	2x8	2x8	3x8	3x8	3x8	3x8
ONE-ARM KETTLEBELL SWINGS	20	20, 15	20, 15, 10	20, 15, 10, 5	20, 15, 10, 5	20, 15, 10, 5

Do three workouts per week, in numerical order. Week one, do workouts 1, 2, and 3. Week two, do workouts 4, 5, and 6. Use this sheet as a tracker to write down the weight used for each exercise in the box for that workout, underneath the sets and reps.

ADVANCED HIGH VOLUME—MONTH ONE, ODD WORKOUTS

	WORKOUT 1	WORKOUT 3	WORKOUT 5	WORKOUT 7	WORKOUT 9	WORKOUT 11
BALL BODY SAWS	2x8	2x8	2x8	3x8	3x8	3x8
DEADLIFT VARIATIONS	Romanian 2x12	Barbell 2x5	Trap Bar 3x5	Romanian 3x12	Barbell 4x5	Trap Bar 4x5
HIP FLEXOR STRETCHES	2x8	2x8	3x8	3x8	4x8	4x8
PUSHUPS	2x max	3x max	3x max	3x max	4x max	4x max
SINGLE-LEG DEADLIFTS	2x10	3X5	3x15	3x10	4X5	4X15
T-SPINE ROTATIONS	2x8	3x8	3x8	3x8	4x8	4x8
SINGLE-CABLE ROWS	2x10	3X5	3x15	3x10	4X5	4X15
DOUBLE KETTLEBELL FRONT SQUATS	2x10	3X5	3x15	3x10	4X5	4X15
BRETZEL STRETCHES	2x8	3x8	3x8	3x8	4x8	4x8
ONE-ARM KETTLEBELL SWINGS	20	20, 15	20, 15, 10	20, 15, 10, 5	20, 15, 10, 5	20, 15, 10, 5

When three exercises are grouped together, do those back-to-back as a tri-set. For exercises on one leg or one arm, sets listed are for each side.

ADVANCED HIGH VOLUME—MONTH ONE, EVEN WORKOUTS

	WORKOUT 2	WORKOUT 4	WORKOUT 6	WORKOUT 8	WORKOUT 10	WORKOUT 12
HORIZONTAL CABLE ROTATIONS	2x8	2x8	2x8	3x8	3x8	3x8
CHIN-UPS VARIATIONS	Single-Arm Lat Pulldown 2x12	Chin-Ups 2x5–15	Chin-ups 3x3–5	Single-Arm Lat Pulldown 3x12	Chin-ups 4x5–15	Chin-ups 4x3–5
T-SPINE ROTATIONS	2x8	2x8	3x8	3x8	4x8	4x8
DOUBLE KETTLEBELL FRONT SQUATS	2x15	3X10	3X5	3x15	4X10	4X5
DUMBBELL ROWS	2x15	3X10	3X5	3x15	4X10	4X5
HIP FLEXOR STRETCHES	2x8	2x8	3x8	3x8	4x8	4x8
SINGLE-KETTLEBELL MILITARY PRESSES	2x15	3X10	3X5	3x15	4X10	4X5
ONE-KETTLEBELL COSSACK DEADLIFTS	2x15	3X10	3X5	3x15	4X10	4X5
BRETZEL STRETCHES	2x8	2x8	3x8	3x8	4x8	4x8
ONE-ARM KETTLEBELL SWINGS	20	20, 15	20, 15, 10	20, 15, 10, 5	20, 15, 10, 5	20, 15, 10, 5

Do three workouts per week, in numerical order. Week one, do workouts 1, 2, and 3. Week two, do workouts 4, 5, and 6. Use this sheet as a tracker to write down the weight used for each exercise in the box for that workout, underneath the sets and reps.

ADVANCED HIGH VOLUME—MONTH TWO, ODD WORKOUTS

	WORKOUT 1	WORKOUT 3	WORKOUT 5	WORKOUT 7	WORKOUT 9	WORKOUT 11
KETTLEBELL DEAD BUGS	2x10	2x10	2x10	3x10	3x10	3x10
DEADLIFT VARIATIONS	Romanian 2x12	Barbell 2x5	Trap Bar 3x5	Romanian 3x12	Barbell 4x5	Trap Bar 4x5
HIP FLEXOR STRETCHES	2x8	2x8	3x8	3x8	4x8	4x8
DUMBBELL BENCH PRESS	2X12	3x8	3x20	3x12	4x8	4x20
SINGLE-LEG DUMBBELL HIP BRIDGES	2X12	3x8	3x20	3x12	4x8	4x20
T-SPINE ROTATIONS	2x8	3x8	3x8	3x8	4x8	4x8
DUMBBELL ROWS	2X12	3x8	3x20	3x12	4x8	4x20
DOUBLE KETTLEBELL FRONT SQUATS	2X12	3x8	3x20	3x12	4x8	4x20
BRETZEL STRETCHES	2x8	3x8	3x8	3x8	4x8	4x8
ONE-ARM KETTLEBELL SWINGS	1x10	2x10	3x10	4x10	5x10	5x10

When three exercises are grouped together, do those back-to-back as a tri-set. For exercises on one leg or one arm, sets listed are for each side.

ADVANCED HIGH VOLUME—MONTH TWO, EVEN WORKOUTS

	WORKOUT 2	WORKOUT 4	WORKOUT 6	WORKOUT 8	WORKOUT 10	WORKOUT 12
HIGH TO LOW ROTATIONS	2x10	2x10	2x10	3x10	3x10	3x10
CHIN-UPS VARIATIONS	Single-Arm Lat Pulldown 2x12	Chin-Ups 3x5–15	Chin-Ups 3x3–5	Single-Arm Lat Pulldown 3x12	Chin-Ups 4x5–15	Chin-Ups 4x3–5
T-SPINE ROTATIONS	2x8	3x8	3x8	3x8	4x8	4x8
WALKING LUNGES	2x20	3X12	3X8	3x20	4X12	4x8
SINGLE-CABLE ROWS	2x20	3X12	3X8	3x20	4X12	4x8
HIP FLEXOR STRETCHES	2x8	2x8	3x8	3x8	4x8	4x8
45° INCLINE DOUBLE-DUMBBELL BENCH PRESSES	2x20	3X12	3X8	3x20	4X12	4x8
ROMANIAN DEADLIFTS	2x20	3X12	3x8	3x20	4X12	4x8
BRETZEL STRETCHES	2x8	3x8	3x8	3x8	4x8	4x8
ONE-ARM KETTLEBELL SWINGS	1x10	2x10	3x10	4x10	5x10	5x10

Do three workouts per week, in numerical order. Week one, do workouts 1, 2, and 3. Week two, do workouts 4, 5, and 6. Use this sheet as a tracker to write down the weight used for each exercise in the box for that workout, underneath the sets and reps.

ADVANCED HIGH VOLUME—MONTH THREE, ODD WORKOUTS

	WORKOUT 1	WORKOUT 3	WORKOUT 5	WORKOUT 7	WORKOUT 9	WORKOUT 11
BALL BODY SAWS	2x12	2x12	2x12	3x12	3x12	3x12
DEADLIFT VARIATIONS	Romanian 2x12	Barbell 2x5	Trap Bar 3x5	Romanian 3x12	Barbell 4x5	Trap Bar 4x5
HIP FLEXOR STRETCHES	2x8	2x8	3x8	3x8	4x8	4x8
SINGLE-KETTLEBELL MILITARY PRESSES	2x8	3x4	3x12	3x8	4x4	4x12
SINGLE-LEG DEADLIFTS	2x8	3x4	3x12	3x8	4x4	4x12
T-SPINE ROTATIONS	2x8	3x8	3x8	3x8	4x8	4x8
BARBELL SQUATS	2x8	3x4	3x12	3x8	4x4	4x12
DUMBBELL ROWS	2x8	3x4	3x12	3x8	4x4	4x12
BRETZEL STRETCHES	2x8	3x8	3x8	3x8	4x8	4x8
ONE-ARM KETTLEBELL SWINGS	:30 work :30 rest x2 minutes	:30 work :30 rest x3 minutes	:30 work :30 rest x4 minutes	:30 work :30 rest x5 minutes	:30 work :30 rest x5 minutes	:30 work :30 rest x5 minutes

When three exercises are grouped together, do those back-to-back as a tri-set. For exercises on one leg or one arm, sets listed are for each side.

ADVANCED HIGH VOLUME—MONTH THREE, EVEN WORKOUTS

	WORKOUT 2	WORKOUT 4	WORKOUT 6	WORKOUT 8	WORKOUT 10	WORKOUT 12
LOW TO HIGH CABLE ROTATIONS	2x12	2x12	2x12	3x12	3x12	3x12
CHIN-UPS VARIATIONS	Single-Arm Lat Pulldown 2x12	Chin-Ups 2x5–15	Chin-Ups 3x3–5	Single-Arm Lat Pulldown 3x12	Chin-Ups 4x5–15	Chin-Ups 4x3–5
T-SPINE ROTATIONS	2x8	2x8	3x8	3x8	4x8	4x8
BARBELL SQUATS	2x12	3x8	3x4	3x12	3x8	4x4
DUMBBELL ROWS	2x12	3x8	3x4	3x12	3x8	4x4
HIP FLEXOR STRETCHES	2x8	3x8	3x8	3x8	3x8	4x8
SINGLE-KETTLEBELL MILITARY PRESSES	2x12	3x8	3x4	3x12	3x8	4x4
SPLIT-STANCE DEADLIFTS	2x12	3x8	3x4	3x12	3x8	4x4
BRETZEL STRETCHES	2x8	3x8	3x8	3x8	3x8	4x8
ONE-ARM KETTLEBELL SWINGS	:30 work :30 rest x2 minutes	:30 work :30 rest x3 minutes	:30 work :30 rest x4 minutes	:30 work :30 rest x5 minutes	:30 work :30 rest x5 minutes	:30 work :30 rest x5 minutes

APPENDIX SIX
EXERCISE DESCRIPTIONS

The exercises are grouped together with other similar exercises. Many of the exercises share the same things to focus on. For this reason, multiple exercises will be shown in photos, with only one set of instructions for all of them listed at the bottom of the page.

For example, look at the instructions for all of the kettlebell and dumbbell press variations:

- Lower the dumbbells
- Flex your butt
- Brace your abs
- Drive your shoes into the floor
- Press the dumbbell(s) up the ceiling

There are multiple exercises in this book that are variations of each other. One of the best ways to learn is to practice the same skill in multiple variations and multiple contexts. A really important lesson for beginner and intermediate trainees is noticing how groups of movements are similar and different, where skills generalize and where they do not.

Most of this book is devoted to skills, Meta-skills, Turning Points, and psychology related to both food and movement; this book doesn't have the most detailed exercise descriptions of all time. Exercise wise, this book mostly is focusing on movement related mindfulness skills you might not have seen before. To dive a little deeper, you can check the exercise-specific mindfulness section on page 130.

This is just to give you sense of what movements you are doing, assuming you have some background in lifting. If you need more detailed explanations that will generalize to most of these movements, check out my first book, *Fat Loss Happens on Monday*. If you want a really in-depth treatise on deadlifting, read Pavel Tsatsouline's *Power to the People*, or for kettlebell swings, cleans, and military presses, *Enter the Kettlebell*.

HOME WORKOUT SWAPS

This workout program was designed to be done in a gym. *Fat Loss Happens on Monday* has a really great program you can do at home with just bodyweight and kettlebells. The idea here is to show what else you could do if you had access to more equipment, like cables, dumbbells, and a bench.

One option for a home trainee would be to buy an adjustable bench and add pairs of dumbbells as you go. If you have tight shoulders and military presses don't feel good, getting a bench to do incline presses instead is a great investment.

You can even get home pulley systems that attach to a doorway pull-up bar from Spud Inc. so you could do single-cable lat-pulldowns and high to low cable rotations. If you want to really deck out your home gym or really struggle with assisted chin-ups, that's an option.

Let's take a look substitutions we could make to do this program with a minimal amount of equipment.

GYM	HOME
Pallof Presses	Pallof Presses with a band
Horizontal Cable Rotations High to Low Cable Rotations Low to High Cable Rotations	Pallof Presses with a band
Double-Dumbbell Bench Presses Single-Dumbbell Bench Presses	Single-kettlebell Floor Presses or the Pushup Progression from Fat Loss Happens on Monday
45° Double-dumbbell Bench Presses 75° Single-dumbbell Bench Presses	Single-kettlebell Military Presses
Single-Cable Rows Double Cable Rows	Dumbbell Bent Over Rows
Single-cable Lat Pulldowns	Assisted Chin-ups or Dumbbell Bent Over Rows
Battling Ropes	Single-kettlebell Swings
Barbell Squats (advanced program only)	Rear-foot-elevated Split-squats
Trap Bar Deadlifts Barbell Deadlifts (advanced program only)	Staggered Stance Deadlifts

With these substitutions, you could do the whole program
with only a doorway pullup bar, kettlebells, bands, and a stability ball.

DOUBLE-DUMBBELL BENCH PRESS

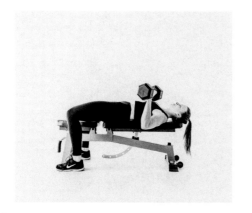

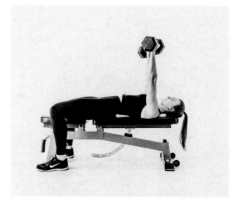

Start

Finish

SINGLE-KETTLEBELL FLOOR PRESS

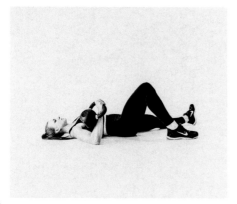

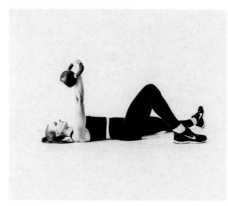

Start

Finish

- Keep your shoulders away from your ears
- Flex your butt
- Brace your abs

- Drive your shoes into the floor
- Press the dumbbells or kettlebell up the ceiling

45° DOUBLE-DUMBBELL INCLINE PRESS

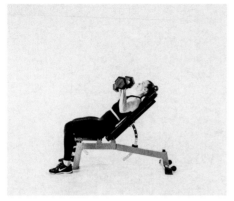

Start

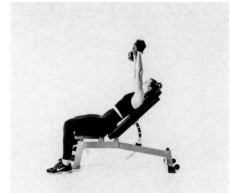

Finish

75° SINGLE-DUMBBELL INCLINE PRESS

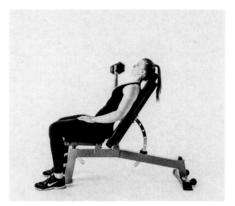

Start

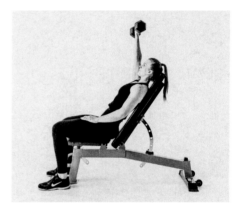

Finish

SINGLE-KETTLEBELL MILITARY PRESS

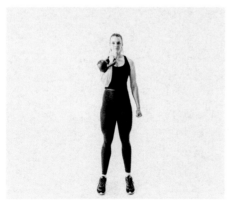

Start

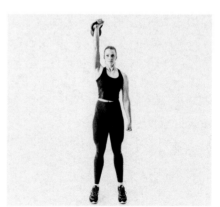

Finish

- Keep your shoulders away from your ears
- Flex your butt
- Brace your abs

- Drive your shoes into the floor
- Press the dumbbell(s) or kettlebell up the ceiling

DUMBBELL ROW

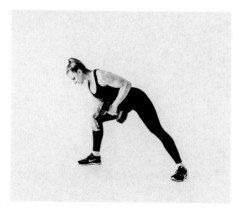

Start

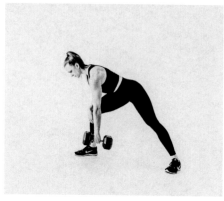

Finish

SINGLE-CABLE ROW

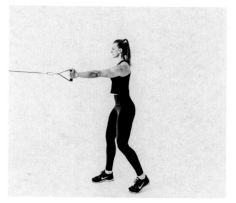

Start

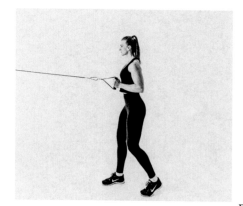

Finish

DOUBLE-CABLE ROW

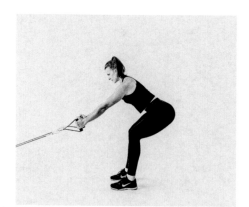

Start

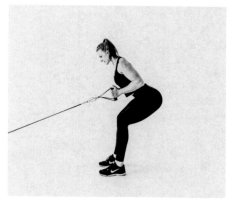

Finish

- Flex your butt
- Brace your abs
- Pull your shoulders back and down

- Pull the dumbbell away from the floor, or the handles away from the machine

SINGLE-ARM LAT PULLDOWN

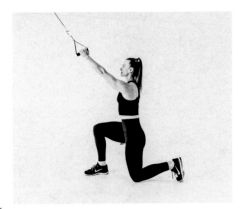
Start

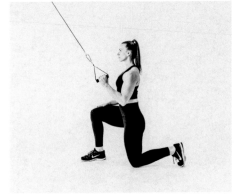
Finish

ASSISTED CHIN-UP

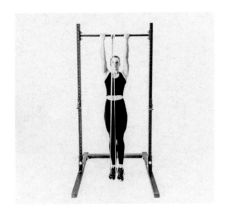
Start

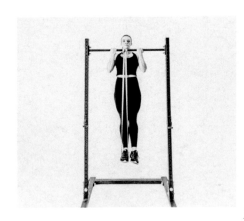
Finish

CHIN-UP

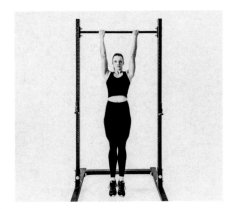
Start

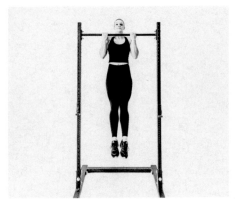
Finish

- Flex your butt
- Brace your abs
- Pull your shoulders back and down

- Pull the bar to your shirt

GOBLET SQUAT

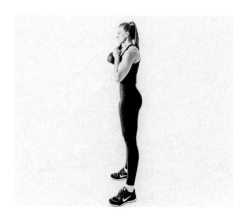

Start

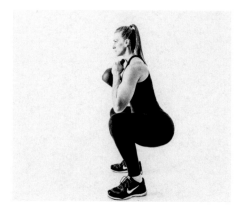

Finish

TWO-KETTLEBELL SQUAT

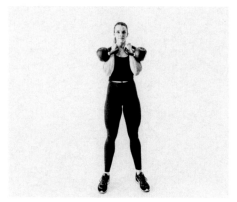

Start

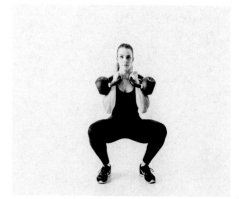

Finish

BARBELL SQUAT

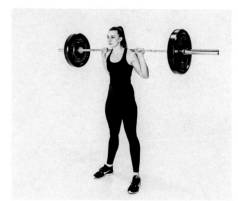

Start

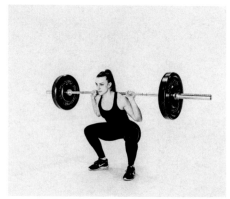

Finish

- Pull your back pockets toward the heels of your shoes

- Flex your butt
- Brace your abs
- Push the ground away

SPLIT SQUAT

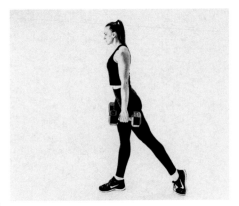

Start

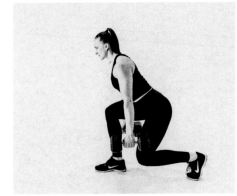

Finish

REAR-FOOT-ELEVATED SPLIT SQUAT

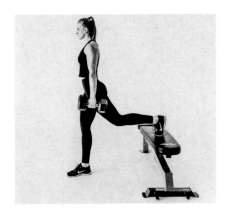

Start

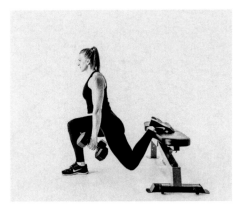

Finish

WALKING LUNGE

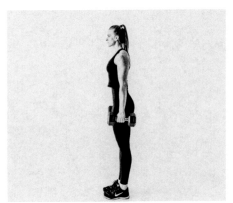

Start

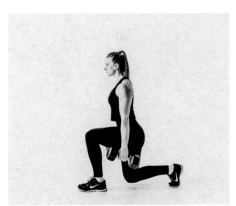

Finish

- Put most of the weight on your front leg

- With the front leg, push the ground away (split squats and rear-foot-elevated split-squats) or push up to standing (walking lunges)

ONE-ARM KETTLEBELL SWING

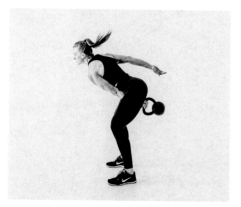

Start

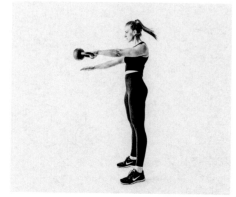

Finish

TWO-ARM KETTLEBELL SWING

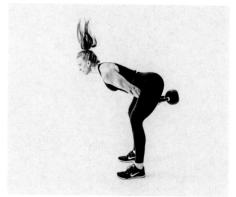

Start

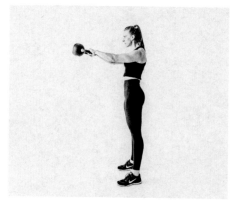

Finish

- Hike the kettlebell back behind your butt

- Drive your shoes into the floor
- Pop your hips forward
- Flex your butt

*Your arms shouldn't do any of the work; it should be all glutes and hamstrings.

DEADLIFT

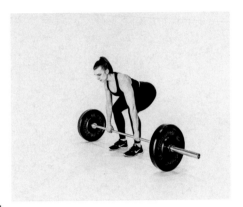

Start

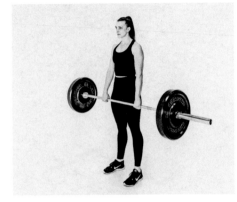

Finish

TRAP BAR DEADLIFT

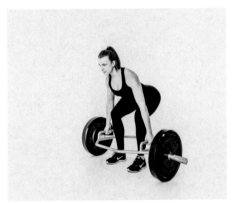

Start

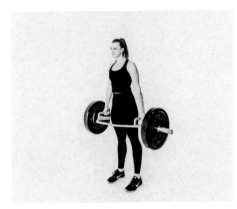

Finish

ROMANIAN DEADLIFT

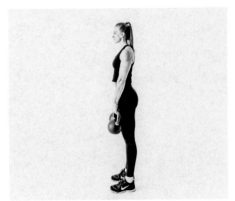

Start

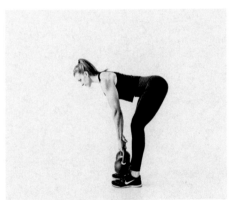

Finish

- Reach your back pockets to the back wall

- Squeeze the bar
- Flex your butt
- Push the ground away

COSSACK DEADLIFT

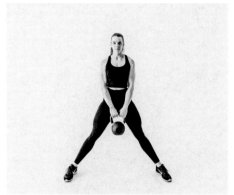

Start

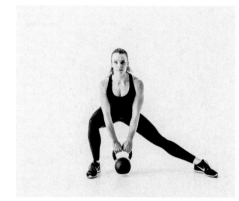

Finish

STAGGERED DEADLIFT

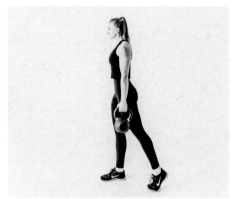

Start

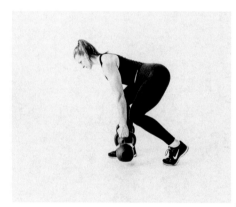

Finish

SINGLE-LEG DEADLIFT

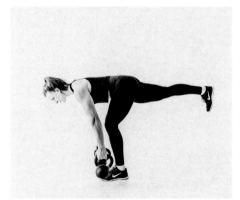

Start

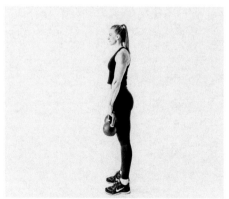

Finish

- Reach your back pockets to the back wall

- Squeeze the kettlebell handles
- Flex your butt
- Push the ground away

SINGLE-LEG DUMBBELL HIP BRIDGE

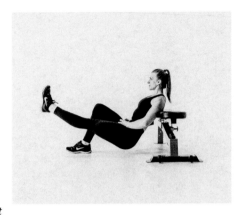

Start

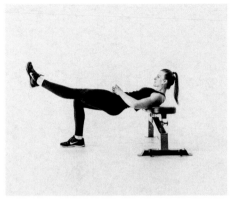

Finish

- Lower hips
- Flex your butt

- Drive the dumbbell up to the ceiling

PALLOF PRESS

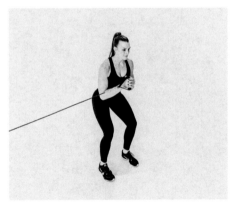

Start

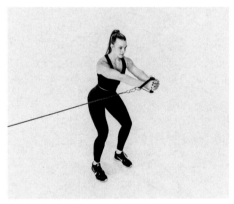

Finish

- Flex your butt
- Brace your abs

- Press the handle out
- Hold for a count at that hardest spot
- Don't let the weight rotate you

BAND DEAD BUG

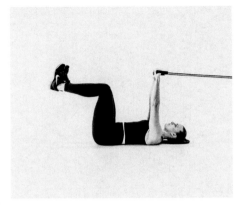

Start

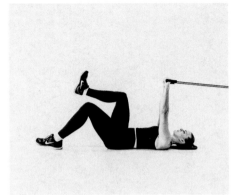

Finish

KETTLEBELL DEAD BUG

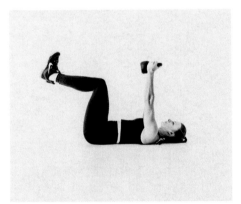

Start

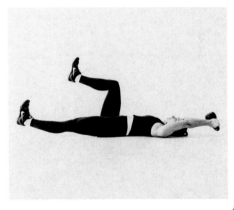

Finish

- Brace your abs
- Press your low back towards the ground

- Extend your leg out to have your heel an inch off the ground, alternating legs

BALL BODY SAW

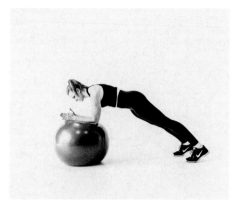

Start

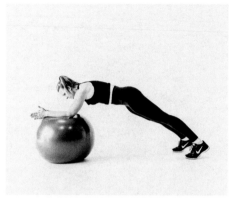

Finish

- Brace abs like a crunch
- Tuck hips under
- Get tall from your heels to the top of your head, just like good posture standing
- Push the ball away with your shoulders

- Roll the ball forward
- If you only roll the ball forward a little, it's easier. If you roll the ball farther forward, it's hard.
- If you do quick rolls (one second out, one second back), it's easier. If you do slower rolls (four seconds out, four seconds back), it's harder.

PUSHUP

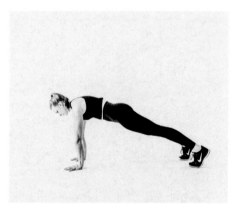

Start

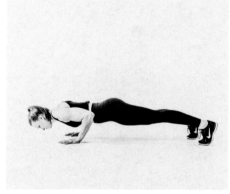

Finish

- Brace abs like a crunch
- Tuck hips under
- Get tall from your heels to the top of your head, just like good posture standing

- Push the ground away

HORIZONTAL CABLE ROTATION

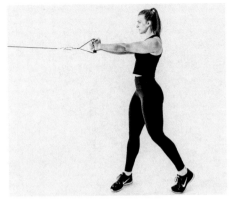

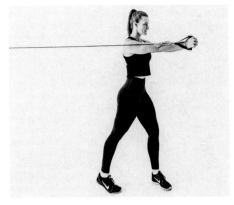

Start

Finish

HIGH TO LOW CABLE ROTATION

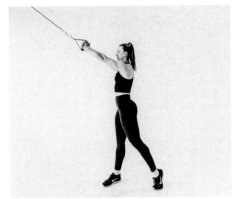

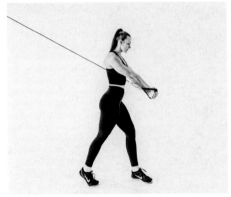

Start

Finish

LOW TO HIGH CABLE ROTATION

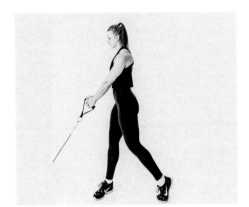

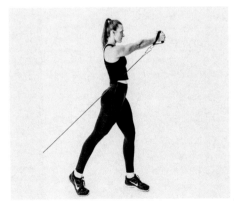

Start

Finish

- Belt buckle faces the machine
- Back shoelaces face the machine
- Flex your butt, and brace your abs

- Turn your hips around
- Turn your belt buckle to face the front wall
- Turn your back shoe around

BATTLING ROPES

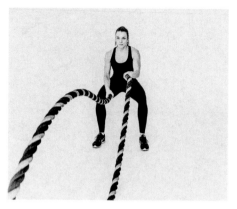

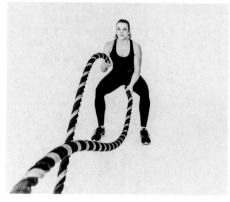

Start

Finish

- Stay in a quarter-squat position
- Lift the ropes up

- Snap the ropes down

BEAR CRAWL

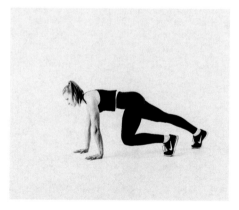

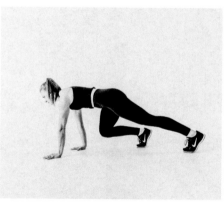

Start

Finish

- Left hand forward
- Left foot back
- Right hand back
- Right foot forward

- Reach right hand forward
- Take a small step with left foot so left foot is forward

HIP FLEXOR STRETCH

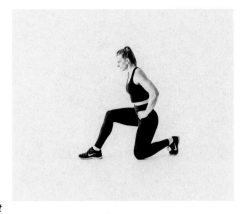

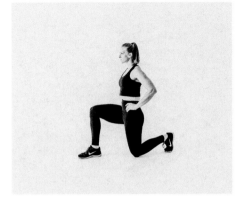

Start   *Finish*

- Pull your belt buckle up, like you're doing a crunch

- Flex your butt
- Push your hips forward into the stretch

T-SPINE ROTATION

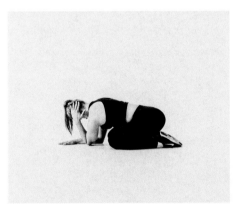

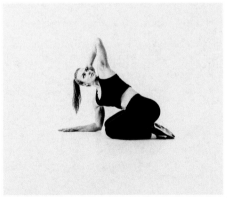

Start   *Finish*

- Sit your butt back towards your heels

- Rotate at your upper back so your elbow moves toward the ceiling
- Follow your elbow with your eyes and head

BRETZEL

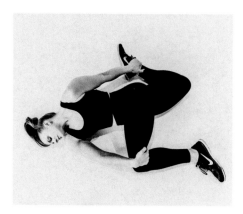

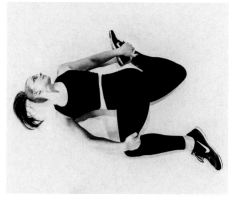

Start

Finish

- Lie on your side, with the top knee forward and on the ground
- Grab your top knee and bottom foot

- Grab your top knee
- Bend your bottom knee so your back foot comes toward you, then grab your bottom foot
- Rotate your chest toward the wall behind you

*You can modify the Bretzel to have less of a stretch by putting a bolster under your head and/or under your top knee.

**Alternately, you can substitute the hip flexor stretch and the t-spine rotation until you have the mobility to get into the Bretzel position. That's why the Bretzel only shows up in the intermediate high-volume program and the advanced medium and high-volume programs—it's a fairly advanced position.

REFERENCES

1 Butler, A. C., & Roediger, H. L. (2008). Feedback enhances the positive effects and reduces the negative effects of multiple-choice testing. *Memory & Cognition*, 36(3), 604-616.

2 Karpicke, J. D., Butler, A. C., & Roediger III, H. L. (2009). Metacognitive strategies in student learning: do students practise retrieval when they study on their own?. *Memory*, 17(4), 471-479.

3 Leeming, F. C. (2002). The exam-a-day procedure improves performance in psychology classes. *Teaching of Psychology*, 29(3), 210-212.

4 McDaniel, M. A., Agarwal, P. K., Huelser, B. J., McDermott, K. B., & Roediger III, H. L. (2011). Test-enhanced learning in a middle school science classroom: The effects of quiz frequency and placement. *Journal of Educational Psychology*, 103(2), 399.

5 Roediger III, H. L., & Karpicke, J. D. (2006). Test-enhanced learning: Taking memory tests improves long-term retention. *Psychological science*, 17(3), 249-255.

6 Thompson, Wenger & Bartling, 1978

7 Wheeler, M. A., & Roediger III, H. L. (1992). Disparate effects of repeated testing: Reconciling Ballard's (1913) and Bartlett's (1932) results. *Psychological Science*, 3(4), 240-246.

8 Smith, J. K. (2015). Brown, PC, Roediger III, HL, & McDaniel, MA (2014). Make It Stick. The Science of Successful Learning.

9 Gollwitzer, P. M., & Sheeran, P. (2006). Implementation intentions and goal achievement: A meta-analysis of effects and processes. *Advances in experimental social psychology*, 38, 69-119.

10 Scholz, U., Schüz, B., Ziegelmann, J. P., Lippke, S., & Schwarzer, R. (2008). Beyond behavioural intentions: Planning mediates between intentions and physical activity. *British journal of health psychology*, 13(3), 479-494.

11 Sniehotta, F. F. (2009). Towards a theory of intentional behaviour change: Plans, planning, and self-regulation. *British journal of health psychology*, 14(2), 261-273.

12 Wiedemann, A. U., Lippke, S., Reuter, T., Ziegelmann, J. P., & Schwarzer, R. (2011). How planning facilitates behaviour change: Additive and interactive effects of a randomized controlled trial. *European Journal of Social Psychology*, 41(1), 42-51.

13 Wiedemann, A. U., Schüz, B., Sniehotta, F., Scholz, U., & Schwarzer, R. (2009). Disentangling the relation between intentions, planning, and behaviour: A moderated mediation analysis. *Psychology and Health*, 24(1), 67-79.

14 Ferrari, M., Yap, K., Scott, N., Einstein, D. A., & Ciarrochi, J. (2018). Self-compassion moderates the perfectionism and depression link in both adolescence and adulthood. *PloS one*, 13(2), e0192022.

15 Fong, C. J., Zaleski, D. J., & Leach, J. K. (2015). The challenge–skill balance and antecedents of flow: A meta-analytic investigation. *The Journal of Positive Psychology*, 10(5), 425-446.

16 Teixeira, P. J., Carraça, E. V., Markland, D., Silva, M. N., & Ryan, R. M. (2012). Exercise, physical activity, and self-determination theory: a systematic review. *International journal of behavioral nutrition and physical activity*, 9(1), 78.

17 Ng, J. Y., Ntoumanis, N., Thøgersen-Ntoumani, C., Deci, E. L., Ryan, R. M., Duda, J. L., & Williams, G. C. (2012). Self-determination theory applied to health contexts: A meta-analysis. *Perspectives on Psychological Science*, 7(4), 325-340.

18 Lekes, N., Hope, N. H., Gouveia, L., Koestner, R., & Philippe, F. L. (2012). Influencing value priorities and increasing wellbeing: The effects of reflecting on intrinsic values. *The Journal of Positive Psychology*, 7(3), 249-261.

19 Lowe, M. R., Doshi, S. D., Katterman, S. N., & Feig, E. H. (2013). Dieting and restrained eating as prospective predictors of weight gain. *Frontiers in psychology*, 4, 577.

20 Dulloo, A. G., & Montani, J. P. (2015). Pathways from dieting to weight regain, to obesity and to the metabolic syndrome: an overview. *Obesity reviews*, 16, 1-6.

21 Hall, K. D., Chen, K. Y., Guo, J., Lam, Y. Y., Leibel, R. L., Mayer, L. E., ... & Ravussin, E. (2016). Energy expenditure and body composition changes after an isocaloric ketogenic diet in overweight and obese men. The American journal of clinical nutrition, 104(2), 324-333.

22 Gardner, C. D., Trepanowski, J. F., Del Gobbo, L. C., Hauser, M. E., Rigdon, J., Ioannidis, J. P., ... & King, A. C. (2018). Effect of low fat vs low carbohydrate diet on 12-month weight loss in overweight adults and the association with genotype pattern or insulin secretion: the DIETFITS randomized clinical trial. *Jama*, 319(7), 667-679.

23 Dansinger, M. L., Gleason, J. A., Griffith, J. L., Selker, H. P., & Schaefer, E. J. (2005). Comparison of the Atkins, Ornish, Weight Watchers, and Zone diets for weight loss and heart disease risk reduction: a randomized trial. *Jama*, 293(1), 43-53.

24 Sacks, F. M., Bray, G. A., Carey, V. J., Smith, S. R., Ryan, D. H., Anton, S. D., ... & Leboff, M. S. (2009). Comparison of weight-loss diets with different compositions of fat, protein, and carbohydrates. *New England Journal of Medicine*, 360(9), 859-873.

25 Johnston, B. C., Kanters, S., Bandayrel, K., Wu, P., Naji, F., Siemieniuk, R. A., ... & Jansen, J. P. (2014). Comparison of weight loss among named diet programs in overweight and obese adults: a meta-analysis. *Jama*, 312(9), 923-933.

26 Wroble, K. A., Trott, M. N., Schweitzer, G. G., Rahman, R. S., Kelly, P. V., & Weiss, E. P. (2019). Low carbohydrate, ketogenic diet impairs anaerobic exercise performance in exercise-trained women and men: a randomized-sequence crossover trial. *The Journal of Sports Medicine and Physical Fitness*, 59(4).

27 Wilson, J. M., Lowery, R. P., Roberts, M. D., Sharp, M. H., Joy, J. M., Shields, K. A., ... & D'Agostino, D. (2017). The Effects of Ketogenic Dieting on Body Composition, Strength, Power, and Hormonal Profiles in Resistance Training Males. *Journal of strength and conditioning research*.

28   Escobar, K. A., Morales, J., & Vandusseldorp, T. A. (2016). The Effect of a Moderately Low and High Carbohydrate Intake on Crossfit Performance. *International journal of exercise science*, 9(4), 460.

29   Maughan, R. J., & Shirreffs, S. M. (2013). IOC consensus statement on sports nutrition 2010. In Food, *Nutrition and Sports Performance III* (pp. 11-12). Routledge

30   Rodriguez, N. R., DiMarco, N. M., & Langley, S. (2009). Position of the American Dietetic Association, Dietitians of Canada, and the American College of Sports Medicine: Nutrition and athletic performance. *Journal of the American Dietetic Association*, 109(3), 509-527.

31   Hall, K.D., Ayuketah, A., Brychta, R., Cai, H., Cassimatis, T., Chen, K. Y. …Zhou, M. (2019). Ultra-processed diets cause excess calorie intake and weight gain: A one-month inpatient randomized controlled trial of ad libitum food intake. *Cell metabolism*.

32   Meule, A., Westenhöfer, J., & Kübler, A. (2011). Food cravings mediate the relationship between rigid, but not flexible control of eating behavior and dieting success. *Appetite*, 57(3), 582-584.

33   Palascha, A., van Kleef, E., & van Trijp, H. C. (2015). How does thinking in Black and White terms relate to eating behavior and weight regain?. *Journal of health psychology*, 20(5), 638-648.

34   Sairanen, E., Lappalainen, R., Lapveteläinen, A., Tolvanen, A., & Karhunen, L. (2014). Flexibility in weight management. *Eating behaviors*, 15(2), 218-224.

35   Smith, C. F., Williamson, D. A., Bray, G. A., & Ryan, D. H. (1999). Flexible vs. rigid dieting strategies: Relationship with adverse behavioral outcomes. *Appetite*, 32(3), 295-305.

36   Westenhoefer, J., Stunkard, A. J., & Pudel, V. (1999). Validation of the flexible and rigid control dimensions of dietary restraint. International Journal of Eating Disorders, 26(1), 53-64Rhea, M. R., & Alderman, B. L. (2004). A meta-analysis of periodized versus nonperiodized strength and power training programs. *Research quarterly for exercise and sport*, 75(4), 413-422.

37   Timko, C. A., & Perone, J. (2005). Rigid and flexible control of eating behavior in a college population. *Eating behaviors*, 6(2), 119-125.

38   Stewart, T. M., Williamson, D. A., & White, M. A. (2002). Rigid vs. flexible dieting: association with eating disorder symptoms in nonobese women. *Appetite*, 38(1), 39-44.

39   Simpson, C. C., & Mazzeo, S. E. (2017). Calorie counting and fitness tracking technology: Associations with eating disorder symptomatology. *Eating behaviors*, 26, 89-92.

40   Linardon, J., & Messer, M. (2019). My fitness pal usage in men: Associations with eating disorder symptoms and psychosocial impairment. *Eating Behaviors*

41   Byrne, S. M., Cooper, Z., & Fairburn, C. G. (2004). Psychological predictors of weight regain in obesity. *Behaviour research and therapy*, 42(11), 1341-1356.

42   Forman, E. M., Hoffman, K. L., Juarascio, A. S., Butryn, M. L., & Herbert, J. D. (2013). Comparison of acceptance-based and standard cognitive-based coping strategies for craving sweets in overweight and obese women. *Eating Behaviors*, 14, 64-68. doi: 10.1016/j.eatbeh.2012.10.016

43   Forman, E. M., Hoffman, K. L., McGrath, K. B., Herbert, J. D., Brandsma, L. L., & Lowe, M. R. (2007). A comparison of acceptance-and control-based strategies for coping with food cravings: An analog study. *Behaviour research and therapy*, 45(10), 2372-2386. doi: 10.1016/j.brat.2007.04.004

44   Forman, E. M., Shaw, J. A., Goldstein, S. P., Butryn, M. L., Martin, L. M., Meiran, N., …Manasse, S. M. (2016). Mindful decision making and inhibitory control training as complementary means to decrease snack consumption. *Appetite*, 103, 176-183. doi: 10.1016/j.appet.2016.04.014

45   Hooper, N., Sandoz, E. K., Ashton, J., Clarke, A., & McHugh, L. (2012). Comparing thought suppression and acceptance as coping techniques for food cravings. *Eating behaviors*, 13(1), 62-64.

46   Hulbert-Williams, L., Hulbert-Williams, N. J., Nicholls, W., Williamson, S., Poonia, J., & Hochard, K. D. (2017). Ultra-brief non-expert-delivered defusion and acceptance exercises for food cravings: A partial replication study. *Journal of health psychology*, 1359105317695424.

47   Rhea, M. R., & Alderman, B. L. (2004). A meta-analysis of periodized versus nonperiodized strength and power training programs. *Research quarterly for exercise and sport*, 75(4), 413-422.

48   Williams, T. D., Tolusso, D. V., Fedewa, M. V., & Esco, M. R. (2017). Comparison of periodized and non-periodized resistance training on maximal strength: a meta-analysis. *Sports medicine*, 47(10), 2083-2100.

49   Willoughby, D. S. (1993). The Effects of Mesocycle-Length Weight Training Programs Involving Periodization and Partially Equated Volumes on Upper and Lower Body Strength. *The Journal of Strength & Conditioning Research*, 7(1), 2-8

50   Eifler, C. (2016). Short-term effects of different loading schemes in fitness-related resistance training. *Journal of strength and conditioning research*, 30(7), 1880-1889.

51   Kok, L. Y., Hamer, P. W., & Bishop, D. J. (2009). Enhancing muscular qualities in untrained women: linear versus undulating periodization. *Medicine and science in sports and* exercise, 41(9), 1797-1807.

52   Buchanan, K., & Sheffield, J. (2017). Why do diets fail? An exploration of dieters' experiences using thematic analysis. *Journal of health psychology*, 22(7), 906-915

53   Denny, K. N., Loth, K., Eisenberg, M. E., & Neumark-Sztainer, D. (2013). Intuitive eating in young adults. Who is doing it, and how is it related to disordered eating behaviors?. *Appetite*, 60, 13-19.

54   Avalos, L. C., & Tylka, T. L. (2006). Exploring a model of intuitive eating with college women. *Journal of Counseling Psychology*, 53(4), 486.

55   Tylka, T. L., & Wilcox, J. A. (2006). Are intuitive eating and eating disorder symptomatology opposite poles of the same construct?. *Journal of Counseling Psychology*, 53(4), 474.

56   Boucher, S., Edwards, O., Gray, A., Nada-Raja, S., Lillis, J., Tylka, T. L., & Horwath, C. C. (2016). Teaching intuitive eating and acceptance and commitment therapy skills via a web-based intervention: a pilot single-arm intervention study. *JMIR research protocols*, 5(4).

57   Tylka, T. L., & Kroon Van Diest, A. M. (2013). The Intuitive Eating Scale–2: Item refinement and psychometric evaluation with college women and men. *Journal of Counseling Psychology*, 60(1), 137.

58   Ibid. Denny, Loth, Eisenberg, and Neumark-Sztainer (2013)

59 Madden, C. E., Leong, S. L., Gray, A., & Horwath, C. C. (2012). Eating in response to hunger and satiety signals is related to BMI in a nationwide sample of 1601 mid-age New Zealand women. *Public Health Nutrition*, 15(12), 2272-2279.

60 Anglin, J. C. (2012). Assessing the effectiveness of intuitive eating for weight loss–pilot study. *Nutrition and health*, 21(2), 107-115.

61 Warren, J. M., Smith, N., & Ashwell, M. (2017). A structured literature review on the role of mindfulness, mindful eating and intuitive eating in changing eating behaviours: effectiveness and associated potential mechanisms. *Nutrition research reviews*, 30(2), 272-283.

62 ibid. Martin et al., (2017)

63 Mantzios, M., & Wilson, J. C. (2014). Making concrete construals mindful: a novel approach for developing mindfulness and self-compassion to assist weight loss. *Psychology & health*, 29(4), 422-441.

64 Luszczynska, A., Sobczyk, A., & Abraham, C. (2007). Planning to lose weight: Randomized controlled trial of an implementation intention prompt to enhance weight reduction among overweight and obese women. *Health Psychology*, 26(4), 507.

65 Teixeira, P. J., Silva, M. N., Coutinho, S. R., Palmeira, A. L., Mata, J., Vieira, P. N., ... & Sardinha, L. B. (2010). Mediators of weight loss and weight loss maintenance in middle-aged women. Obesity, 18(4), 725-735.

66 Mela, D. J. (2001). Determinants of food choice: relationships with obesity and weight control. *Obesity research*, 9(S11), 249S-255S.

67 Andrade, A. M., Coutinho, S. R., Silva, M. N., Mata, J., Vieira, P. N., Minderico, C. S., ... & Teixeira, P. J. (2010). The effect of physical activity on weight loss is mediated by eating self-regulation. *Patient Education and Counseling*, 79(3), 320-326.

68 Ibid. Sairanen, Lappalainen, Lapveteläinen, Tolvanen, and Karhunen, (2014)

69 Ibid. Timko and Perone, (2005)

70 Carper, J. L., Fisher, J. O., & Birch, L. L. (2000). Young girls' emerging dietary restraint and disinhibition are related to parental control in child feeding. *Appetite*, 35(2), 121-129.

71 Faith, M. S., Scanlon, K. S., Birch, L. L., Francis, L. A., & Sherry, B. (2004). Parent-child feeding strategies and their relationships to child eating and weight status. *Obesity research*, 12(11), 1711-1722.

72 Polivy, J., & Herman, C. P. (1999). Distress and eating: why do dieters overeat?. *International Journal of Eating Disorders*, 26(2), 153-164.

73 Tribole, E., & Resch, E. (2012). *Intuitive eating: A revolutionary program that works* . New York: St.

74 Tylka, T. L. (2006). Development and psychometric evaluation of a measure of intuitive eating. *Journal of Counseling Psychology*, 53(2), 226.

75 Ibid. Anglin (2012)

76 Ibid. Anderson, Schaumberg, Anderson, and Reilly (2015)

77 Ibid. Tylka, Calogero & Daníelsdóttir (2015)

78 Linardon, J., & Mitchell, S. (2017). Rigid dietary control, flexible dietary control, and intuitive eating: Evidence for their differential relationship to disordered eating and body image concerns. *Eating behaviors*, 26, 16-22.

79 Duffey, K. J., & Popkin, B. M. (2011). Energy density, portion size, and eating occasions: contributions to increased energy intake in the United States, 1977–2006. *PLoS medicine*, 8(6), e1001050.

80 Keski-Rahkonen, A., Bulik, C. M., Pietiläinen, K. H., Rose, R. J., Kaprio, J., & Rissanen, A. (2007). Eating styles, overweight and obesity in young adult twins. *European journal of clinical nutrition*, 61(7), 822.

81 Hess, J. M., Jonnalagadda, S. S., & Slavin, J. L. (2016). What is a snack, why do we snack, and how can we choose better snacks? A review of the definitions of snacking, motivations to snack, contributions to dietary intake, and recommendations for improvement. *Advances in Nutrition*, 7(3), 466-475.

82 Leech, R. M., Livingstone, K. M., Worsley, A., Timperio, A., & McNaughton, S. A. (2016). Meal frequency but not snack frequency is associated with micronutrient intakes and overall diet quality in Australian men and women. *The Journal of nutrition*, 146(10), 2027-2034.

83 Murakami, K., & Livingstone, M. B. E. (2015). Eating frequency is positively associated with overweight and central obesity in US adults. *The Journal of nutrition*, 145(12), 2715-2724.

84 Mattes, R. (2014). Energy intake and obesity: ingestive frequency outweighs portion size. *Physiology & behavior*, 134, 110-118.

85 Leidy, H. J., & Campbell, W. W. (2010). The effect of eating frequency on appetite control and food intake: brief synopsis of controlled feeding studies. *The Journal of nutrition*, 141(1), 154-157.

86 Ogden, J., Wood, C., Payne, E., Fouracre, H., & Lammyman, F. (2018). 'Snack'versus 'meal': The impact of label and place on food intake. *Appetite*, 120, 666-672.

87 Chapelot, D. (2010). The role of snacking in energy balance: a biobehavioral approach. *The Journal of nutrition*, 141(1), 158-162.

88 Njike, V. Y., Smith, T. M., Shuval, O., Shuval, K., Edshteyn, I., Kalantari, V., & Yaroch, A. L. (2016). Snack food, satiety, and weight. *Advances in Nutrition*, 7(5), 866-878.

89 Bellisle, F. (2014). Meals and snacking, diet quality and energy balance. *Physiology & behavior*, 134, 38-43.

90 Al Khatib, H. K., Harding, S. V., Darzi, J., & Pot, G. K. (2017). The effects of partial sleep deprivation on energy balance: a systematic review and meta-analysis. *European journal of clinical nutrition*, 71(5), 614.

91 Chapman, C. D., Benedict, C., Brooks, S. J., & Birgir Schiöth, H. (2012). Lifestyle determinants of the drive to eat: a meta-analysis. *The American journal of clinical nutrition*, 96(3), 492-497.

92 Kahn, M., Sheppes, G., & Sadeh, A. (2013). Sleep and emotions: bidirectional links and underlying mechanisms. *International Journal of Psychophysiology*, 89(2), 218-228.

93 Beattie, L., Kyle, S. D., Espie, C. A., & Biello, S. M. (2015). Social interactions, emotion and sleep: A systematic review and research agenda. *Sleep medicine reviews*, 24, 83-100.

94 Carter, B., Rees, P., Hale, L., Bhattacharjee, D., & Paradkar, M. S. (2016). Association between portable screen-based media device access or use and sleep outcomes: a systematic review and meta-analysis. *JAMA pediatrics*, 170(12), 1202-1208.

95 Chambers, L., McCrickerd, K., & Yeomans, M. R. (2015). Optimising foods for satiety. *Trends in Food Science & Technology*, 41(2), 149-160.

96   Nielsen, L., Kristensen, M., Klingenberg, L., Ritz, C., Belza, A., Astrup, A., & Raben, A. (2018). Protein from Meat or Vegetable Sources in Meals Matched for Fiber Content has Similar Effects on Subjective *Appetite* Sensations and Energy Intake—A Randomized Acute Cross-Over Meal Test Study. Nutrients, 10(1), 96.

97   Lissner, L., Levitsky, D. A., Strupp, B. J., Kalkwarf, H. J., & Roe, D. A. (1987). Dietary fat and the regulation of energy intake in human subjects. *The American journal of clinical nutrition*, 46(6), 886-892.

98   Blundell, J. E., Burley, V. J., Cotton, J. R., & Lawton, C. L. (1993). Dietary fat and the control of energy intake: evaluating the effects of fat on meal size and postmeal satiety. *The American journal of clinical nutrition*, 57(5), 772S-778S.

99   Leibel, R. L., Hirsch, J., Appel, B. E., & Checani, G. C. (1992). Energy intake required to maintain bodyweight is not affected by wide variation in diet composition. *The American journal of clinical nutrition*, 55(2), 350-355.

100   Paddon-Jones, D., Westman, E., Mattes, R. D., Wolfe, R. R., Astrup, A., & Westerterp-Plantenga, M. (2008). Protein, weight management, and satiety. *The American journal of clinical nutrition*, 87(5), 1558S-1561S.

101   Barkeling, B., Rössner, S., & Björvell, H. (1990). Effects of a high-protein meal (meat) and a high-carbohydrate meal (vegetarian) on satiety measured by automated computerized monitoring of subsequent food intake, motivation to eat and food preferences. *International journal of obesity*, 14(9), 743-751.

102   Crovetti, R., Porrini, M., Santangelo, A., & Testolin, G. (1998). The influence of thermic effect of food on satiety. *European journal of clinical nutrition*, 52(7), 482.

103   Poppitt, S. D., McCormack, D., & Buffenstein, R. (1998). Short-term effects of macronutrient preloads on appetite and energy intake in lean women. *Physiology & behavior*, 64(3), 279-285.

104   Porrini, M., Santangelo, A., Crovetti, R., Riso, P., Testolin, G., & Blundell, J. E. (1997). Weight, protein, fat, and timing of preloads affect food intake. *Physiology & behavior*, 62(3), 563-570.

105   Rolls, B. J., Hetherington, M., & Burley, V. J. (1988). The specificity of satiety: the influence of foods of different macronutrient content on the development of satiety. *Physiology & behavior*, 43(2), 145-153.

106   Stubbs, R. J., Johnstone, A. M., & Harbron, C. G. (1996). Breakfasts high in protein, fat or carbohydrate: effect on within-day appetite and energy balance. *European journal of clinical nutrition*, 50(7), 409-417

107   Due, A., Toubro, S., Skov, A. R., & Astrup, A. (2004). Effect of normal-fat diets, either medium or high in protein, on bodyweight in overweight subjects: a randomised 1-year trial. *International journal of obesity*, 28(10), 1283.

108   Rolls, B. J., Ello-Martin, J. A., & Tohill, B. C. (2004). What can intervention studies tell us about the relationship between fruit and vegetable consumption and weight management?. *Nutrition reviews*, 62(1), 1-17.

109   Ledoux, T. A., Hingle, M. D., & Baranowski, T. (2011). Relationship of fruit and vegetable intake with adiposity: a systematic review. *Obesity reviews*, 12(5), e143-e150.

110   Wildman, R., Kerksick, C., & Campbell, B. (2010). Carbohydrates, physical training, and sport performance. *Strength & Conditioning Journal*, 32(1), 21-29.

111   Wroble, K. A., Trott, M. N., Schweitzer, G. G., Rahman, R. S., Kelly, P. V., & Weiss, E. P. (2019). Low carbohydrate, ketogenic diet impairs anaerobic exercise performance in exercise-trained women and men: A randomized-sequence crossover trial. *The Journal of Sports Medicine and Physical Fitness*, 59(4). doi:10.23736/s0022-4707.18.08318-4

112   Maughan, R., Greenhaff, P. L., Leiper, J. B., Ball, D., Lambert, C. P., & Gleeson, M. (1997). Diet composition and the performance of high intensity exercise. *Journal of sports sciences*, 15(3), 265-275.

113   Schoenfeld, B. J., Aragon, A. A., & Krieger, J. W. (2013). The effect of protein timing on muscle strength and hypertrophy: a meta-analysis. *Journal of the International Society of Sports Nutrition*, 10(1), 53.

114   Morton, R. W., Murphy, K. T., McKellar, S. R., Schoenfeld, B. J., Henselmans, M., Helms, E., ... & Phillips, S. M. (2018). A systematic review, meta-analysis and meta-regression of the effect of protein supplementation on resistance training-induced gains in muscle mass and strength in healthy adults. *Br J Sports Med*, 52(6), 376-384.

115   Pasiakos, S. M., McLellan, T. M., & Lieberman, H. R. (2015). The effects of protein supplements on muscle mass, strength, and aerobic and anaerobic power in healthy adults: a systematic review. *Sports Medicine*, 45(1), 111-131.

116   Lemon, P. W. (2000). Beyond the zone: protein needs of active individuals. Journal of the American College of Nutrition, 19(sup5), 513S-521S.

117   Phillips, S. M., Moore, D. R., & Tang, J. E. (2007). A critical examination of dietary protein requirements, benefits, and excesses in athletes. *International journal of sport nutrition and exercise metabolism*, 17(s1), S58-S76.

118   Geier, A. B., Rozin, P., & Doros, G. (2006). Unit bias: A new heuristic that helps explain the effect of portion size on food intake. *Psychological Science*, 17(6), 521-525.

119   Lewis, H. B., Ahern, A. L., Solis-Trapala, I., Walker, C. G., Reimann, F., Gribble, F. M., & Jebb, S. A. (2015). Effect of reducing portion size at a compulsory meal on later energy intake, gut hormones, and appetite in overweight adults. *Obesity*, 23(7), 1362-1370.)

120   Haynes, A., Hardman, C. A., Makin, A. D., Halford, J. C., Jebb, S. A., & Robinson, E. (2019). Visual perceptions of portion size normality and intended food consumption: A norm range model. *Food quality and preference*, 72, 77.

121   Bellisle, F., Dalix, A. M., & Slama, G. (2004). Non food-related environmental stimuli induce increased meal intake in healthy women: comparison of television viewing versus listening to a recorded story in laboratory settings. *Appetite*, 43(2), 175-180.

122   Braude, L., & Stevenson, R. J. (2014). Watching television while eating increases energy intake. Examining the mechanisms in female participants. *Appetite*, 76, 9–16.

123   Ogden, J., Coop, N., Cousins, C., Crump, R., Field, L., Hughes, S., & Woodger, N. (2013). Distraction, the desire to eat and food intake. Towards an expanded model of mindless eating. *Appetite*, 62, 119-126.

124   Blass, E. M., Anderson, D. R., Kirkorian, H. L., Pempek, T. A., Price, I., & Koleini, M. F. (2006). On the road to obesity: Television viewing increases intake of high-density foods. *Physiology & Behavior*, 88(4-5), 597–604.

125   Higgs, S., & Woodward, M. (2009). Television watching during lunch increases afternoon snack intake of young women. *Appetite*, 52(1), 39–43

126 Mittal, D., Stevenson, R. J., Oaten, M. J., & Miller, L. A. (2011). Snacking while watching TV impairs food recall and promotes food intake on a later TV free test meal. *Applied Cognitive Psychology*, 25(6), 871-877.

127 Scheibehenne, B., Todd, P. M., & Wansink, B. (2010). Dining in the dark. The importance of visual cues for food consumption and satiety. *Appetite*, 55(3), 710-713.

128 Bellisle, F., & Dalix, A. M. (2001). Cognitive restraint can be offset by distraction, leading to increased meal intake in women. *The American journal of clinical nutrition*, 74(2), 197-200.

129 Higgs, S., Williamson, A. C., Rotshtein, P., & Humphreys, G. W. (2008). Sensory-specific satiety is intact in amnesics who eat multiple meals. *Psychological Science*, 19(7), 623-628.

130 Robinson, E., Aveyard, P., Daley, A., Jolly, K., Lewis, A., Lycett, D., & Higgs, S. (2013). Eating attentively: a systematic review and meta-analysis of the effect of food intake memory and awareness on eating. *The American journal of clinical nutrition*, ajcn-045245.

131 Tanihara, S., Imatoh, T., Miyazaki, M., Babazono, A., Momose, Y., Baba, M., ... & Une, H. (2011). Retrospective longitudinal study on the relationship between 8-year weight change and current eating speed. *Appetite*, 57(1), 179-183.

132 Andrade, A. M., Greene, G. W., & Melanson, K. J. (2008). Eating slowly led to decreases in energy intake within meals in healthy women. *Journal of the American Dietetic Association*, 108(7), 1186-1191.

133 Leong, S. L., Madden, C., Gray, A., Waters, D., & Horwath, C. (2011). Faster self-reported speed of eating is related to higher body mass index in a nationwide survey of middle-aged women. *Journal of the American Dietetic Association,* 111(8), 1192-1197.

134 Ibid. Madden, Leong, Gray, and Horwath (2012)

135 Ciampolini, M., Lovell-Smith, H. D., Kenealy, T., & Bianchi, R. (2013). Hunger can be taught: hunger recognition regulates eating and improves energy balance. International journal of general medicine, 6, 465.

136 Schaefer, J. T., & Magnuson, A. B. (2014). A review of interventions that promote eating by internal cues. *Journal of the Academy of Nutrition and Dietetics*, 114(5), 734-760.

137 Hayes, S. C. (2005). *Get out of your mind and into your life: The new acceptance and commitment therapy.* New Harbinger Publications.

138 Moffitt, R., Haynes, A., & Mohr, P. (2015). Treatment beliefs and preferences for psychological therapies for weight management. *Journal of clinical psychology*, 71(6), 584-596.

139 Moffitt, R., Brinkworth, G., Noakes, M., & Mohr, P. (2012). A comparison of cognitive restructuring and cognitive defusion as strategies for resisting a craved food. *Psychology & health*, 27(sup2), 74-90.

140 Ibid. Forman, Hoffman, Juarascio, Butryn, and Herbert (2013)

141 Ibid. Forman, Hoffman, McGrath, Herbert, Brandsma, and Lowe (2007)

142 Ibid. Hooper, Sandoz, Ashton, Clarke, and McHugh (2012)

143 Harris, R., *The happiness trap: how to stop struggling and start living.* 2008. Trumpeter, Boston, 27.

144 Kalokerinos, E. K., Erbas, Y., Ceulemans, E., & Kuppens, P. (2019). Differentiate to Regulate: Low Negative Emotion Differentiation Is Associated With Ineffective Use but Not Selection of Emotion-Regulation Strategies. *Psychological scienc*e, 0956797619838763.

145 Forman, E. M., Butryn, M. L., Juarascio, A. S., Bradley, L. E., Lowe, M. R., Herbert, J. D., & Shaw, J. A. (2013). The mind your health project: a randomized controlled trial of an innovative behavioral treatment for obesity. *Obesity*, 21(6), 1119-1126.

146 Lillis, J., Niemeier, H. M., Thomas, J. G., Unick, J., Ross, K. M., Leahey, T. M., ... & Wing, R. R. (2016). A randomized trial of an acceptance-based behavioral intervention for weight loss in people with high internal disinhibition. *Obesity*, 24(12), 2509-2514.

147 Forman, E. M., Butryn, M. L., Manasse, S. M., Crosby, R. D., Goldstein, S. P., Wyckoff, E. P., & Thomas, J. G. (2016). Acceptance-based versus standard behavioral treatment for obesity: Results from the mind your health randomized controlled trial. *Obesity*, 24(10), 2050-2056.

148 Elder, R. S., & Mohr, G. S. (2016). The crunch effect: food sound salience as a consumption monitoring cue. *Food quality and Preference*, 51, 39-46.

149 Robinson, E., Aveyard, P., Daley, A., Jolly, K., Lewis, A., Lycett, D., & Higgs, S. (2013). Eating attentively: a systematic review and meta-analysis of the effect of food intake memory and awareness on eating–. *The American journal of clinical nutrition*, 97(4), 728-742.

150 Higgs, S., & Donohoe, J. E. (2011). Focusing on food during lunch enhances lunch memory and decreases later snack intake. *Appetite*, 57(1), 202-206.

151 Beshara, M., Hutchinson, A. D., & Wilson, C. (2013). Does mindfulness matter? Everyday mindfulness, mindful eating and self-reported serving size of energy dense foods among a sample of South Australian adults. *Appetite*, 67, 25-29.

152 Ibid. Martin et al., 2017

153 Ibid. Tylka and Wilcox (2006)

154 Ibid. Schaefer and Magnuson (2014)

155 Ibid. Mantzios and Wilson (2013)

156 Ibid. Anglin (2012)

157 Anglin, J. C., Borchardt, N., Ramos, E., & Mhoon, K. (2013). Diet quality of adults using intuitive eating for weight loss–pilot study. *Nutrition and health*, 22(3-4), 255-264.

158 Brown, P. (2014). *Make it stick.* Cambridge, Massachusetts: The Belknap Press of Harvard University Press.

159 Usman, E. A. (2016). Making legal education stick: using cognitive science to foster long-term learning in the legal writing classroom. *Geo. J. Legal Ethics*, 29, 355.

160 Wulf, G. (2013). Attentional focus and motor learning: a review of 15 years. International Review of sport and *Exercise psychology*, 6(1), 77-104.

161 Schoenfeld, B. J., Vigotsky, A., Contreras, B., Golden, S., Alto, A., Larson, R., ... & Paoli, A. (2018). Differential effects of attentional focus strategies during long-term resistance training. *European journal of sport* science, 18(5), 705-712.

162 Davies, T., Orr, R., Halaki, M., & Hackett, D. (2016). Effect of training leading to repetition failure on muscular strength: a systematic review and meta-analysis. *Sports medicine*, 46(4), 487-502.

163   Helms, E. R., Byrnes, R. K., Cooke, D. M., Haischer, M. H., Carzoli, J. P., Johnson, T. K., ... & Zourdos, M. C. (2018). RPE vs. Percentage 1RM loading in periodized programs matched for sets and repetitions. *Frontiers in physiology*, 9, 247.

164   Izquierdo, M., Ibanez, J., González-Badillo, J. J., Hakkinen, K., Ratamess, N. A., Kraemer, W. J., ... & Gorostiaga, E. M. (2006). Differential effects of strength training leading to failure versus not to failure on hormonal responses, strength, and muscle power gains. *Journal of applied physiology*, 100(5), 1647-1656.

165   Schoenfeld, B. J. (2010). The mechanisms of muscle hypertrophy and their application to resistance training. *The Journal of Strength & Conditioning Research*, 24(10), 2857-2872.

166   Sheeran, P., Webb, T. L., & Gollwitzer, P. M. (2005). The interplay between goal intentions and implementation intentions. *Personality and Social Psychology Bulletin*, 31(1), 87-98.

167   Ibid. Gollwitzer, and Sheeran (2006)

168   Adriaanse, M. A. (2010). Planning to break habits: Efficacy, mechanisms, and boundary conditions of implementation intentions targeting unhealthy snacking habits. Utrecht University.

169   DeWitte, S., Verguts, T., & Lens, W. (2003). Implementation intentions do not enhance all types of goals: The moderating role of goal difficulty. *Current Psychology*, 22(1), 73-89.

170   Gollwitzer, P. M., & Brandstätter, V. (1997). Implementation intentions and effective goal pursuit. *Journal of personality and social psychology*, 73(1), 186.

171   Bayer, U. C., Gollwitzer, P. M., & Achtziger, A. (2010). Staying on track: Planned goal striving is protected from disruptive internal states. *Journal of Experimental Social Psychology*, 46(3), 505-514.

172   Ibid. Rhea and Alderman (2004)

173   Ibid. **Willoughby (1993)**

174   Kraemer, W. J., Ratamess, N., Fry, A. C., Triplett-McBride, T., Koziris, L. P., Bauer, J. A., ... & Fleck, S. J. (2000). Influence of resistance training volume and periodization on physiological and performance adaptations in collegiate women tennis players. *The American Journal of Sports Medicine*, 28(5), 626-633

175   Kraemer, W. J., Hakkinen, K., Triplett-McBride, N. T., Fry, A. C., Koziris, L. P., Ratamess, N. A., ... & Gordon, S. E. (2003). Physiological changes with periodized resistance training in women tennis players. *Medicine and science in sports and exercise*, 35(1), 157-168.

176   Strohacker, K., Fazzino, D., Breslin, W. L., & Xu, X. (2015). The use of periodization in exercise prescriptions for inactive adults: A systematic review. *Preventive medicine reports*, 2, 385-396

177   De Lima, C., Boullosa, D. A., Frollini, A. B., Donatto, F. F., Leite, R. D., Gonelli, P. R. G., ... & Cesar, M. C. (2012). Linear and daily undulating resistance training periodizations have differential beneficial effects in young sedentary women. *International journal of sports medicine*, 33(09), 723-727.

178   Campos, G. E., Luecke, T. J., Wendeln, H. K., Toma, K., Hagerman, F. C., Murray, T. F., ... & Staron, R. S. (2002). Muscular adaptations in response to three different resistance-training regimens: specificity of repetition maximum training zones. *European journal of applied physiology*, 88(1-2), 50-60.

179   Stone, W. J., & Coulter, S. P. (1994). Strength/Endurance Effects From Three Resistance Training Protocols With Women. *The Journal of Strength & Conditioning Research*, 8(4), 231-234.

180   Schoenfeld, B. J., Peterson, M. D., Ogborn, D., Contreras, B., & Sonmez, G. T. (2015). Effects of low-vs. high-load resistance training on muscle strength and hypertrophy in well-trained men. *The Journal of Strength & Conditioning Research*,29(10), 2954-2963.

181   O'Shea, P. (1966). Effects of selected weight training programs on the development of strength and muscle hypertrophy. Research Quarterly. *American Association for Health, Physical Education and Recreation*, 37(1), 95-102.

182   Boyer, B. T. (1990). A Comparison of the Effects of Three Strength Training Programs on Women. *The Journal of Strength & Conditioning Research*, 4(3), 88-94.

183   Beaven, C. M., Cook, C. J., & Gill, N. D. (2008). Significant strength gains observed in rugby players after specific resistance exercise protocols based on individual salivary testosterone responses. *The Journal of Strength & Conditioning Research*, 22(2), 419-425.

184   Lorenz, D. S., Reiman, M. P., & Walker, J. C. (2010). Periodization Current review and suggested implementation for athletic rehabilitation. *Sports Health: A Multidisciplinary Approach*, 2(6), 509-518.

185   Lorenz, D., & Morrison, S. (2015). Current concepts in periodization of strength and conditioning for the sports physical therapist. *International journal of sports physical therapy*,10(6), 734.

186   Bartolomei, S., Stout, J. R., Fukuda, D. H., Hoffman, J. R., & Merni, F. (2015). Block vs. weekly undulating periodized resistance training programs in women. *The Journal of Strength & Conditioning Research*, 29(10), 2679-2687.

187   Apel, J. M., Lacey, R. M., & Kell, R. T. (2011). A comparison of traditional and weekly undulating periodized strength training programs with total volume and intensity equated. *The Journal of Strength & Conditioning Research*, 25(3), 694-703.

188   Painter, K. B., Haff, G. G., Ramsey, M. W., McBride, J., Triplett, T., Sands, W. A., ... & Stone, M. H. (2012). Strength gains: Block versus daily undulating periodization weight training among track and field athletes. *International journal of sports physiology and performance*, 7(2), 161-169.

189   Ralston, G. W., Kilgore, L., Wyatt, F. B., & Baker, J. S. (2017). The effect of weekly set volume on strength gain: a meta-analysis. *Sports Medicine*, 47(12), 2585-2601.

190   Schoenfeld, B. J., Ogborn, D., & Krieger, J. W. (2017). Dose-response relationship between weekly resistance training volume and increases in muscle mass: A systematic review and meta-analysis. *Journal of sports sciences*, 35(11), 1073-1082.

191   Radaelli, R., Fleck, S. J., Leite, T., Leite, R. D., Pinto, R. S., Fernandes, L., & Simão, R. (2015). Dose-response of 1, 3, and 5 sets of resistance exercise on strength, local muscular endurance, and hypertrophy. *The Journal of Strength & Conditioning Research*, 29(5), 1349-1358.

192   Marx, J. O., Ratamess, N. A., Nindl, B. C., Gotshalk, L. A., Volek, J. S., Dohi, K., ... Kraemer, W. J. (2001). Low-volume circuit versus high-volume periodized resistance training in women. *Medicine and Science in Sports and Exercise*, 635–643.

193   Peterson, M. D., Rhea, M. R., & Alvar, B. A. (2005). Applications of the dose-response for muscular strength development: a review of meta-analytic efficacy and reliability for designing training prescription. *The Journal of Strength & Conditioning Research*, 19(4), 950-958.

194 Alghadir, A. H., Gabr, S. A., & Aly, F. A. (2015). The effects of four weeks aerobic training on saliva cortisol and testosterone in young healthy persons. *Journal of physical therapy science*, 27(7), 2029-2033.

195 Focht, B. C. (2009). Brief walks in outdoor and laboratory environments: effects on affective responses, enjoyment, and intentions to walk for exercise. *Research quarterly for exercise and sport*, 80(3), 611-620.

196 Marselle, M., Irvine, K., Lorenzo-Arribas, A., & Warber, S. (2015). Moving beyond green: Exploring the relationship of environment type and indicators of perceived environmental quality on emotional wellbeing following group walks. *International journal of environmental research and public health*, 12(1), 106-130

197 Ledochowski, L., Ruedl, G., Taylor, A. H., & Kopp, M. (2015). Acute effects of brisk walking on sugary snack cravings in overweight people, affect and responses to a manipulated stress situation and to a sugary snack cue: A crossover study. *PloS one*, 10(3), e0119278.

198 Milkman, H. B., Sunderwirth, S. G. & Hil K. G. (2019). *Craving for ecstasy and natural highs: A positive approach to mood alteration.* Cognella.

199 Mikkelsen, K., Stojanovska, L., Polenakovic, M., Bosevski, M., & Apostolopoulos, V. (2017). Exercise and mental health. *Maturitas*, 106, 48-56.

200 Sheldon, K. M., & Elliot, A. J. (1999). Goal striving, need satisfaction, and longitudinal wellbeing: the self-concordance model. *Journal of personality and social psychology*, 76(3), 482.

201 Parks, L., & Guay, R. P. (2009). Personality, values, and motivation. *Personality and individual differences*, 47(7), 675-684.

202 Ryan, R. M., & Deci, E. L. (2000). Self-determination theory and the facilitation of intrinsic motivation, social development, and wellbeing. *American psychologist*, 55(1), 68.

203 Patrick, H., & Williams, G. C. (2012). Self-determination theory: its application to health behavior and complementarity with motivational interviewing. International *Journal of behavioral nutrition and physical Activity*, 9(1), 18

204 Ibid. Forman et al. (2016)

205 Ibid. Forman et al. (2019)

206 Lillis, J., Thomas, J. G., Niemeier, H. M., & Wing, R. R. (2017). Exploring process variables through which acceptance-based behavioral interventions may improve weight loss maintenance. *Journal of contextual behavioral science*, 6(4), 398-403.

207 Lillis, J., Niemeier, H. M., Thomas, J. G., Unick, J., Ross, K. M., Leahey, T. M., ... & Wing, R. R. (2016). A randomized trial of an acceptance-based behavioral intervention for weight loss in people with high internal disinhibition. *Obesity*, 24(12), 2509-2514.

208 Manasse, S. M., Flack, D., Dochat, C., Zhang, F., Butryn, M. L., & Forman, E. M. (2017). Not so fast: The impact of impulsivity on weight loss varies by treatment type. *Appetite*, 113, 193-199.

209 210. Forman, E. M., & Butryn, M. L. (2016). *Effective weight loss: An acceptance-based behavioral approach: Clinician guide.* New York, NY, United States of America: Oxford University Press.

210 Dahl, J., Lundgren, T., Plumb, J., & Stewart, I. (2009). *The Art and Science of Valuing in Psychotherapy: Helping Clients Discover, Explore, and Commit to Valued Action Using Acceptance and Commitment Therapy.* New Harbinger Publications

211 Hardcastle, S. J., Hancox, J., Hattar, A., Maxwell-Smith, C., Thøgersen-Ntoumani, C., & Hagger, M. S. (2015). Motivating the unmotivated: how can health behavior be changed in those unwilling to change?. *Frontiers in psychology*, 6, 835.

212 Ibid. Fedewa, Burns, and Gomez (2005)

213 Ibid. Stoeber and Otto (2006)

214 Hill, A. P., & Curran, T. (2016). Multidimensional perfectionism and burnout: A meta-analysis. *Personality and Social Psychology Review*, 20(3), 269-288.

215 Sherry, S. B., & Hall, P. A. (2009). The perfectionism model of binge eating: Tests of an integrative model. *Journal of Personality and Social Psychology*, 96(3), 690.

216 Peck, L. D., & Lightsey Jr, O. R. (2008). The eating disorders continuum, self-esteem, and perfectionism. *Journal of Counseling & Development*, 86(2), 184-192.

217 Haase, A. M., Prapavessis, H., & Owens, R. G. (2002). Perfectionism, social physique anxiety and disordered eating: A comparison of male and female elite athletes. *Psychology of sport and Exercise*, 3(3), 209-222.

218 Urquhart, C. S., & Mihalynuk, T. V. (2011). Disordered eating in women: implications for the obesity pandemic. *Canadian Journal of Dietetic Practice and Research*, 72(1), e115-e125.

219 Boone, L., Vansteenkiste, M., Soenens, B., der Kaap-Deeder, V., & Verstuyf, J. (2014). Self-critical perfectionism and binge eating symptoms: A longitudinal test of the intervening role of psychological need frustration. *Journal of counseling psychology*, 61(3), 363.

220 Ibid. Ferrari, Yap, Scott, Einstein, and Ciarrochi (2018)

221 Neff, K. D. (2011). Self-compassion, self-esteem, and well-being. *Social and personality psychology compass*, 5(1), 1-12.

222 Ibid. Ferrari, Yap, Scott, Einstein and Ciarrochi (2018)

223 Fryar, C. D., Gu, Q., & Ogden, C. L. (2012). Anthropometric reference data for children and adults; United States, 2007-2010.

224 Augustus-Horvath, C. L., & Tylka, T. L. (2011). The acceptance model of intuitive eating: A comparison of women in emerging adulthood, early adulthood, and middle adulthood. *Journal of counseling psychology*, 58(1), 110.

225 Oh, K. H., Wiseman, M. C., Hendrickson, J., Phillips, J. C., & Hayden, E. W. (2012). Testing the acceptance model of intuitive eating with college women athletes. *Psychology of Women Quarterly*, 36(1), 88-98.

226 Andrew, R., Tiggemann, M., & Clark, L. (2015). Predictors of intuitive eating in adolescent girls. *Journal of Adolescent Health*, 56(2), 209-214.

227 Ibid. Avalos and Tylka (2006)

228 Wegner, D. M., Schneider, D. J., Carter, S. R., & White, T. L. (1987). Paradoxical effects of thought suppression. *Journal of personality and social psychology*, 53(1), 5.

229 Davies, M. I., & Clark, D. M. (1998). Thought suppression produces a rebound effect with analogue post-traumatic intrusions. *Behaviour Research and Therapy*, 36(6), 571-582.

230   Clark, D. M., Ball, S., & Pape, D. (1991). An experimental investigation of thought suppression. *Behaviour Research and Therapy*, 29(3), 253-257.

231   Ibid. Hooper, Sandoz, Ashton, Clarke, and McHugh (2012)

232   Ibid. Hulbert-Williams, Hulbert-Williams, Nicholls, Williamson, Poonia, and Hochard, (2017)

233   Ibid. Forman, Hoffman, Juarascio, Butryn, and Herbert, (2013)

234   Rose, J. P. (2012). Debiasing comparative optimism and increasing worry for health outcomes. *Journal of health psychology*, 17(8), 1121-1131.

235   Fowler, S. L., & Geers, A. L. (2015). Dispositional and comparative optimism interact to predict avoidance of a looming health threat. *Psychology & health*, 30(4), 456-474.

236   Davidson, K., & Prkachin, K. (1997). Optimism and unrealistic optimism have an interacting impact on health-promoting behavior and knowledge changes. *Personality and social psychology bulletin*, 23(6), 617-625.

237   Newby-Clark, I. R., Ross, M., Buehler, R., Koehler, D. J., & Griffin, D. (2000). People focus on optimistic scenarios and disregard pessimistic scenarios while predicting task completion times. *Journal of Experimental Psychology*: Applied, 6(3), 171.

238   Kashdan, T. B., & Rottenberg, J. (2010). Psychological flexibility as a fundamental aspect of health. *Clinical psychology review, 30*(7), 865-878.

239   Fledderus, M., Bohlmeijer, E. T., Smit, F., & Westerhof, G. J. (2010). Mental health promotion as a new goal in public mental health care: A randomized controlled trial of an intervention enhancing psychological flexibility. *American journal of public health*, 100(12), 2372-2372.

240   Ivtzan, I., Lomas, T., Hefferon, K., & Worth, P. (2015). *Second wave positive psychology: Embracing the dark side of life*. Routledge.

241   Ibid. Lekes, Hope, Gouveia, Koestner, and Philippe (2012)

242   Huldtgren, A., Wiggers, P., & Jonker, C. M. (2013). Designing for self-reflection on values for improved life decision. *Interacting with Computers*, 26(1), 27-45.

243   Gillison, F. B., Rouse, P., Standage, M., Sebire, S. J., & Ryan, R. M. (2019). A meta-analysis of techniques to promote motivation for health behaviour change from a self-determination theory perspective. *Health psychology review*, 13(1), 110-130

244   Ryan, R. M., & Deci, E. L. (2019). Brick by Brick: The Origins, Development, and Future of Self-Determination Theory. *Advances in Motivation Science*, 6, 111.

245   Deci, E. L., & Ryan, R. M. (2008). Self-determination theory: A macrotheory of human motivation, development, and health. *Canadian psychology/ Psychologie canadienne*, 49(3), 182.

246   Teixeira, P. J., Carraça, E. V., Markland, D., Silva, M. N., & Ryan, R. M. (2012). Exercise, physical activity, and self-determination theory: a systematic review. *International journal of behavioral nutrition and physical activity*, 9(1), 78

247   Deci, E. L., Koestner, R., & Ryan, R. M. (1999). A meta-analytic review of experiments examining the effects of extrinsic rewards on intrinsic motivation. *Psychological bulletin*, 125(6), 627.

248   Crocker, J., & Park, L. E. (2004). The costly pursuit of self-esteem. *Psychological bulletin*, 130(3), 392.

249   Dweck, C. S. (2000). *Self-theories: Their role in motivation, personality, and development*. Psychology press.

250   Grant, H., & Dweck, C. S. (2003). Clarifying achievement goals and their impact. *Journal of personality and social psychology*, 85(3), 541.

251   Souza, L. K. D., & Hutz, C. S. (2016). Self-compassion in relation to self-esteem, self-efficacy and demographical aspects. *Paidéia (Ribeirão Preto)*, 26(64), 181-188.

252   Khanzadeh, A. H., Taher, M., Zeenat Fallah Morteza Nejad, & Noori, Z. S. (2016). Prediction of self-efficacy and self-esteem based on self-compassion. CPAP. 2016; 14 (1) :33-42.

253   Ibid. Neff (2011)

254   Moffitt, R. L., Neumann, D. L., & Williamson, S. P. (2018). Comparing the efficacy of a brief self-esteem and self-compassion intervention for state body dissatisfaction and self-improvement motivation. *Body image*, 27, 67-76.

255   Seekis, V., Bradley, G. L., & Duffy, A. (2017). The effectiveness of self-compassion and self-esteem writing tasks in reducing body image concerns. *Body image*, 23, 206-213.

256   Crocker, J., & Park, L. E. (2004). The costly pursuit of self-esteem. *Psychological bulletin*, 130(3), 392.

257   Fardouly, J., & Vartanian, L. R. (2016). Social media and body image concerns: Current research and future directions. *Current opinion in psychology*, 9, 1-5.

258   Prichard, I., McLachlan, A. C., Lavis, T., & Tiggemann, M. (2018). The impact of different forms of# fitspiration imagery on body image, mood, and self-objectification among young women. *Sex Roles*, 78(11-12), 789-798.

259   Kasser, T., & Ryan, R. M. (1996). Further examining the American dream: Differential correlates of intrinsic and extrinsic goals. *Personality and social psychology bulletin*, 22(3), 280-287.

260   Mask, L., Blanchard, C. M., & Baker, A. (2014). Do portrayals of women in action convey another ideal that women with little self-determination feel obligated to live up to? Viewing effects on body image evaluations and eating behaviors. *Appetite*, 83, 277-286.

261   Pinquart, M., & Sörensen, S. (2000). Influences of socioeconomic status, social network, and competence on subjective wellbeing in later life: a meta-analysis. *Psychology and aging*, 15(2), 187.

262   Anderson, C., & Kilduff, G. J. (2009). The pursuit of status in social groups. *Current Directions in Psychological Science,* 18(5), 295-298.

263   Ibid. Milkman, Sunderwirth & Hil (2019)

264   Ibid. Harris (2008)

265   Held, B. S. (2002). The tyranny of the positive attitude in America: Observation and speculation. *Journal of clinical psychology*, 58(9), 965-991.

266   Wong, P. T. (2011). *Positive psychology 2.0: Towards a balanced interactive model of the good life*. Canadian Psychology/Psychologie Canadienne, 52(2), 69.

267   Ibid. Ivtzan, Lomas, Hefferon & Worth (2015)

268   Evers, C., Marijn Stok, F., & de Ridder, D. T. (2010). Feeding your feelings: Emotion regulation strategies and emotional eating. *Personality and Social Psychology Bulletin*, 36(6), 792-804.

269 Hayes, S. C. (2004). Acceptance and commitment therapy, relational frame theory, and the third wave of behavioral and cognitive therapies. *Behavior therapy*, 35(4), 639-665.

270 Ibid. Hulbert-Williams, Hulbert-Williams, Nicholls, Williamson, Poonia, and Hochard (2017)

271 Ibid. Forman, Hoffman, McGrath, Herbert, Brandsma, and Lowe (2007)

272 Ibid.Manasse, Flack, Dochat, Zhang, Butryn, and Forman (2017)

273 Ibid. Moffitt, Brinkworth, Noakes, and Mohr (2012)

274 Ibid. Hooper, Sandoz, Ashton, Clarke, and McHugh (2012)

275 Ibid. Lillis et al. (2016)

276 Ibid. Forman, Hoffman, Juarascio, Butryn, and Herbert (2013)

277 Ibid. Forman et al. (2016)

278 Ibid. Lillis, Thomas, Niemeier, and Wing (2017)*

279 Iibid. Forman, Manasse, Butryn, Crosby, Dallal, and Crochiere (2019)

280 Ford, B. Q., Lam, P., John, O. P., & Mauss, I. B. (2018). The psychological health benefits of accepting negative emotions and thoughts: Laboratory, diary, and longitudinal evidence. *Journal of personality and social psychology*, 115(6), 1075.

281 Flett, G. L., & Hewitt, P. L. (2006). Positive versus negative perfectionism in psychopathology a comment on Slade and Owens's dual process model. Behavior modification, 30(4), 472-495.

282 Fedewa, B. A., Burns, L. R., & Gomez, A. A. (2005). Positive and negative perfectionism and the shame/guilt distinction: Adaptive and maladaptive characteristics. Personality and individual differences, 38(7), 1609-1619.

283 Stoeber, J., & Otto, K. (2006). Positive conceptions of perfectionism: Approaches, evidence, challenges. Personality and social psychology review,10(4), 295-319.

284 Kobori, O., & Tanno, Y. (2005). Self-oriented perfectionism and its relationship to positive and negative affect: The mediation of positive and negative perfectionism cognitions. Cognitive Therapy and Research, 29(5), 555-567.

285 Andrews, D. M., Burns, L. R., & Dueling, J. K. (2014). Positive perfectionism: Seeking the healthy "should", or should we?. Open Journal of Social Sciences, 2(08), 27.

286 Egan, S., Piek, J., Dyck, M., & Kane, R. (2011). The reliability and validity of the positive and negative perfectionism scale. Clinical Psychologist, 15(3), 121-132.

287 Smith, C. F., Williamson, D. A., Bray, G. A., & Ryan, D. H. (1999). Flexible vs. rigid dieting strategies: Relationship with adverse behavioral outcomes. Appetite, 32(3), 295-305

INDEX